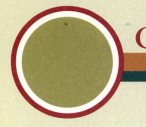

CASE STUDIES IN

DENTAL HYGIENE

Second Edition

Evelyn M. Thomson, BSDH, MS

Senior Lecturer
Gene W. Hirschfeld School of Dental Hygiene
Old Dominion University
Norfolk, Virginia

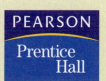

PEARSON

Prentice
Hall

Upper Saddle River, New Jersey 07458

Thomson, Evelyn M.
    Case studies in dental hygiene / Evelyn M.
Thomson—2nd ed.
       p. cm.
    ISBN 978-0-13-158994-0
    Book (Print, Microform, Electronic, etc.)
    0131589946   2007039696

Publisher: Julie Levin Alexander
Publisher's Assistant: Regina Bruno
Executive Editor: Mark Cohen
Associate Editor: Melissa Kerian
Editorial Assistant: Nicole Ragonese
Senior Marketing Manager: Harper Coles
Marketing Specialist: Michael Sirinides
Marketing Assistant: Lauren Castellano
Managing Editor: Patrick Walsh
Senior Operations Manager: Ilene Sanford
Operations Specialist: Pat Brown
Cover Art Director: Jayne Conte
Cover Design: Bruce Kenselaar
Full-Service Project Management: Lynn Steines, S4Carlisle Publishing Services
Printer/Binder: C. J. Krehbiel
Cover Printer: Phoenix Color Corporation
Typeface: 10/12 Minion

Pearson Education Ltd., London   Pearson Education North Asia Ltd.
Pearson Education Singapore, Pte. Ltd.   Pearson Educación de Mexico, S.A. de C.V.
Pearson Education Canada, Inc.   Pearson Education Malaysia, Pte. Ltd.
Pearson Education—Japan   Pearson Education, Inc., Upper Saddle River, New Jersey
Pearson Education Australia PTY, Limited

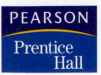

10 9 8 7 6 5 4 3
ISBN-13: 978-0-13-158994-0
ISBN-10:   0-13-158994-6

CONTENTS

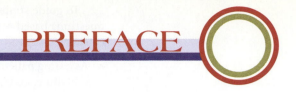

Within the educational environment exists the goal to assist students in linking basic knowledge to dental hygiene care that is evidence based and patient centered. With the constantly evolving knowledge base and changing technologies, dental hygiene faculty are challenged to incorporate educational technologies that exceed knowledge acquisition and focus on critical decision making. This book is intended to provide dental hygiene educators with a ready-made bank of cases upon which to build meaningful learning activities for the student.

Health care educators are fully cognizant that effective clinical judgment comes from experience. It is the use of real-life situations that encourages student analysis and decision making in areas relevant to professional practice. During the course of their formal education, dental hygiene students may be exposed to only a small spectrum of cases they might encounter in the real world. The diversity of the cases in this text provides an avenue for simulating experiences students might not encounter in their education.

Case Studies in Dental Hygiene, Second Edition, is designed to guide the development of critical-thinking skills and the application of theory to care at all levels of dental hygiene education—from beginning to advanced students. This textbook is designed to be used throughout the dental hygiene curriculum. Because the questions and decisions regarding treatment of each case span the dental hygiene sciences and clinical practice protocols, this book will find a place in enhancing every course required of dental hygiene students. Introducing this text at the beginning of the educational experience may help the student realize early on the link between theory and patient care. Students then progress through the program with a heightened awareness of evidence-based practice.

Students also perceive an increase in confidence regarding preparation for board examinations when they have been given the opportunity to practice case-based decision making. *Case Studies in Dental Hygiene*, Second Edition, is a viable study guide to help students prepare for success on national, regional, and state examinations with a patient care focus. This revised edition also is an excellent review text for the graduating dental hygiene student who is preparing to take the National Board Dental Hygiene Examination.

FEATURES

Case Studies in Dental Hygiene, Second Edition, presents oral health case situations representing a variety of patients that would typically be encountered in clinical settings. Of the 15 cases, 3 each represent the following patient types.

- Pediatric
- Adult-Periodontal
- Geriatric
- Special Needs
- Medically Compromised

Each case contains the following patient information.

- Medical history
- Vital signs
- Dental history
- Dental and periodontal charting
- Intraoral photographs
- Radiographs

To guide student learning and to meet the needs of instructors who desire to assign questions based on the topic being taught, questions are subdivided into the following categories.

- Assessing patient characteristics
- Obtaining and interpreting radiographs
- Planning and managing dental hygiene care
- Performing periodontal procedures
- Using preventive agents
- Providing supportive treatment services
- Demonstrating professional responsibility

Learning objectives help the student realize key concepts. Each learning objective is evaluated through the use of multiple-choice questions expertly written in the format used for the National Board Dental Hygiene Examination. Each question is identified as a basic knowledge level or as a competency level question, further guiding educators and students to use each case to maximum benefit at all levels of student learning. Correct answers and descriptive rationales for responses are provided for all questions, thus allowing the student and instructor to assess learning outcomes.

What sets *Case Studies in Dental Hygiene*, Second Edition, apart from a basic board examination review book is the inclusion of treatment planning exercises and reflective activities that challenge the student to develop decision-making skills regarding patient care and treatment recommendations that promote oral health and prevent oral diseases. Students usually respond favorably to the opportunity to apply knowledge gained in the classroom to fictional cases, and *Case Studies in Dental Hygiene*, Second Edition, provides a stress-free environment in which to learn how to make increasingly competent decisions.

SUGGESTIONS FOR EDUCATORS

In case-based teaching, a frequent faculty concern is that students have difficulty integrating information from various courses within the discipline to make competent, evidence-based decisions regarding dental hygiene care planning. Although there are a variety of ways to use *Case Studies in Dental Hygiene*, Second Edition, in the dental hygiene curriculum, educators may benefit from the suggestions discussed here.

Because each case is contained in a stand-alone chapter, the cases can be introduced in any order and at any time during the curriculum. Students who have the opportunity to simulate clinical treatment planning and decision making report increased confidence when faced with treatment planning and implementation decisions regarding patients in the clinical setting. For this reason, it is suggested that students be introduced to case scenarios early in the curriculum. For example, one of the adult-periodontal patient cases could be used as required reading for the preclinical student to introduce the dental hygiene process of care. The pediatric patient cases can provide an opportunity for the beginning student to identify eruption patterns. As the student progresses through the curriculum, other cases that correspond with coursework may be introduced. For example, the pharmacology instructor may use the medically compromised patient cases to provide a realistic setting to assist students in linking drug interactions with dental hygiene care planning and managing patient treatment.

Another feature of *Case Studies in Dental Hygiene*, Second Edition, that makes it ideally suited for use throughout the curriculum is the division of basic and competency levels of questions in each of the 15 cases. Because the questions for each case are subdivided and labeled, instructors can readily identify introductory knowledge questions that can be introduced at the beginning of the term and those questions which test the student's comprehensive knowledge of the subject. The beginning student may be directed to answer the basic level questions, leaving the competency level questions until later in the curriculum. For example, the radiology instructor may assign students to complete the basic level questions of all the cases under the subheading "Obtaining and Interpreting Radiographs" during the first half of the term; then direct the students to complete the competency level questions during the second half of the term. Applying theory and knowledge gained in the classroom to solve problems encountered through case-based questioning allows the student to become actively involved in the learning process. *Case Studies in Dental Hygiene,* Second Edition, advances with students as they progress through the curriculum. As students progress through the curriculum, the same cases may be revisited by directing the student to answer the competency level questions.

Instructors may use this revised edition to compliment and enhance material learned in other textbooks. For example, students learning instrument design from a theory book may link application of this knowledge when challenged by case photographs and charts to choose an appropriate instrument for scaling a specific area; and radiographic problem-solving skills are enhanced by examination of the case radiographs, challenging the student to identify technique and processing errors and to recommend corrective actions.

Case Studies in Dental Hygiene, Second Edition, is invaluable in the classroom. Discussion of answers to complex questions, presentations of student-developed dental hygiene care plans, and use of the suggested reflective activities can increase the incidence of critical-thinking skills and reinforce and facilitate learning in a dynamic, stimulating manner, thus motivating the student to more fully participate in the learning process.

ABOUT THE SECOND EDITON

To provide a valuable resource for comprehensive cases that educators may use to guide students in developing critical decision-making skills continues to be the goal of *Case Studies in Dental Hygiene,* Second Edition. This book was designed specifically to encourage dental hygiene students to base patient care decisions on knowledge gained in theory, thus fostering in students an appreciation of the link between theory and clinical practice. The following enhance this revised edition.

- Five new cases represent important health issues the dental hygienist will encounter in today's population.
- Continuing the theme of the first edition, the new cases represent a cross section of today's population, representing diverse age groups, ethnicity, and cultures.
- Reorganized pages place the patient situation and questions with the charting data, photographs, and radiographs for ease of reference.
- Facial profiles have been added to each case to provide a "snapshot" of patient characteristics.
- Completely updated questions are based on new research since the publication of the first edition.
- Addition of questions pertaining to ethical decision making and professional responsibility reflect the addition of this category to the National Board Dental Hygiene Examination since publication of the first edition.
- Each case has 5 additional questions for a total of 25.
- Enhanced answer section provides comprehensive rationales for correct answers and a detailed explanation of why an answer is incorrect.
- Updated reference section at the end of each case with publication page numbers provides students and instructors easy access to more information about a subject.
- Enhanced care planning exercises prompt the student to identify patient needs and to develop comprehensive dental hygiene care plans.
- A cross-referenced index to all questions by topic areas guides instructors looking to use questions that pertain to their course subjects.

ACKNOWLEDGMENTS

This second edition of *Case Studies in Dental Hygiene* builds on the original ideas put together for the first edition with my colleagues Deborah Blythe Bauman, BSDH, MS; Deanne Shuman, BSDH, MS, PhD; and Esther K. Andrews, CDA, RDA, RDH, MA. I would like to recognize their contributions, which laid the foundation for the continued success of this edition. I especially appreciate Debbie Bauman's co-authorship of the first drafts of the five new cases. Her efforts in securing the new cases, brainstorming the scenarios, and her expert contributions as a dental hygiene clinical educator were invaluable.

As was true for the first edition, this book would not have been possible without the support and assistance of the students, faculty, and staff at Old Dominion University's Gene W. Hirschfeld School of Dental Hygiene and the patients at the school's Sofia and David Konikoff Dental Hygiene Care Facility who consented to donate personal data to be part of this book. I would like to thank adjunct clinical instructors Walter Milnichuk, DDS; Anne Pennington, RDH, MS; and Margaret Lemaster, BSDH. Wally's enthusiastic response to the need for clinical assistance in securing patients that represent the health issues facing today's population played a significant role in the selection of the new cases; Anne's affiliation with the Hampton Virginia Veterans Affairs Medical Center helped secure volunteer patients for the new cases; and Meg was instrumental in assistance with the clinical photography.

I am particularly grateful to dental hygiene graduate students Ann Poindexter and Joyce Downs for their efforts and the time they devoted to preparing and proofreading the manuscript for publication. I am particularly grateful to undergraduate dental hygiene students Rachel Gray, Sonia Melton, Laura Rowe, Bindiya Shah, Carrie Teague, Elif Thompson, and Heather Vaughan who recognized challenging cases and volunteered to share their learning experiences.

I would like to acknowledge the expert opinions of my colleagues Michele Darby, BSDH, MS; Lynn Tolle, BSDH, MS; and Irene Connolly, BSDH, MS who provided feedback on the accuracy of information included in this second edition.

And, I would like to express appreciation to Mark Cohen, Executive Editor, and to Melissa Kerian, Associate Editor, at Prentice Hall, and to Amy Gehl, Manager Editorial Services, and Lynn Steines, Senior Project Editor at S4Carlisle Publishing Services, for their feedback, contributions, and guidance.

A very special thank you goes to my husband, Hu Odom, for his support and patience throughout the process, and to my good friend Virginia Beach City Public Schools educator Darcy Mahler for her assistance with the photographic images.

Evie Thomson

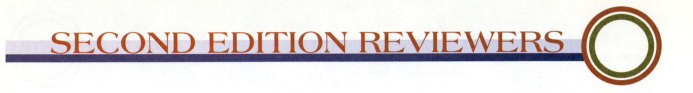

Jill Benetti, RDH, BSDH
Second Year Coordinator and Instructor,
    Dental Hygiene
Yakima Valley Community College
Yakima, Washington

Kristie Boatz, RDH, BS
Instructor, Dental Hygiene
Minnesota State Community and Technical
    College
Moorhead, Minnesota

Marsha E. Bower, CDA, RDH, MA
Associate Professor, Dental Studies
Monroe Community College
Rochester, New York

Valerie L. Carter, RDH, BS, MSDH
Associate Professor, Dental Hygiene
St. Petersburg College
Pinellas Park, Florida

Wanda Cloet, RDH, MS
Director, Dental Hygiene Program
Central Community College
Hastings, Nebraska

Joan M. Davis, RDH, MS
Assistant Professor, Dental Hygiene
Southern Illinois University
Carbondale, Illinois

Barbara Ebert, RDH, MA
Program Director, Dental Hygiene
Wallace State Community College
Hanceville, Alabama

Charmaine P. Godwin, AS, BA, MEd
Assistant Professor, Dental Programs
Santa Fe Community College
Gainesville, Florida

Kimberly Grubka, RDH, AS, BS, MEd
Faculty, Dental Hygiene
Kalamazoo Valley Community College
Kalamazoo, Michigan

Judith A. Hall, RDH, BS
Department Chair, Dental Hygiene
Delaware Technical & Community College
Wilmington, Delaware

Karen Wynn Herrin, RDH, MEd
Professor, Allied Dental Education
New Hampshire Technical Institute
Concord, New Hampshire

Joan L. McClintock, RDH, MEd
Professor, Dental Hygiene
Montgomery County Community College
Blue Bell, Pennsylvania

David C. Reff, BS, DDS
Program Director, Dental Hygiene
Apollo College
Boise, Idaho

Barbara M. Sidel, RDH, MA
Instructor, Dental Hygiene
Delaware Technical & Community College
Dover, Delaware

Julie A. Stage, RDH, BS
Professor, Dental Hygiene
Truckee Meadows Community College
Reno, Nevada

Sharon Struminger, RDH, BS, MPS, MA
Professor, Dental Hygiene
Farmingdale State College
Farmingdale, New York

Joanne N Wylie, RDH, MA
First Year Clinic Coordinator, Dental
    Hygiene
Cabrillo College
Aptos, California

FIRST EDITION REVIEWERS

Pamela Brilowski, RDH, MS
Director, Dental Hygiene Program
Waukesha County Technical College
Pewaukee, Wisconsin

Judith A. Hall, RDH, BS
Department Chair, Dental Hygiene
Delaware Technical & Community College
Wilmington, Delaware

Janet L. Hillis, RDH, MA
Program Chair, Dental Hygiene
Iowa Western Community College
Council Bluffs, Iowa

Julia E. Jevack, BSDH, MS
Assistant Professor, Dental Hygiene
The Ohio State University
Columbus, Ohio

Wendy Kerschbaum, RDH, MA, MPH
Associate Professor and Program Director,
   Dental Hygiene
University of Michigan
Ann Arbor, Michigan

Ulla E. Lemborn, MS
Professor and Director, Dental Hygiene
West Los Angeles College
Culver City, California

Elaine Satin, RDH, MS
Professor, Dental Hygiene
Bergen Community College
Paramus, New Jersey

Rebecca L. Stolberg, RDH, MS
Chairperson, Dental Hygiene
Eastern Washington University
Spokane, Washington

CASE A

Maya Patel

SITUATION

Maya Patel's mother brought her to the dental office today for her 6 months' oral prophylaxis. Maya appears unnaturally stiff and short of breath. She seems to have some difficulty answering when questioned about her self-care. Maya does, however, appear overly willing to cooperate and is opening and closing a poetry journal she has brought with her.

LEARNING GOALS

Following integration of core scientific concepts and application of dental hygiene theory to the care of this patient, you will be able to

1. **Assess patient characteristics.**
   A. Identify developmental normalities and ab-normalities of the dentition.
   B. Identify the normal range of vital signs in the pediatric patient.
   C. Recognize oral conditions of the tongue.
   D. Identify side effects of medications used to treat asthma.

2. **Obtain and interpret radiographs.**
   A. Identify anatomic structures radiographically.
   B. Determine the recommended oral radiographic projection for a pediatric patient.
   C. Recognize the cause of radiographic image distortion.

3. **Plan and manage dental hygiene care.**
   A. Appropriately manage the pediatric patient for successful completion of treatment.
   B. Individualize oral health care instructions for the pediatric patient.
   C. Recognize the signs of an emergency situation and initiate appropriate management actions.

4. **Perform periodontal procedures.**
   A. Recognize microorganisms associated with gingivitis.
   B. Select the most appropriate instruments for subgingival deplaquing for the pediatric patient with gingivitis.

5. **Use preventive agents.**
   A. Select teeth for sealant placement.
   B. Recommend the appropriate preventive agent for the pediatric patient.
   C. Select professionally applied topical fluoride treatment based on patient's needs.

6. **Provide supportive treatment services.**
   A. Determine the appropriate method of stain removal.
   B. Demonstrate knowledge of impression-taking procedure.
   C. Identify nutritional data critical to oral health.

7. **Demonstrate professional responsibility.**
   A. Differentiate between protocols that protect and actions that violate privacy rights of the patient.
   B. Maintain patient health data to reduce the risk of legal implications for the practice.

PEDIATRIC PATIENT—*Maya Patel*
PATIENT HISTORY SYNOPSIS

VITAL STATISTICS

Age	*9 years*	Blood Pressure	*100/60 mm Hg*
Gender	*female*	Pulse Rate	*110 bpm*
Height	*4' 5"*	Respiration	*20 rpm*
Weight	*70 lbs.*		

1. Under care of physician
   Yes ☒   No ☐   Condition: *asthma*

2. Hospitalized within the last 5 years
   Yes ☐   No ☒   Reason: _____

3. Has or had the following conditions
   none

4. Current medications
   montelukast sodium (Singulair) — leukotriene receptor antagonist albuterol (Proventil HFA) — bronchodilator inhaler

5. Smokes or uses tobacco products
   Yes ☐   No ☒

6. Is pregnant
   Yes ☐   No ☒   N/A ☐

MEDICAL HISTORY
Has had several emergency room visits for breathing difficulty.

DENTAL HISTORY
Keeps regular 6-month appointments for oral prophylaxis. Exaggerated gag reflex and mouth breathing. Impressions for study casts have been indicated to evaluate occlusion.

SOCIAL HISTORY
Lives with both parents and 5-year-old younger brother. Both parents work outside the home and they enjoy a middle-class lifestyle. The family moved to the United States from India 6 years ago and they practice the Hindu religion. Maya is a good student in the fourth grade. Her favorite subject is math and she enjoys poetry.

CHIEF COMPLAINT
Nervous about dental treatment

CURRENT ORAL HYGIENE STATUS
Generalized marginal plaque with slight bleeding on probing
Slight supragingival calculus lingual surfaces of the mandibular anterior teeth
Slight generalized brown stain
Flosses occasionally

SUPPLEMENTAL ORAL EXAMINATION FINDINGS
Slight tongue thrust
Slight gingival sensitivity distal to the mandibular left permanent canine
Maxillary left primary first molar is mobile.

ADULT CLINICAL EXAMINATION

	Tooth	Probe 1 / Probe 2
Maxillary R→L (1–16) Probe 1 (upper)	2: 213, 7: 212, 8: 213, 9: 312, 10: 212, 14: 323
Maxillary Probe 1 (lower)	2: 213, 7: 212, 8: 212, 9: 212, 10: 212, 14: 323
Mandibular Probe 1 (upper)	31: 213, 26: 212, 25: 212, 24: 212, 23: 212, 22: 213, 19: 323
Mandibular Probe 1 (lower)	31: 213, 27: 323, 26: 323, 25: 323, 24: 323, 23: 323, 22: 223, 19: 323

🦷 Clinically visible carious lesion

✗ Clinically missing tooth

△ Furcation

▲ "Through and through" furcation

Probe 1: Initial probing depth

Probe 2: Probing depth 6 weeks after periodontal therapy

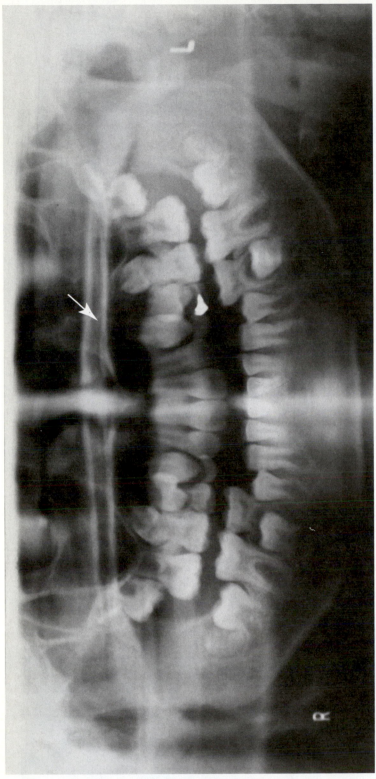

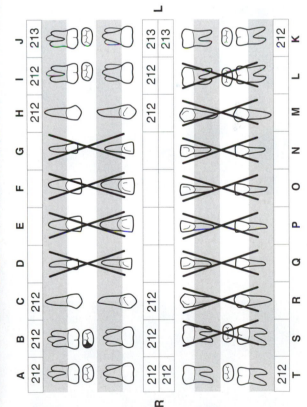

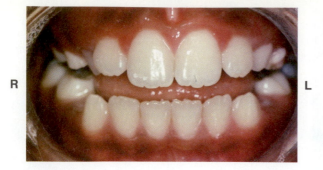

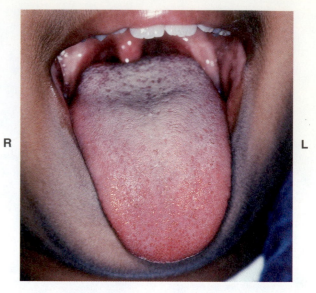

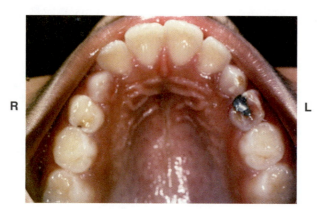

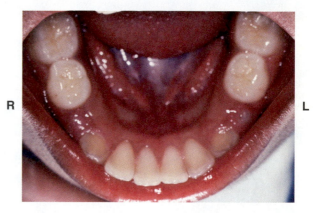

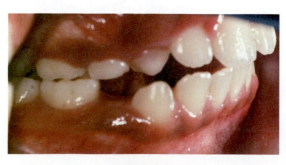

Right side

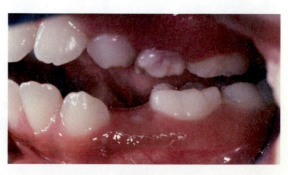

Left side

CASE QUESTIONS

ASSESSING PATIENT CHARACTERISTICS
Basic Level Questions

1. The anterior teeth exhibit which of the following conditions?
   A. Perikymata
   B. Hypoplasia
   C. Fluorosis
   D. Mamelons
   E. Attrition

2. Which of the following best describes this patient's vital signs?
   A. Respiration rate is considered high.
   B. Respiration rate is considered low.
   C. Pulse rate is considered high.
   D. Pulse rate is considered within normal range.
   E. Blood pressure is considered high.

Competency Level Questions

3. The raised, white finding that appears between the mandibular left permanent canine and the mandibular left primary second molar is most likely a(n)
   A. Aphthous ulcer
   B. Mandibular torus
   C. Developmental cyst
   D. Retained primary root tip
   E. Erupting permanent premolar

4. Which of the following is the correct assessment of the appearance of this patient's tongue?
   A. Coated
   B. Fissured
   C. Lymphangioma
   D. Macroglossia
   E. Ulcerated

5. Which of the following is NOT an adverse effect of this patient's medications?
   A. Xerostomia
   B. Taste changes
   C. Increased anxiety
   D. Sore throat
   E. Gingival bleeding

OBTAINING AND INTERPRETING RADIOGRAPHS
Basic Level Questions

6. What is the name of the anatomic structure seen as a horizontal radiopacity above the maxillary teeth (arrow) in the panoramic radiograph?
   A. Incisive foramen
   B. Hard palate
   C. Nasal fossae
   D. Nasal septum
   E. Median palatine suture

Competency Level Questions

7. Which of the following is the best reason why the panoramic radiograph was chosen over intraoral radiographs for this patient?
   A. Possibility of asthma attack
   B. Patient must remain in an upright position.
   C. Hypersensitive gag reflex
   D. Lower radiation dosage
   E. Patient is nervous about treatment.

8. What is the reason for the shortened appearance of the mandibular incisors on the panoramic radiograph?
   A. Teeth tipped out of the focal trough
   B. External physiologic resorption
   C. Apices have not fully formed.
   D. Microdontia of the central and lateral incisors
   E. Incorrect vertical angulation of the x-ray beam

PLANNING AND MANAGING DENTAL HYGIENE CARE
Basic Level Questions

9. This patient's behavior today may be clinical signs of each of the following EXCEPT one. Which one is the EXCEPTION?
   A. Asthma attack onset
   B. Cultural background
   C. Moderate anxiety
   D. Medication side effects

10. Each of the following will help to manage this patient's hypersensitive gag reflex during the taking of impressions EXCEPT one. Which one is the EXCEPTION?
    A. Select a tray size to accommodate the size of the arches by trying the tray in the mouth before loading with impression material.
    B. Direct the patient to quietly hum her favorite song while the tray is in place.
    C. Ask the patient to breath deeply through the nose during the procedure.
    D. Press down on the anterior region of the tray first when seating in the mouth.
    E. Explain the procedure to the patient with empathetic rapport, while maintaining confidence and authority.

11. What method of tongue debridement is recommended for this patient?
    A. Rinse the mouth daily with an oxygenating mouth rinse.
    B. Scrape the tongue with a tongue scraper.
    C. Brush the tongue with a toothbrush.
    D. Irrigate the tongue with an oral irrigator.
    E. Recommend the use of a sugarless gum with xylitol.

12. What method of patient management would best serve this patient?
    A. Show-tell-do
    B. Oral sedation
    C. Papoose board restriction
    D. Hypnosis
    E. Biofeedback

Competency Level Questions

13. Which of the following will assist in managing a possible emergency medical situation regarding this patient?
    A. Premedicate with oral antibiotics.
    B. Monitor vital signs during dental hygiene treatment.
    C. Request a recent prothrombin time.

D. Require that her mother remain in the room during treatment.

E. Place Proventil HFA inhaler on the bracket table ready for use.

14. Approximately halfway through the appointment, this patient complains of trouble breathing. The clinician should do each of the following EXCEPT one. Which one is the EXCEPTION?

A. Continue conversation that calms the patient.

B. Terminate the dental procedure at once.

C. Remove all instruments from the patient's mouth.

D. Place the patient in the Trendelenberg position.

E. Administer a bronchodilator.

PERFORMING PERIODONTAL PROCEDURES
Basic Level Questions

15. Which of the following microorganisms is/are associated with this patient's periodontal condition?

A. *Streptococcus salivaris*

B. Actinomyces, Streptococcus, and Fusobacterium

C. *Fusobacterium nucleatum* and *Prevotella intermedia*

D. *Streptococcus mutans* and lactobaccilli

E. *Actinobacillus actinomycetemcomitans*

16. Which of the following would be the best instrument for subgingival deplaquing this patient's bleeding sites?

A. Ultrasonic scaling device

B. Anterior sickle scaler

C. Area-specific curets

D. Universal sickle scaler

E. Universal curet

USING PREVENTIVE AGENTS
Basic Level Questions

17. Which of this patient's teeth should be indicated for sealants?

A. Primary first molars

B. Primary second molars

C. Permanent first premolars

D. Permanent first molars

E. Permanent second molars

Competency Level Questions

18. Which of the following chemotherapeutics and preventive agents should be recommended for daily use for this patient?

A. Self-applied fluoride

B. Phenolic-related essential oils

C. Oxygenating agents

D. Quaternary ammonium compounds

E. Chlorhexidine gluconate

19. Which of the following is the best choice for a professionally applied topical fluoride treatment for this patient?

A. Acidulated phosphate fluoride

B. Neutral sodium fluoride

C. Stannous fluoride

D. Sodium monofluorophosphate fluoride

PROVIDING SUPPORTIVE TREATMENT SERVICES
Basic Level Questions

20. Which of the following is the method of choice for extrinsic stain removal for this patient?
    A. Rubber cup coronal polishing
    B. Air-powder abrasive
    C. Scaling and toothbrush prophylaxis
    D. Toothbrushing with commercial prophylaxis paste
    E. Ultrasonic scaling

21. Which of the following will most likely cause difficulty when taking impressions on this patient?
    A. Sensitive gingiva
    B. Tongue thrust
    C. Pronounced overjet
    D. Occlusal open bite
    E. Hypersensitive gag reflex

Competency Level Questions

22. Each of the following is considered critical to nutritional counseling for this patient EXCEPT one. Which one is the EXCEPTION?
    A. Cultural food preferences
    B. Inclusion of person responsible for meal preparation
    C. Medication interference with metabolism
    D. Frequency of carbohydrate intake
    E. Number of servings from food groups

DEMONSTRATING PROFESSIONAL RESPONSIBILITY
Basic Level Questions

23. How long should this patient's panoramic radiograph be retained by the practice?
    A. For 5 years from the date of exposure
    B. Until the patient turns 18 years of age
    C. Until a new radiograph is taken to update this survey
    D. Until the patient ceases to be a client of this practice
    E. Indefinitely

Competency Level Questions

24. Discussing this patient's personal oral self-care habits, dental hygiene treatment plan, and goals for achieving oral health with her mother is in violation of HIPAA (Health Insurance Portability and Accountability Act).

    Protecting this patient's privacy is a HIPAA regulation.
    A. The first statement is true, the second statement is false.
    B. The first statement is false, the second statement is true.
    C. Both statements are true.
    D. Both statements are false.

25. Placing a red sticker on this patient's dental record indicating that she is asthmatic is a good risk management strategy.

    Tagging the patient record in this manner is acceptable because only oral health care personnel will handle the charts.
    A. The first statement is true, the second statement is false.
    B. The first statement is false, the second statement is true.
    C. Both statements are true.
    D. Both statements are false.

SETTING PATIENT GOALS

ESTABLISHING A DENTAL HYGIENE CARE PLAN

To assist this patient in meeting her needs, develop a dental hygiene care plan that establishes a framework within which to help her and her caregiver identify goals for obtaining oral health. In addition to the clinical assessment, a well-prepared dental hygiene care plan should take into account the patient's age, gender, lifestyle, culture, attitudes, health beliefs, and knowledge level. To help link this patient's needs for overall well-being with her oral conditions, and to provide motivation for achieving better health, the following is a partial list of possible deficits based on the Human Needs Conceptual Model to Dental Hygiene Practice. (See the appendix for an explanation of the Human Needs Conceptual Model to Dental Hygiene Practice to help you identify additional unmet needs.) Use this partial list of unmet needs or deficits as a guide in preparing a dental hygiene care plan for this patient. One set of goals and dental hygiene actions/implications has been completed as an example.

Deficit identified in Protection from Health Risks

Due to: risk for an asthma attack
Evidenced by: potential for a medical emergency

Goals: _____

Dental hygiene actions/implications: _____

Deficit identified in Freedom from Anxiety and Stress

Due to: fear related to dental treatment
Evidenced by: parent report and anxious behaviors
Goals: *to avoid an emergency situation involving an acute asthma attack; anticipate dental hygiene appointments without anxiety*

Dental hygiene actions/implications: *communicate on the patient's level of understanding; use child-friendly techniques and equipment; use show-tell-do and modeling, when possible, so the child can observe the procedure being performed on a parent*

Deficit identified in Skin and Mucous Membrane Integrity of the Head and Neck

Due to: bacterial plaque and inadequate oral health behaviors
Evidenced by: presence of gingival inflammation and bleeding

Goals: _____

Dental hygiene actions/implications: _____

Deficit identified in Biologically Sound Dentition

Due to: future caries risk
Evidenced by: existing carious lesion

Goals: _____

Dental hygiene actions/implications: _____

Deficit identified in Responsibility for Oral Health

Due to: inadequate oral health behaviors and parental supervision
Evidenced by: gingivitis and caries

Goals: _____

Dental hygiene actions/implications: _____

REFLECTIVE ACTIVITIES

1. People from India who practice the Hindu religion consider cows sacred and do not eat beef. Review the nutrients available from the consumption of beef and recommend other nutritional sources for these nutrients to improve oral health.

2. Examine the ethnic, cultural, or regional dietary practices and/or problems present in the population in your area. Plan a 3-day menu that would fulfill the recommended dietary allowance and incorporate food preferences for this population.

3. Discuss preappointment dental hygiene interventions that will create a child-centered, nonthreatening environment to minimize this patient's anxiety.

REFERENCES

Bird DL, Robinson DS: *Torres and Ehrlich Modern Dental Assisting,* 7th ed. St. Louis: Saunders (Elsevier), 2002, pp. 735–739.

Darby ML, Walsh MM: *Dental Hygiene Theory and Practice,* 2nd ed. St. Louis: Saunders (Elsevier), 2003, pp. 54–56, 252–255, 373–376, 529–561.

Davis JR, Stegeman CA: *The Dental Hygienist's Guide to Nutritional Care,* 2nd ed. St. Louis: Saunders (Elsevier), 2005, pp. 447–470.

Davison JA: *Legal and Ethical Considerations for Dental Hygienists and Assistants.* St. Louis: Mosby, 2000, p. 159.

Ibsen AOC, Phelan JA: *Oral Pathology for the Dental Hygienist,* 4th ed. St. Louis: Saunders (Elsevier), 2004, pp. 95–98, 173.

Johnson ON, Thomson EM: *Essentials of Dental Radiography for Dental Assistants and Hygienists,* 8th ed. Upper Saddle River, NJ: Prentice Hall, 2007, pp. 387–403.

Kimbrough VJ, Lautar CJ: *Ethics, Jurisprudence, and Practice Management in Dental Hygiene,* 2nd ed. Upper Saddle River, NJ: Prentice Hall, 2007, pp. 100–102.

Malamed SF: *Medical Emergencies in the Dental Office,* 5th ed. St. Louis: Mosby, 2000, pp. 36, 39–49, 214–221.

McDonald RE, Avery DR, Dean JA: *Dentistry for the Child and Adolescent,* 8th ed. St. Louis: Mosby (Elsevier), 2004, pp. 33–49, 354–363.

Nazario B (ed.): Recognizing an asthma attack. WebMD. 2006. http://www.webmd.com/content/article/72/81592.htm. Accessed February 8, 2007.

Neuenfeldt E: The use of pit and fissure sealants in preventive dentistry. *Access,* 20(10), 34–37, 2006.

Perry DA, Beemsterboer P, Taggart EJ: *Periodontology for the Dental Hygienist,* 3rd ed. St. Louis: Saunders (Elsevier), 2007, pp. 62–76.

Pickett FA, Gurenlian JR: *The Medical History: Clinical Implications and Emergency Prevention in Dental Settings.* Baltimore: Lippincott Williams & Wilkins, 2005, pp. 46, 142–143, 174–176.

Pickett FA, Terezhalmy GT: *Lippincott Williams & Wilkins' Dental Drug Reference with Clinical Implications.* Baltimore: Lippincott Williams & Wilkins, 2006, pp. 188–190, 559.

Pinkham JR, Casamassimo PS, Fields HW, McTigue DJ, Nowak AJ: *Pediatric Dentistry: Infancy through Adolescence,* 4th ed. St. Louis: Elsevier (Saunders) 2005, pp. 223–233, 513–519.

Samaranayake L: *Essentials of Microbiology for Dentistry,* 3rd ed. New York: Churchill Livingstone, 2006, p. 227.

Spolarich AE: Drugs used to manage asthma. *Access,* 15(10), 38–41, 2001.

Wilkins EM: *Clinical Practice of the Dental Hygienist,* 9th ed. Philadelphia: Lippincott Williams & Wilkins, 2005, pp. 131, 192, 388–390, 419–420, 444–445, 520–564, 571–572, 729–730.

Woelful JB, Scheid RC: *Dental Anatomy: Its Relevance to Dentistry,* 6th ed. Philadelphia: Lippincott Williams & Wilkins, 2002, pp. 100, 114.

CASE B

Zack Ware

SITUATION

Zack Ware is a physically active sixth grader who spends his free time playing baseball and skateboarding with friends. Although he has always enjoyed the camaraderie of his peers, he has suffered teasing lately as he begins orthodontic treatment. To help maintain his acceptance, Zack has allowed his peers to talk him into trying spit tobacco, suggesting that professional athletes benefit from its use. His mother does not know about the tobacco use.

LEARNING GOALS

Following integration of core scientific concepts and application of dental hygiene theory to the care of this patient, you will be able to

1. **Assess patient characteristics.**
   A. Classify facial profile.
   B. Classify occlusion using Angle's system of malocclusion.
   C. Recognize eruption/exfoliation patterns.
   D. Identify the probable cause of nocturnal bruxism.
   E. Recognize the need for orthodontic evaluation.
   F. Differentiate dental fluorosis from other white spot lesions.

2. **Obtain and interpret radiographs.**
   A. Interpret radiopaque findings commonly present on radiographic images.
   B. Identify oral conditions indicating the need for a cephalometric radiograph.
   C. Identify radiographic artifacts commonly found on a cephalometric radiograph.
   D. Identify anatomic planes used to position a patient for a cephalometric radiograph.

3. **Plan and manage dental hygiene care.**
   A. Make oral self-care recommendations based on individual needs of the patient.
   B. Recognize the cognitive development stages of adolescent patients.
   C. Communicate effectively with the pediatric patient to improve motivation for oral self-care.

4. **Perform periodontal procedures.**
   A. Use appropriate terminology when describing gingival appearance.
   B. Identify the causes of gingival tissue changes.

5. **Use preventive agents.**
   A. Utilize preventive agents based on patient assessment.
   B. Select the appropriate type of fluoride based on patient assessment.

6. **Provide supportive treatment services.**
   A. Select the appropriate stain removal method based on patient assessment.
   B. Evaluate the quality of study cast models.
   C. Determine the reasons for spit tobacco use among adolescents.
   D. Plan oral health instruction for an adolescent using spit tobacco.
   E. Determine the need for mouthguard protection.

7. **Demonstrate professional responsibility.**
   A. Implement strategies that will elicit a thorough and complete health history.
   B. Identify legal responsibilities of treating the adolescent patient.

PEDIATRIC PATIENT—*Zack Ware*
PATIENT HISTORY SYNOPSIS

Age	*12 years*
Gender	*male*
Height	*5' 1"*
Weight	*90 lbs.*

VITAL STATISTICS

Blood Pressure	*112/68 mm Hg*
Pulse Rate	*74 bpm*
Respiration	*14 rpm*

1. Under care of physician
   Yes ☐   No ☒   Condition: _____
   _____

2. Hospitalized within the last 5 years
   Yes ☐   No ☒   Reason: _____
   _____

3. Has or had the following conditions
   none _____
   _____
   _____

4. Current medications
   none _____
   _____
   _____
   _____

5. Smokes or uses tobacco products
   Yes ☒   No ☐

6. Is pregnant
   Yes ☐   No ☐   N/A ☒

MEDICAL HISTORY
Good health

DENTAL HISTORY
Patient grew up in a region with a water supply that contained a high fluoride concentration (greater than 2 ppm). Currently in maxillary orthodontics. His mother reports that he has started to grind his teeth at night.

SOCIAL HISTORY
Patient lives with his mother, who works many hours in the restaurant business. He is unsupervised from 3:00 p.m. until 6:30 p.m. Monday through Friday. Drinks several bottles of sports drinks throughout the day. When asked, he admits to trying spit tobacco.

CHIEF COMPLAINT
Patient is just getting used to the braces recently placed on his maxillary teeth. He is not happy about having to brush better or longer and expresses that he is angry about having to give up chewing bubble gum while in orthodontic treatment.

ADULT CLINICAL EXAMINATION

	1	2	3	4	5	6	7	8	9	10	11	12	13	14	15	16
Probe 2																
Probe 1	X	323	323	323	312	212	222	323	323	222	223	323	X	323	323	X
Probe 1	X	323	323	323	323	312	212	212	212	212	213	323	X	323	323	X
Probe 2																

R | | | | | | | | | | | | | | | | | L

	32	31	30	29	28	27	26	25	24	23	22	21	20	19	18	17
Probe 2																
Probe 1	X	323	323	212	212	212	212	212	212	212	212	X	X	323	323	X
Probe 1	X	323	323	212	212	212	212	213	312	212	213	212	X	323	323	X
Probe 2																

CURRENT ORAL HYGIENE STATUS
Generalized marginal plaque accumulation with slight bleeding on probing

SUPPLEMENTAL ORAL EXAMINATION FINDINGS
Breathes through his mouth
Mandibular left primary molar is mobile

⬜ Clinically visible carious lesion
✗ Clinically missing tooth
△ Furcation
▲ "Through and through" furcation
Probe 1: Initial probing depth
Probe 2: Probing depth 6 weeks after periodontal therapy

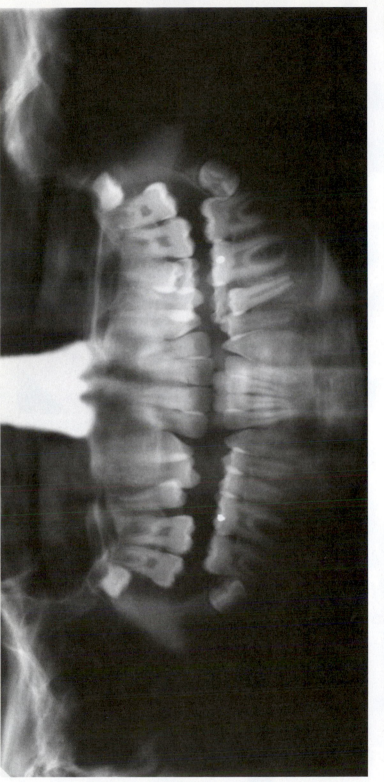

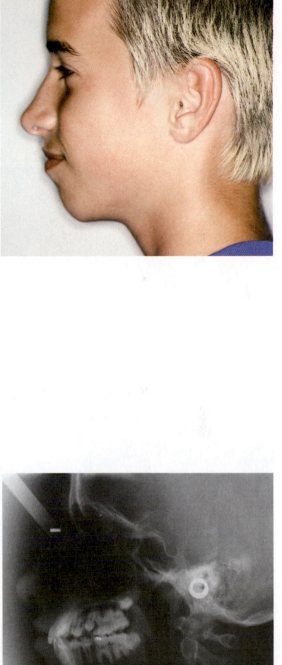

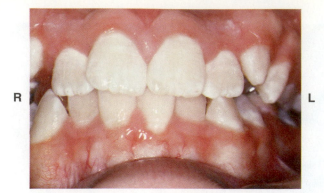

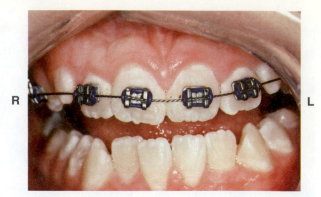

**1 month prior to placement of
orthodontic bands**

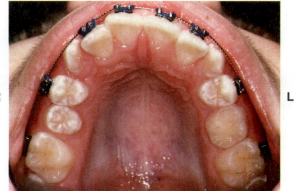

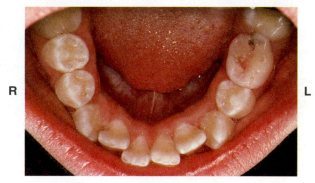

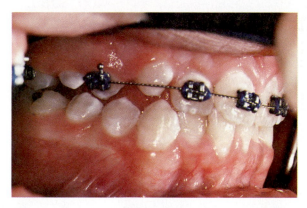

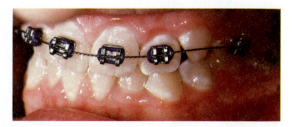

Left side

Right side

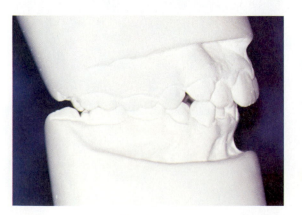

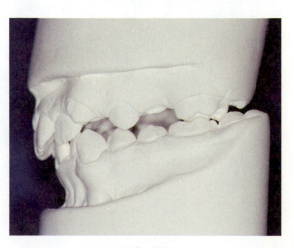

Right side

Left side

CASE QUESTIONS

ASSESSING PATIENT CHARACTERISTICS
Basic Level Questions

1. Which of the following terms best describes this patient's facial profile?
   A. Mesognathic
   B. Retrognathic
   C. Prognathic
   D. Orthognathic

2. What is Angle's classification of malocclusion for this patient?
   A. Class I
   B. Class II, Division 1
   C. Class II, Division 2
   D. Class III

3. The primary mandibular left second molar will most likely be the next tooth exfoliated.

   The mandibular left second premolar will erupt into this position.
   A. The first statement is true, the second statement is false.
   B. The first statement is false, the second statement is true.
   C. Both statements are true.
   D. Both statements are false.

Competency Level Questions

4. Which of the following would be the most likely explanation for the nocturnal bruxism reported by his mother?
   A. Stress of being teased by peers
   B. Uneven incisal edges of the anterior teeth
   C. Chewing bubble gum
   D. Occlusal interferences
   E. Retained primary teeth

5. All of this patient's permanent teeth are developing normally.

   This patient's arch space is adequate for the eruption of the permanent teeth.
   A. The first statement is true, the second statement is false.
   B. The first statement is false, the second statement is true.
   C. Both statements are true.
   D. Both statements are false.

6. What is the most likely assessment of the white spots observed on the anterior teeth?
   A. Caries
   B. Remineralization
   C. Abrasion
   D. Fluorosis
   E. Wear facets

OBTAINING AND INTERPRETING RADIOGRAPHS
Basic Level Questions

7. The radiopacities on the permanent mandibular first molars, visible on the panoramic radiograph, are most likely
   A. Carious lesions
   B. Enamel pearls
   C. Processor artifacts
   D. Orthodontic brackets
   E. Amalgam restorations

8. The cephalometric radiograph was exposed on this patient to assess which one of the following?
   A. Periodontal status
   B. Growth and development
   C. Presence of caries
   D. Sinus cavity congestion
   E. Detection of precancerous lesions

Competency Level Questions

9. What is the radiopaque circle-shaped object that appears on the cephalometric radiograph near the external auditory meatus?
   A. Metal earring stud
   B. Orthodontic bracket
   C. Cephalostat ear rod
   D. Fixer contamination
   E. Film label

10. The radiopaque object visible at the patient's nasion on the cephalometric radiograph is used to align the
    A. Midsaggital plane
    B. Frankfort plane
    C. Occlusal plane
    D. Vertical plane
    E. Mandibular plane

11. Which of the following is the most likely reason for the widened appearance of the pulp chambers of the mandibular canines visible on the panoramic radiograph?
    A. Internal resorption
    B. External resorption
    C. Cervical burnout
    D. Incomplete root formation
    E. Nocturnal bruxism

PLANNING AND MANAGING DENTAL HYGIENE CARE
Basic Level Questions

12. Which of the following would be the best recommendation for oral self-care for this patient?
    A. Power toothbrush
    B. Oral irrigation device
    C. Floss threader
    D. Sulcus brush
    E. Wooden wedge

Competency Level Questions

13. Which of the following characteristics of development is relevant to this patient's age group and managing his preventive oral health self-care instruction?
    A. Incomplete development of a sense of logic will limit an explanation of the disease process.
    B. Continued dependence on his mother will necessitate parental influence to achieve optimal oral health self-care.
    C. A heightened sense of imagination may increase anxiety related to his lack of adequate self-care behaviors.

    D. Orientation to future possibilities will enhance acceptance of preventive regimens discussed today.

    E. An overriding sense of invincibility will promote a lack of concern for developing good oral health care habits now.

14. Which of the following paired actions will most likely result in an increase in successful oral health education for this patient?

    A. Consult his mother to complete a dental history and determine her role in his oral home self-care.

    B. Assess the patient's oral conditions and document oral problems to show him a visual progression of his developing oral conditions.

    C. Investigate his personal interests to determine what motivates him and present him with a new oral hygiene aid.

    D. Determine his current self-care regimen and suggest he increase the time spent performing self-care techniques.

PERFORMING PERIODONTAL PROCEDURES
Basic Level Questions

15. Which of the following terms best describes the appearance of the maxillary facial gingiva before orthodontic intervention?

    A. Knife-like

    B. Rolled

    C. Cratered

    D. Clefting

    E. Blunted

Competency Level Questions

16. Which of the following is the most likely explanation for the appearance of the maxillary facial gingiva before orthodontic intervention?

    A. Erupting teeth

    B. Subgingival calculus

    C. Spit tobacco use

    D. Mouth breathing

    E. Carbohydrate drinks

USING PREVENTIVE AGENTS
Competency Level Questions

17. Each of the following should be recommended for this patient EXCEPT one. Which one is the EXCEPTION?

    A. Sealants

    B. Fluoride varnish

    C. Enamel microabrasion

    D. Oral irrigation

    E. Dietary counseling

18. It is highly likely that this patient will consume another sports drink immediately upon leaving the office following his fluoride treatment. Anticipating this, which of the following professionally applied fluoride treatments would be recommended?

    A. 2% NaF gel

    B. 5% NaF varnish

    C. 1.23% APF foam

    D. 1.23% APF aqueous solution

    E. 8% SnF aqueous solution

PROVIDING SUPPORTIVE TREATMENT SERVICES
Basic Level Questions

19. Which of the following extrinsic stain removal polishing methods is indicated for this patient?
    A. Rubber cup
    B. Manual toothbrush
    C. Air-powder abrasive
    D. Porte polisher

20. Which of the following criteria for an acceptable cast applies to this patient's finished casts?
    A. Mean occlusal planes are parallel to the bases.
    B. Posterior borders are at right angles to the bases.
    C. If stood on the posterior base, the casts would rest together naturally.
    D. Anterior border of the mandibular cast is cut arc shaped.
    E. Proportions are two-thirds anatomic and one-third art.

Competency Level Questions

21. This patient is too young to get addicted to tobacco use.

    Adolescents may experiment with tobacco because of insecurity, rebelliousness, and identification with role models.
    A. The first statement is true, the second statement is false.
    B. The first statement is false, the second statement is true.
    C. Both statements are true.
    D. Both statements are false.

22. Each of these statements is accurate and can be used to assist this patient in making his decision to use spit tobacco EXCEPT one. Which one is the EXCEPTION?
    A. Highly addictive
    B. Contains nicotine
    C. Helps athletic performance
    D. Not a safe alternative to cigarettes
    E. Contributes to oral diseases

23. A hard plastic thermoset resin mouthguard is indicated for this patient, because skateboarding increases his risk of oral injury.
    A. Both the statement and reason are correct and related.
    B. Both the statement and reason are correct but not related.
    C. The statement is correct but the reason is not.
    D. The statement is not correct but the reason is accurate.
    E. Neither the statement nor reason is correct.

DEMONSTRATING PROFESSIONAL RESPONSIBILITY
Competency Level Questions

24. Each of the following will help to obtain an accurate medical history and to deal appropriately with conditions and concerns regarding this patient EXCEPT one. Which one is the EXCEPTION?
    A. This patient can give informed consent to undergo treatment.
    B. This patient's parent should be encouraged to complete his health history *with* her son and not *for* him.
    C. The dental hygienist should explain oral health findings and the care plan to both the patient and his parent.
    D. The dental hygienist should provide an opportunity for the patient to contribute to the health history alone, away from his parent.
    E. The health history of the adolescent patient is constantly changing and should be updated regularly.

25. The dental hygienist has a responsibility to report this patient's tobacco use to his mother.

   Reporting his tobacco use is a form of paternalism.
   A. The first statement is true, the second statement is false.
   B. The first statement is false, the second statement is true.
   C. Both statements are true.
   D. Both statements are false.

SETTING PATIENT GOALS

ESTABLISHING A DENTAL HYGIENE CARE PLAN

To assist this patient in meeting his needs, develop a dental hygiene care plan that establishes a framework within which to help him and his caregiver identify goals for obtaining oral health. In addition to the clinical assessment, a well-prepared dental hygiene care plan should take into account the patient's age, gender, lifestyle, culture, attitudes, health beliefs, and knowledge level. To help link this patient's needs for overall well-being with his oral conditions, and to provide motivation for achieving better health, the following is a partial list of possible deficits based on the Human Needs Conceptual Model to Dental Hygiene Practice. (See the appendix for an explanation of the Human Needs Conceptual Model to Dental Hygiene Practice to help you identify additional unmet needs.) Use this partial list of unmet needs or deficits as a guide in preparing a dental hygiene care plan for this patient. One set of goals and dental hygiene actions/implications has been completed as an example.

Deficit identified in Protection from Health Risks

Due to: increased risk for oral injury
Evidenced by: self-reported skateboarding

Goals: _____

Dental hygiene actions/implications: _____

Deficit identified in Biologically Sound Dentition

Due to: future caries risk
Evidenced by: existing caries; consuming carbohydrate drinks

Goals: _____

Dental hygiene actions/implications: _____

Deficit identified in Conceptualization and Problem Solving

Due to: lack of knowledge regarding the link of spit tobacco and health
Evidenced by: self-report that athletes use it, so it must be beneficial

Goals: _____

Dental hygiene actions/implications: _____

Deficit identified in Responsibility for Oral Health

Due to: inadequate oral health behaviors and parental supervision
Evidenced by: gingivitis and caries; use of spit tobacco

Goals: _____

Dental hygiene actions/implications: _____

Deficit identified in Wholesome Facial Image

Due to: presence of braces

Evidenced by: lack of understanding and acceptance of orthodontic bands in improving functionality and appearance

Goals: *to understand and accept that the outcomes of orthodontic intervention will include multiple benefits; to assist the success of orthodontic intervention by improving oral self-care*

Dental hygiene actions/implications: *develop a rapport on the patient's level of understanding to obtain answers to questions regarding why he is dissatisfied/embarrassed by wearing braces; assist the patient in developing strategies to deal with the perceived inconvenience of wearing braces; educate the patient on the benefits of orthodontic intervention and the failures that may result if self-care instructions are not followed*

REFLECTIVE ACTIVITIES

1. Divide into small groups of three to five students. Each group should list one patient-centered goal for each dental hygiene diagnosis for this patient. Compile the goals as a group and report to the class. Goals may be written for the cognitive, psychomotor, or affective domains or for oral health status improvement. Each goal should have a subject, verb, criteria for measurement, and a time line for when the subject is to have achieved the goal.

2. Applying a cotherapeutic, collaborative, patient-centered view of the dental hygiene process of care, list strategies that can be utilized to involve and motivate the adolescent patient in the care planning process.

REFERENCES

Academy for Sports Dentistry: Mouthguards essential for today's female athlete. 1999. http://www.ada.org/public/media/newsrel/9910/nr-13.html. Accessed April 9, 2002.

American Dental Association: Do you need a mouth guard? *Journal of the American Dental Association*, 132, 2001. http://jada.ada.org. Accessed February 10, 2007.

American Dental Association: Protecting teeth with mouth guards. *Journal of the American Dental Association*, 137, 2006. http://jada.ada.org. Accessed February 10, 2007.

Darby ML, Walsh MM: *Dental Hygiene Theory and Practice*, 2nd ed. St. Louis: Saunders (Elsevier), 2003, pp. 245–255, 343, 354–357.

Ellison J, Mansell C, Hoika L, MacDougall W, Gansky S, Walsh M: Characteristics of adolescent smoking in high school students in California. *Journal of Dental Hygiene*, 80(2), 1–16, 2006.

Horowitz HS, Driscoll WS, Meyers RJ, Heifetz SB, Kingman AK: A new method for assessing the prevalence of dental fluorosis. The tooth surface index of fluorosis. *Journal of the American Dental Association*, 109(7), 37, 1984.

Kimbrough VJ, Henderson K: *Oral Health Education*. Upper Saddle River, NJ: Prentice Hall, 2006, pp. 27–29, 57–59.

Johnson ON, Thomson EM: *Essentials of Dental Radiography for Dental Assistants and Hygienists*, 8th ed. Upper Saddle River, NJ: Prentice Hall, 2007, pp. 368–380.

Mayo Foundation for Medical Education and Research: Chewing tobacco. Not a risk-free alternative to cigarettes. http://www.mayoclinic.com. Accessed February 10, 2007.

McDonald RE, Avery DR, Dean JA: *Dentistry for the Child and Adolescent*, 8th ed. St. Louis: Mosby (Elsevier), 2004, pp. 205–207, 251–254, 646–648.

Morris DW: Using evidence-based tobacco cessation therapies in dental hygiene practice. *Contemporary Dental Hygiene*, 6(9), 20–25, 2006.

National Cancer Institute and National Institute of Dental Research: *Spitting into the Wind: The Facts about Dip and Chew.* Washington, DC: U.S. Department of Health and Human Services, 1996.

National Institute of Dental and Craniofacial Research: Spit tobacco. A guide for quitting. http://www.nidcr.nih.gov. Accessed February 10, 2007.

Neuenfeldt E: The use of pit and fissure sealants in preventive dentistry. *Access*, 20(10), 34–37, 2006.

Pinkham JR, Casamassimo PS, Fields HW, McTigue DJ, Nowak AJ: *Pediatric Dentistry: Infancy through Adolescence*, 4th ed. St. Louis: Elsevier (Saunders) 2005, pp. 431–439, 499–506, 674–675, 703.

Wilkins EM: *Clinical Practice of the Dental Hygienist*, 9th ed. Philadelphia: Lippincott Williams & Wilkins, 2005, pp. 200–204, 278–287, 458, 546, 726–740, 817–819.

Woelful JB, Scheid RC: *Dental Anatomy: Its Relevance to Dentistry*, 6th ed. Philadelphia: Lippincott Williams & Wilkins, 2002, pp. 100, 114.

CASE C

Andrew Christianson

SITUATION

Andrew Christianson appears to be having difficulty paying attention to what is expected of him during today's appointment. His mother says that he has been particularly "spacey" the last couple of days. When asked to demonstrate what he has just learned following self-care instructions, he seems to lack an understanding of what he is supposed to do and makes frequent mistakes. He is cooperating with the treatment today, sitting quietly, unobtrusively, but appears to not be fully attending to or understanding the task and the instructions.

LEARNING GOALS

Following integration of core scientific concepts and application of dental hygiene theory to the care of this patient, you will be able to

1. **Assess patient characteristics.**
   A. Distinguish between oral conditions encountered during an intraoral examination.
   B. Identify various conditions of the teeth.
   C. Describe caries observed clinically.
   D. Classify tooth stains.
   E. List possible adverse effects of medications.

2. **Obtain and interpret radiographs.**
   A. Identify the cause of radiographic errors.
   B. Demonstrate knowledge of the radiographic appearance of normal anatomical conditions of the developing tooth.
   C. Interpret radiographs for deviations from the normal and pathologic conditions.
   D. Distinguish normal tooth development from pathologic conditions.

3. **Plan and manage dental hygiene care.**
   A. Recognize potential triggers of a gag reflex.
   B. Provide dental hygiene treatment based on the patient's needs.
   C. Recognize conditions of the oral cavity that may contraindicate treatment.
   D. Utilize a communication style that meets the needs of the pediatric patient.

4. **Perform periodontal procedures.**
   A. Differentiate between various soft and hard deposits found on the teeth.

5. **Use preventive agents.**
   A. Select appropriate teeth for sealant placement.
   B. Prescribe appropriate home fluoride therapy.

6. **Provide supportive treatment services.**
   A. Select the appropriate stain removal technique based on patient needs.
   B. Counsel the pediatric patient for improved nutrition.

7. **Demonstrate professional responsibility.**
   A. Apply ALARA philosophy when exposing radiographs on pediatric patients.
   B. Recognize dental neglect and its link to child abuse.
   C. Utilize effective communication techniques to educate the pediatric patient's caregiver on the importance of the child's oral health.

PEDIATRIC PATIENT—_Andrew Christianson_
PATIENT HISTORY SYNOPSIS

VITAL STATISTICS

Age	_8 years_
Gender	_male_
Height	_4' 3"_
Weight	_58 lbs._

Blood Pressure	_108/62 mm Hg_
Pulse Rate	_80 bpm_
Respiration	_16 rpm_

1. Under care of physician
   Yes [X] No [ ]
   Condition: _attention deficit_
   hyperactivity disorder
   (ADHD)

2. Hospitalized within the last 5 years
   Yes [ ] No [X]
   Reason: _____
   _____

3. Has or had the following conditions
   seasonal allergies
   _____
   _____

4. Current medications
   amphetamine (Adderall)
   _____
   _____
   _____

5. Smokes or uses tobacco products
   Yes [ ] No [X]

6. Is pregnant
   Yes [ ] No [ ] N/A [X]

MEDICAL HISTORY
Under physician's care for ADHD since age 5. Andrew's predominately inattentive type ADHD (as opposed to hyperactive-impulsive type) makes it more difficult for him to process information as quickly and accurately as other children. Seldom acting impulsive or hyperactive, he often appears to be daydreaming, slow moving, and lethargic as a result of this disorder. Physician has recently changed his medication.

DENTAL HISTORY
No history of professional dental or dental hygiene treatment. His mother reports that he may have participated in oral screenings and school fluoride treatments in the past.

SOCIAL HISTORY
Has one older brother and two younger sisters. Attends an after school program at the neighborhood recreation center where his favorite activity is playing video games. He has access to snack vending machines and loves to drink soda.

ADULT CLINICAL EXAMINATION

CURRENT ORAL HYGIENE STATUS
Moderate anterior plaque
Materia alba accumulating around large caries

He brushes up and down in the morning and before bed, when he remembers.

SUPPLEMENTAL ORAL EXAMINATION FINDINGS
Mouth breather

 Clinically visible carious lesion

 Clinically missing tooth

△ Furcation

▲ "Through and through" furcation

Probe 1: Initial probing depth

Probe 2: Probing depth 6 weeks after periodontal therapy

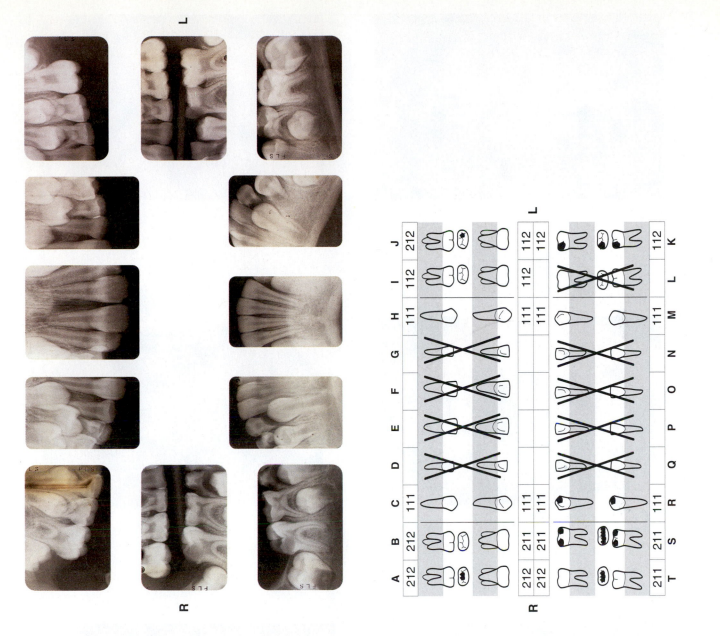

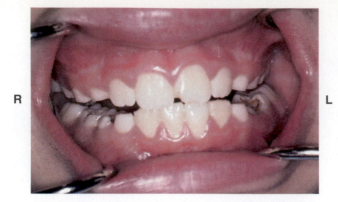

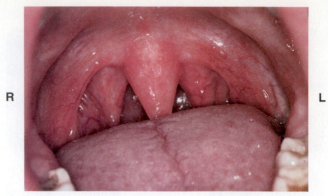

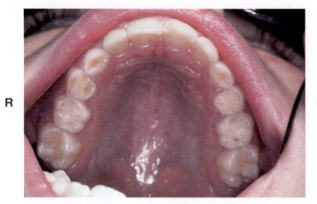

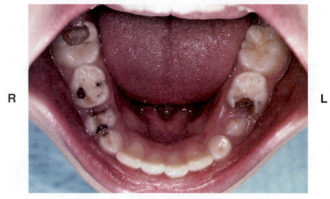

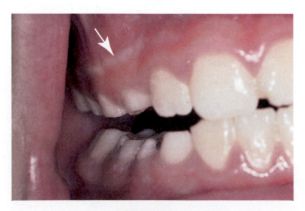

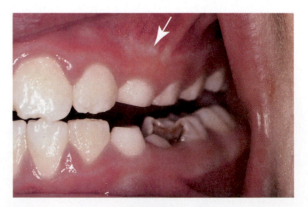

Right side   **Left side**

CASE QUESTIONS

ASSESSING PATIENT CHARACTERISTICS
Basic Level Questions

1. Which of the following is the most likely assessment of the bilateral white lines (arrows) observed on the right and left facial side of the arches?
   A. Linea alba
   B. Mucogingival line
   C. Free gingival margin
   D. Exotosis
   E. Scarring

2. The yellow spots observed on the occlusal surfaces of the primary maxillary right canine, first molar, and left canine are most likely
   A. Dentin
   B. Caries
   C. Stained enamel
   D. Food debris
   E. Cementum

3. Which of the following accurately describes the defect observed on the incisal edge of the permanent maxillary left central incisor?
   A. Abfraction
   B. Abrasion
   C. Attrition
   D. Erosion
   E. Fracture

Competency Level Questions

4. Which of the following terms best describes this patient's caries?
   A. Hidden or backward
   B. Early childhood
   C. Chronic
   D. Arrested
   E. Recurrent

5. Which of the following terms best describes the stains observed on the facial surfaces of the mandibular anterior teeth?
   A. Intrinsic and endogenous
   B. Intrinsic and exogenous
   C. Extrinsic and endogenous
   D. Extrinsic and exogenous

6. Which of the following is an oral adverse effect of this patient's medication?
   A. Xerostomia
   B. Early tooth loss
   C. Increased risk for congenitally missing teeth
   D. Intrinsic tooth staining
   E. Mouth breathing

OBTAINING AND INTERPRETING RADIOGRAPHS
Basic Level Questions

7. The brown stains on the maxillary right molar periapical radiograph and the left bitewing radiograph indicate that
   A. These two films became overlapped in the automatic processor and stuck together while processing.
   B. These film packets were opened before turning off the white light in the darkroom.
   C. Saliva penetrated the outer protective paper wrapping of these film packets to contaminate the films.
   D. These two films were rubbed together during transport to the darkroom and static electricity created artifacts.

8. The radiographic appearance of the primary mandibular canines indicates
   A. Incomplete developing root structure
   B. Congenitally missing root structure
   C. External resorption
   D. Internal resorption

9. The radiolucency surrounding the permanent mandibular left second molar is most likely
   A. A dentigerous cyst
   B. The dental sac
   C. An abscess
   D. The dental papilla
   E. Sharpey's fibers

Competency Level Questions

10. Which of the following is the most likely reason for the wide appearance of the pulp chambers of the permanent maxillary central incisors?
    A. Hypercementosis
    B. Lack of formation of secondary dentin
    C. Internal resorption
    D. Sclerosis
    E. Pulpal infection

11. The radiographs reveal an abscess on which of the following teeth?
    A. Primary maxillary left first molar
    B. Primary mandibular right canine
    C. Permanent maxillary right canine
    D. Permanent mandibular left second molar
    E. Permanent mandibular right first molar

12. Which of the following primary teeth will most likely be exfoliated next?
    A. Maxillary right first molar
    B. Maxillary right canine
    C. Mandibular left second molar
    D. Mandibular left canine
    E. Mandibular right first molar

PLANNING AND MANAGING DENTAL HYGIENE CARE
Basic Level Questions

13. Which of the following will most likely play a role in influencing this patient's gag reflex?
    A. Shiny, edematous facial gingival tissue
    B. Color and consistency of hard palate rugae
    C. White coating on dorsal surface of tongue
    D. Size and shape of uvula and tonsils
    E. Eruption pattern of transitional dentition

14. Each of the following is recommended for this patient EXCEPT one. Which one is the EXCEPTION?
    A. Short appointments
    B. Professional fluoride treatment
    C. Full-mouth disinfection
    D. Nutritional counseling
    E. Monitoring of vital signs

Competency Level Questions

15. Following examination of the oral pharyngeal area, which of these would be contraindicated for this patient?
    A. Foam dispensed fluoride tray application
    B. Conscious sedation with nitrous oxide
    C. Using compressed air for examining tissues
    D. Cotton roll isolation of teeth for sealant placement
    E. Placing the patient in a supine position during treatment

16. Which of these actions is least likely to motivate this patient to better oral self-care?
    A. Comprehensively explain the causes of caries and what the patient can do to help prevent his adult teeth from ending up the same shape as his decayed primary teeth.
    B. Using disclosing solution, demonstrate brushing technique in the patient's mouth and then have him practice while you observe his ability to use the technique.
    C. Use a lot of positive feedback and compliment the patient on his desire to want to learn better self-care for healthier teeth.
    D. Provide a reward system such as placing a star sticker on the indices you use to score the patient's biofilm accumulation at each appointment.
    E. Repeat the oral hygiene instructions multiple times and use several ways to explain the same message.

PERFORMING PERIODONTAL PROCEDURES
Basic Level Questions

17. Which of the following is observed on the facial surfaces of the mandibular anterior teeth?
    A. Acquired pellicle
    B. Microbial biofilm
    C. Materia alba
    D. Food debris
    E. Calculus

USING PREVENTIVE AGENTS
Basic level questions

18. Which of the following permanent first molars should be recommended for sealant placement?
    A. Maxillary right
    B. Maxillary left
    C. Mandibular right
    D. Mandibular left

Competency Level Questions

19. Which of the following home-use fluorides should be recommended for this patient?
    A. Brush-on gel of 0.4% SnF_2 once daily
    B. Oral rinse with 0.05% NaF once daily
    C. Tray application of 0.5% APF once daily
    D. Oral rinse with 0.2% NaF once weekly
    E. Brush-on dentifrice containing Na_2PO_3F two to three times daily

PROVIDING SUPPORTIVE TREATMENT SERVICES
Basic Level Questions

20. In addition to scaling, which of the following would be recommended for professional stain removal for this patient?
    A. Air-power polishing with sodium bicarbonate
    B. Porte polisher with sodium fluoride
    C. Oral irrigation with chlorhexidine gluconate
    D. Power-driven prophylaxis with pumice
    E. Toothbrushing with tartar control toothpaste

21. Each of the following must be assessed to assist this patient with caries control EXCEPT one. Which one is the EXCEPTION?
    A. Frequency of intake of cariogenic foods
    B. Types of foods selected for snacks
    C. Identification of food consistency (soft, sticky, etc.)
    D. When fermentable carbohydrates are consumed
    E. Number of calories consumed per day

Competency Level Questions

22. Which one of these snacks reported as his favorites by the patient's mother would be least likely to produce acidic plaque precipitating demineralization of enamel?
    A. Cookies
    B. Pretzels
    C. Ice cream
    D. Coke™
    E. Gummy bears

DEMONSTRATING PROFESSIONAL RESPONSIBILITY
Basic Level Questions

23. Which of the following is the ALARA exposure setting for this patient's radiographs?
    A. Equivalent to the exposure setting used for adult radiographs
    B. A reduction by one-fourth of the exposure setting used for adult radiographs
    C. A reduction by one-third of the exposure setting used for adult radiographs
    D. A reduction by one-half of the exposure setting used for adult radiographs

Competency Level Questions

24. Neglect of oral health needs can be considered child abuse.

    This patient's oral condition is most likely the result of child abuse.
    A. The first statement is true, the second statement is false.
    B. The first statement is false, the second statement is true.
    C. Both statements are true.
    D. Both statements are false.

25. Which of the following responses to this patient's mother's concerns regarding the value of dental treatment is most helpful?
    A. "Not accepting the care plan for restoring Andrew's oral health could be considered child neglect."
    B. "We can see that you want the best for Andrew, and now that you understand the role that baby teeth play, we want to assist you with his oral health needs."
    C. "A responsible parent would accept the recommended treatment plan for getting Andrew's mouth back in shape."
    D. "If you do not agree to treatment of Andrew's baby teeth, then he is likely to encounter worse problems down the road."
    E. "We can't believe that you let Andrew's teeth get this bad."

SETTING PATIENT GOALS

ESTABLISHING A DENTAL HYGIENE CARE PLAN

To assist this patient in meeting his needs, develop a dental hygiene care plan that establishes a framework within which to help him and his caregiver identify goals for obtaining oral health. In addition to the clinical assessment, a well-prepared dental hygiene care plan should take into account the patient's age, gender, lifestyle, culture, attitudes, health beliefs, and knowledge level. To help link this patient's needs for overall well-being with his oral conditions, and to provide motivation for achieving better health, the following is a partial list of possible deficits based on the Human Needs Conceptual Model to Dental Hygiene Practice. (See the appendix for an explanation of the Human Needs Conceptual Model to Dental Hygiene Practice to help you identify additional unmet needs.) Use this partial list of unmet needs or deficits as a guide in preparing a dental hygiene care plan for this patient. One set of goals and dental hygiene actions/implications has been completed as an example.

Deficit identified in Protection from Health Risks

Due to: adverse side effects of medication
Evidenced by: elevated readings for vital signs

Goals: _____

Dental hygiene actions/implications: _____

Deficit identified in Biologically Sound Dentition

Due to: future caries risk; premature loss of primary teeth
Evidenced by: multiple, large caries present

Goals: _____

Dental hygiene actions/implications: _____

Deficit identified in Conceptualization and Problem Solving

Due to: mother's lack of preventive actions, knowledge of preventive measures for oral health
Evidenced by: self-report that baby teeth don't need restoration

Goals: *schedule and keep appointments to restore oral health; maintain regular preventive dental hygiene appointments; monitor patient's oral self-care for effectiveness; assist patient with developing lifelong sound nutritional habits*

Dental hygiene actions/implications: *educate the patient's caregiver on the value of primary teeth and their role in future oral health; include caregiver in oral self-care instructions for patient; enlist caregiver's help in keeping a food diary for the patient; use food diary to plan nutritional counseling*

Deficit identified in Responsibility for Oral Health

Due to: lack of professional oral health care
Evidenced by: caries; plaque and stain accumulation

Goals: _____

Dental hygiene actions/implications: _____

REFLECTIVE ACTIVITIES

1. Develop a comprehensive oral hygiene instruction care plan for this patient. Then role-play the presentation with the patient's parent, explaining the value of early professional care, developing good oral self-care habits, and the purpose of introducing preventive agents.

2. List the possible barriers this patient faces to achieving better oral health through altering his dietary habits. Develop suggestions and recommendations to help this patient and his caregiver overcome these barriers.

3. Keep a 5-day food diary. Exchange your diary with a classmate. Each of you should then analyze the data noting the number of servings in each food group, the frequency of meals, and how often cariogenic foods were consumed. Together with your partner, create realistic goals for changes that will lead to improved nutrition.

REFERENCES

Bath-Balogh M, Fehrenbach MJ: *Dental Embryology, Histology, and Anatomy,* 2nd ed. St. Louis: Saunders (Elsevier), 2006, pp. 61–91.

Cooper MD: Nitrous oxide/oxygen sedation in dentistry. *Contemporary Oral Hygiene,* 6(12), 24–29, 2006.

Darby ML, Walsh MM (eds.): *Dental Hygiene Theory and Practice,* 2nd ed. St. Louis: Elsevier, 2003, pp. 238–240, 440–441.

Johnson ON, Thomson EM: *Essentials of Dental Radiography for Dental Assistants and Hygienists,* 8th ed. Upper Saddle River, NJ: Prentice Hall, 2007, pp. 312–313, 337–338.

Kimbrough VJ, Lautar CJ: *Ethics, Jurisprudence, and Practice Management in Dental Hygiene,* 2nd ed. Upper Saddle River, NJ: Prentice Hall, 2007, pp. 104–105.

McDonald RE, Avery DR, Dean JA: *Dentistry for the Child and Adolescent,* 8th ed. St. Louis: Mosby, 2004, pp. 288–289.

Neuenfeldt E: The use of pit and fissure sealants in preventive dentistry. *Access,* 20(10), 34–37, 2006.

Palmer CA: *Diet and Nutrition in Oral Health,* 2nd ed. Upper Saddle River, NJ: Prentice Hall, 2007, pp. 287–302.

Pickett FA, Terezhamlmy GT: *Lippincott Williams & Wilkins' Dental Drug Reference with Clinical Implications.* Baltimore: Lippincott Williams & Wilkins, 2006, p. 214.

Pinkham JR, Casamassimo PS, Fields HW, McTigue DJ, Nowak AJ: *Pediatric Dentistry: Infancy through Adolescence,* 4th ed. St. Louis: Elsevier (Saunders), 2005, pp. 466–476.

Stegeman CA, Davis JR: *The Dental Hygienist's Guide to Nutritional Care,* 2nd ed. St. Louis: Elsevier, 2005, pp. 404–411.

Wilkins EM: *Clinical Practice of the Dental Hygienist,* 9th ed. Philadelphia: Lippincott Williams & Wilkins, 2005, pp. 210–216, 289–303, 522–541, 726–741.

Wright R: *Tough Questions, Great Answers. Responding to Patient Concerns about Today's Dentistry.* Carol Stream, IL: Quintessence Publishing Company, 1997, pp. 89–92, 97.

CASE **D**

Katherine Flynn

SITUATION

Katherine Flynn enjoys her new job in the administrative office at the local community college. She is a petite, attractive woman who always presents for her 4-month periodontal maintenance appointments impeccably dressed in business attire. Today she appears overly enthusiastic about her appointment, which may be indicative of apprehension.

LEARNING GOALS

Following integration of core scientific concepts and application of dental hygiene theory to the care of this patient, you will be able to

1. **Assess patient characteristics.**
   A. Define classification of restorations.
   B. Identify the components of a removable partial denture.
   C. Recognize root caries risk factors.
   D. Identify risks of tissue trauma caused by dentures.

2. **Obtain and interpret radiographs.**
   A. Determine dental materials type by their radiographic appearance.
   B. Identify radiographic artifacts.
   C. Distinguish normal radiographic anatomy and pathosis.
   D. Interpret periodontal pathology radiographically.

3. **Plan and manage dental hygiene care.**
   A. Prepare appropriately to prevent medical emergencies during treatment.
   B. Plan treatment for a periodontal maintenance appointment.
   C. Recognize risk factors for anxiety regarding dental treatment.
   D. Identify contraindications to the use of pain control agents.

4. **Perform periodontal procedures.**
   A. Identify risk and contributing factors for periodontal disease.
   B. Determine clinical attachment levels (CAL).
   C. Identify mucogingival involvement.
   D. Identify when to use local drug delivery.
   E. Select appropriate drug delivery therapy.

5. **Use preventive agents.**
   A. Identify conditions that would benefit from fluoride therapies.
   B. Recommend appropriate self-applied fluoride.

6. **Provide supportive treatment services.**
   A. Select appropriate adjunct therapies for hypersensitive root surfaces.
   B. Recommend appropriate therapy for parafunctional habits.

7. **Demonstrate professional responsibility.**
   A. Identify terms used to describe ethical principles.
   B. Establish ethical priorities for dental hygiene interventions that place the patient's needs first.
   C. Use effective patient communication that encourages patient cooperation with dental hygiene treatment.

ADULT-PERIODONTAL PATIENT—*Katherine Flynn*
PATIENT HISTORY SYNOPSIS

VITAL STATISTICS

Age	*53 years*
Gender	*female*
Height	*5' 2"*
Weight	*105 lbs.*

Blood Pressure	*103/62 mm Hg*
Pulse Rate	*72 bpm*
Respiration	*18 rpm*

1. Under care of physician
   Yes [X]   No [ ]
   Condition: *angina pectoris, rheumatoid arthritis*

2. Hospitalized within the last 5 years
   Yes [X]   No [ ]
   Reason: *shoulder surgery*

3. Has or had the following conditions
   syncope
   hormonal replacement therapy
   tetracycline allergic response

4. Current medications
   acetaminophen (Tylenol)—nonnarcotic analgesic
   diclofenac (Voltaren)—nonsteroidal anti-inflammatory
   diltiazem HCL (Cardizem)—calcium channel antagonist, antianginal
   estrogen (Premarin)—hormone replacement

5. Smokes or uses tobacco products
   Yes [ ]   No [X]

6. Is pregnant
   Yes [ ]   No [X]   N/A [ ]

MEDICAL HISTORY
Although not currently taking nitroglycerin, she does keep a prescription for this drug.

DENTAL HISTORY
Has recently experienced a fainting episode during dental treatment. Reports that her teeth are very sensitive to hot and cold stimulation and that during her last scaling appointment the pain became so intense that she fainted. She was embarrassed by this incident and she appears worried that it will happen today. A lifelong resident in a community with optimal levels of fluoride in the water.

SOCIAL HISTORY
Patient's husband of 33 years passed away about 1.5 years ago. To help cope with her loss, she reentered the workforce after many years as a homemaker and an active life of volunteerism. Her husband's professional career provided her with financial security, but working at the community college adds more structure to her life since his death. She is determined to "make it on her own."

CHIEF COMPLAINT
Hot and cold sensitivity, limiting her ability to enjoy certain foods. She is also concerned about the continuing gum recession along her lower anterior teeth.

CURRENT ORAL HYGIENE STATUS
She is meticulous about her home care and reports "wearing out" her toothbrushes within a "couple of weeks." She uses a scrub method of brushing. She also uses floss, fluoride rinses, and rubber tip stimulators. Slight calculus present on the lingual surfaces of the mandibular anterior teeth; slight interproximal plaque detected especially around restoration margins

SUPPLEMENTAL ORAL EXAMINATION FINDINGS
Nocturnal bruxism
Class I mobility on the mandibular left and right lateral and central incisors; and the maxillary left second premolar
Early demineralization on the facial surfaces of the mandibular canines

🦷 Clinically visible carious lesion
✖ Clinically missing tooth
△ Furcation
▲ "Through and through" furcation
Probe 1: Initial probing depth
Probe 2: Probing depth 6 weeks after periodontal therapy

ADULT CLINICAL EXAMINATION

Maxillary (teeth 1–16)

	1	2	3	4	5	6	7	8	9	10	11	12	13	14	15	16
Probe 2 (F)	X	223	X	213	423	223	312	212	222	223	312	323	312	X	X	X
Probe 1 (F)	X	112	X	212	313	222	212	212	222	112	312	323	312	X	X	X
Probe 1 (P)	X	223	X	324	324	532	333	312	212	212	212	222	223	X	X	X
Probe 2 (P)	X	223	X	333	325	532	333	312	212	212	212	323	323	X	X	X

Mandibular (teeth 32–17)

	32	31	30	29	28	27	26	25	24	23	22	21	20	19	18	17
Probe 2 (L)	X	336	822	213	212	212	212	111	111	111	213	311	X	222	X	X
Probe 1 (L)	X	337	814	413	313	323	323	111	111	111	212	221	X	111	X	X
Probe 1 (F)	X	333	623	423	313	111	321	111	111	123	321	223	X	112	X	X
Probe 2 (F)	X	223	723	313	312	122	222	211	112	113	312	313	X	112	X	X

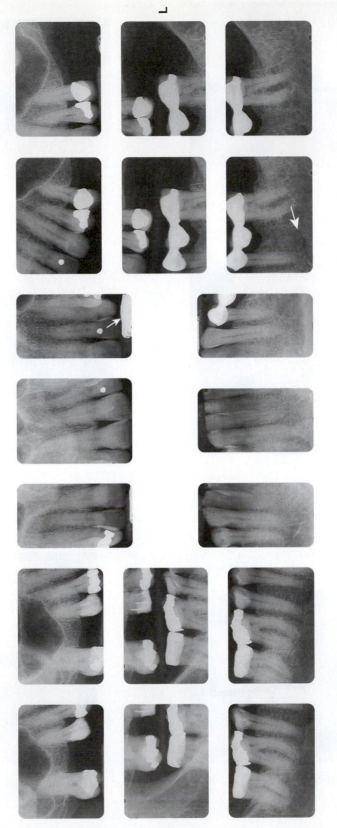

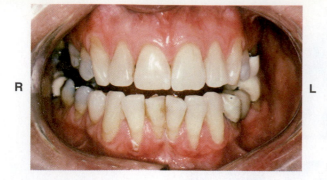

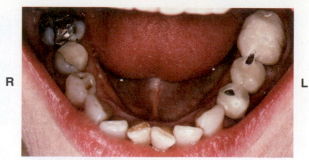

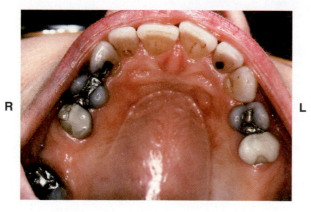

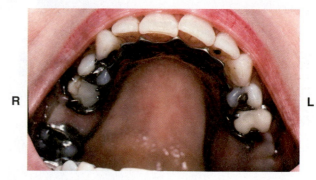

Partial denture in place

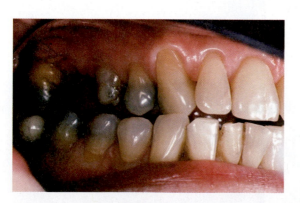

Right side

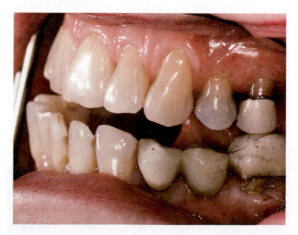

Left side

CASE QUESTIONS

ASSESSING PATIENT CHARACTERISTICS
Basic Level Questions

1. What is the classification of restoration for the maxillary left lateral incisor?
   A. Class I
   B. Class III
   C. Class IV
   D. Class V
   E. Class VI

Competency Level Questions

2. Which of the following abutment teeth support the removable partial denture rest?
   A. Maxillary first molars
   B. Maxillary anterior teeth
   C. Mandibular left first premolar and first molar
   D. Maxillary second premolars

3. Which of these is NOT a risk factor for root caries for this patient?
   A. Prosthetic devices
   B. Medications
   C. Recession
   D. Microbial biofilm
   E. Fluoride history

4. What is the most likely assessment of the appearance of the patient's palate?
   A. Frictional hyperkeratosis
   B. Denture-induced fibrous hyperplasia
   C. Denture stomatitis
   D. Papillary hyperplasia
   E. Squamous cell carcinoma

OBTAINING AND INTERPRETING RADIOGRAPHS
Basic Level Questions

5. In addition to the composite restoration, which of the following dental materials is present on the maxillary right second premolar?
   A. Post and core
   B. Retention pins
   C. Silver points
   D. Gutta percha

6. The large radiopaque artifact present on the maxillary left lateral-canine periapical radiograph and identified by the arrow is
   A. Cone cut error
   B. An image of the partial denture clasp
   C. An amalgam tattoo
   D. An image of the film holding device

7. Which of the following teeth presents with a composite restoration?
   A. Maxillary right first premolar
   B. Maxillary left first premolar
   C. Maxillary left second premolar
   D. Mandibular left first premolar
   E. Mandibular right second premolar

8. The round radiolucency visible near the apex of the mandibular left first premolar (arrow) is interpreted as
   A. The mental foramen
   B. A residual cyst
   C. A periapical abscess
   D. A granuloma

Competency Level Questions

9. The distal aspect of the mandibular right first molar reveals what periodontal condition?
   A. Periodontal abscess
   B. Vertical bone loss
   C. Furcation involvement
   D. Horizontal bone loss

PLANNING AND MANAGING DENTAL HYGIENE CARE
Basic Level Questions

10. Each of the following dental hygiene interventions will prevent the escalation of a medical emergency EXCEPT one. Which one is the EXCEPTION?
    A. Resume upright chair position slowly after treatment.
    B. Set an ammonia capsule within easy reach during treatment.
    C. Provide prophylactic antibiotic premedication.
    D. Request patient bring nitroglycerine to appointment.
    E. Develop patient rapport that conveys warmth and empathy.

Competency Level Questions

11. Each of the following should be planned for this patient's periodontal maintenance appointment EXCEPT one. Which one is the EXCEPTION?
    A. Deplaquing and removing calculus from affected teeth
    B. Scaling the exposed root surfaces
    C. Using subgingival instrumentation to disrupt biofilm
    D. Reprobing the entire dentition
    E. Evaluating and reinforcing oral self-care

12. Each of the following may be a contributing factor to this patient's dental anxiety EXCEPT one. Which one is the EXCEPTION?
    A. Medications taken
    B. Past dental experiences
    C. Desire to appear in control
    D. Fear of pain
    E. Blood pressure

13. Which one of the following options for pain control during instrumentation for this patient has the potential to compromise use of her medications?
    A. Oral conscious sedation (diazepam)
    B. Inhalation sedation (nitrous oxide)
    C. Topical benzocaine (Hurricane)
    D. Noninjectable anesthetic gel (Oraqix)
    E. Injection mepivacaine (Mepivacaine 3%)

PERFORMING PERIODONTAL PROCEDURES
Basic Level Questions

14. Each of the following is a risk or contributing factor for periodontal disease for this patient EXCEPT one. Which one is the EXCEPTION?
    A. Tetracycline allergy
    B. Estrogen therapy
    C. Contour of restorations
    D. Age
    E. Stress

15. The maxillary right canine has 4 mm of recession on the facial surface. What would be the clinical attachment loss for this tooth?
    A. 3 mm
    B. 4 mm
    C. 5 mm
    D. 6 mm
    E. 7 mm

16. Which of the following teeth is most at risk for mucogingival involvement?
    A. Maxillary right first premolar
    B. Maxillary right lateral incisor
    C. Maxillary left second premolar
    D. Mandibular left first molar
    E. Mandibular right lateral incisor

Competency Level Questions

17. Based on the reassessment data at the 6-week reevaluation appointment, which of the following teeth would be an ideal candidate for local drug delivery therapy?
    A. Maxillary right second molar
    B. Maxillary left second premolar
    C. Mandibular left first molar
    D. Mandibular left first premolar
    E. Mandibular right first molar

18. Which of the following locally applied therapeutic agents would be most appropriate for this patient?
    A. Arestin (1 mg minocycline hydrochloride)
    B. Atridox (10% doxycycline hyclate)
    C. PerioChip (2.5 mg chlorhexidine gluconate)
    D. Actisite (25% tetracycline)

USING PREVENTIVE AGENTS
Basic Level Questions

19. Each of the following is a reason to recommend home fluoride use for this patient EXCEPT one. Which one is the EXCEPTION?
    A. Fluoride history
    B. Areas of demineralization
    C. Root exposures
    D. Salivary flow factors
    E. Multiple restorations

Competency Level Questions

20. Which of the following fluoride recommendations would provide this patient with the best therapy?
    A. Use of 1 ppm fluoridated water
    B. Daily 520 ppm fluoride rinse
    C. Weekly 900 ppm fluoride rinse
    D. Brush-on 1,000–1,500 ppm fluoride gel

PROVIDING SUPPORTIVE TREATMENT SERVICES
Basic Level Questions

21. Which of the following chemical agents would be the most appropriate to recommend for at-home therapy to help alleviate the sensitivity of this patient's teeth?
    A. Bonding agent
    B. Potassium nitrate
    C. Sodium fluoride
    D. Ferric oxylate
    E. Potassium oxylate

Competency Level Questions

22. Because of the patient's condition in the mandibular anterior region, which of the following would be the most effective supportive therapy to lessen tooth mobility?
    A. Fabrication of a night guard
    B. Biofeedback to reduce parafunctional habits
    C. Therapeutic massage of tense muscles
    D. Splinting the teeth for stabilization

DEMONSTRATING PROFESSIONAL RESPONSIBILITY
Basic Level Questions

23. To assist with pain control, the dental hygienist who tells the patient he/she will not instrument the sensitive teeth may violate the ethical principle of
    A. Autonomy
    B. Beneficence
    C. Nonmaleficence
    D. Justice
    E. Fidelity

24. Which of the following should be established as a priority when developing the dental hygiene care plan for this patient?
    A. Controlling blood pressure
    B. Reducing tooth sensitivity
    C. Eliminating nocturnal bruxing
    D. Providing a new soft toothbrush
    E. Obtaining vertical bitewing radiographs

Competency Level Questions

25. This patient's anxiety may be managed best by
    A. Allowing the patient to stop the instrumentation process at any time
    B. Introducing relaxation techniques such as deep breathing
    C. Consulting with the dentist to prescribe an antianxiety premedication
    D. Providing the patient with headphones to listen to music during treatment
    E. Correctly and carefully adapting instrumentation

SETTING PATIENT GOALS

ESTABLISHING A DENTAL HYGIENE CARE PLAN

To assist this patient in meeting her needs, develop a dental hygiene care plan that establishes a framework within which to help her identify goals for obtaining oral health. In addition to the clinical assessment, a well-prepared dental hygiene care plan should take into account the patient's age, gender, lifestyle, culture, attitudes, health beliefs, and knowledge level. To help link this patient's needs for overall well-being with her oral conditions, and to provide motivation for achieving better health, the following is a partial list of possible deficits based on the Human Needs Conceptual Model to Dental Hygiene Practice. (See the appendix for an explanation of the Human Needs Conceptual Model to Dental Hygiene Practice to help you identify additional unmet needs.) Use this partial list of unmet needs or deficits as a guide in preparing a dental hygiene care plan for this patient. One set of goals and dental hygiene actions/implications have been completed as an example.

Deficit identified in Protection from Health Risks

Due to: loss of consciousness as a result of sudden fall in blood pressure
Evidenced by: history of syncope and low blood pressure
Goals: *to complete dental hygiene appointments without incidence of syncope; to anticipate dental hygiene appointments without anxiety*
Dental hygiene actions/implications: *record vital signs; document medical alert on patient chart; plan for medical emergency; establish rapport that encourages trust; use listening and communication skills to assist patient with identifying the cause (physical or psychological) and address to help patient gain control*

Deficit identified in Freedom from Head and Neck Pain

Due to: teeth sensitivity
Evidenced by: self-report; exposed root surfaces

Goals: _____

Dental hygiene actions/implications: _____

Deficit identified in Freedom from Stress

Due to: apprehension regarding pain and embarrassment regarding fainting episodes
Evidenced by: rapid speech, nervous laughter, and overt enthusiasm

Goals: _____

Dental hygiene actions/implications: _____

Deficit identified in Skin and Mucous Membrane Integrity of the Head and Neck

Due to: bacterial plaque and trauma from occlusion
Evidenced by: mucogingival involvement

Goals: _____

Dental hygiene actions/implications: _____

Deficit identified in Biologically Sound Dentition

Due to: decreased salivary production and root exposure

Evidenced by: dental caries and dentinal hypersensitivity

Goals: _____

Dental hygiene actions/implications: _____

REFLECTIVE ACTIVITIES

1. Describe methods of anxiety control that could be implemented for this patient.

2. Outline a plan of appointments addressing time needed, services planned, specific instruments, equipment necessary, and reevaluation intervals for each appointment.

3. Identify self-care instructions to address the challenges associated with removable partial dentures, dentinal hypersensitivity, mucogingival involvement, and xerostomia.

REFERENCES

Bader JD, Shugars DA, Bonito AJ: A systematic review of selected caries prevention and management methods. *Community Dentistry and Oral Epidemiology*, 29, 399–411, 2001.

Bennett JD, Rosenberg MB: *Medical Emergencies in Dentistry*. St. Louis: Saunders (Elsevier), 2002, pp. 183–188, 254–256, 313–324.

Blackwell RE: *G. V. Black's Operative Dentistry*, vol. II, 9th ed. Milwaukee: Medico-Dental Publishing, 1955, pp. 1–4.

Collins F, Veis R: Periodontal treatment: The delivery and role of locally applied therapeutics. *Dental CE Digest*, 3(4), 14–20, 2006.

Darby ML: *Mosby's Comprehensive Review of Dental Hygiene*, 6th ed. St. Louis: Mosby (Elsevier), 2006, pp. 586–602, 992–997.

Darby ML, Walsh MM: *Dental Hygiene Theory and Practice*, 2nd ed. St. Louis: Saunders (Elsevier), 2003, pp. 241–242.

Denstply Pharmaceutical: Oraqix prescribing information. http://www.oraqix.com/assets/oraqix/USAOraqixPILv10.pdf . Accessed October 1, 2006.

Gage TW, Little JW: *Mosby's 2007 Dental Drug Consult*. St. Louis: Mosby (Elsevier), 2005, pp. 357–359, 373–375, 462–464.

Genco RJ: Current view of risk factors for periodontal disease. *Journal of Periodontology*, 7, 1041–1049, 1996.

Hatrick CD, Eakle WS, Bird WF: *Dental Materials. Clinical Applications for Dental Assistants and Dental Hygienists*. Philadelphia: Saunders (Elsevier), 2003, pp. 97–100.

Haveles EB: *Applied Pharmacology for the Dental Hygienist*, 5th ed. St. Louis: Mosby (Elsevier), 2007, pp. 199–211.

Johnson L, Stoller N: Rationale for the use of Atridox® therapy for managing periodontal patients. *Compendium of Continuing Education in Dentistry*, 20(4) (Suppl.), 19–25, 1999.

Kimbrough VJ, Henderson K: *Oral Health Education*. Upper Saddle River, NJ: Prentice Hall, 2006, pp. 63–65.

Kimbrough VJ, Lauter CJ: *Ethics, Jurisprudence, & Practice Management*, 2nd ed. Upper Saddle River, NJ: Prentice Hall, 2007, pp. 19–31.

Little JW, Falace DA, Miller CS, Rhodus NL: *Dental Management of the Medically Compromised Patient*, 7th ed. St. Louis: Mosby (Elsevier), 2008, pp. 56–59.

Magnusson I, Geurs N, Harris P, Hefti A, Mariotti A, Mauriello S, Soler L, Offenbacher S: Intrapocket anesthesia for scaling and root planing in pain-sensitive patients. *Journal of Periodontology*, 74(5), 597–602, 2003.

Malamed SF: *Sedation. A Guide to Patient Management*, 4th ed. St. Louis: Mosby (Elsevier), 2003, pp. 103–108, 551–552.

Nield-Gehrig JS, Willmann DE: *Foundations of Periodontics for the Dental Hygienist*, 2nd ed. Philadelphia: Lippincott Williams & Wilkins, 2008, pp. 258–259, 361–364.

Page RC: The microbiological case for adjunctive therapy for periodontitis. *Journal of the International Academy of Periodontology*, 6(4), 143–149, 2004.

Rule JT: *Ethical Questions in Dentistry*, 2nd ed. Chicago: Quintessence Publishing Co., Inc., 2004, pp. 57–72.

Serio FG, Hawley CE: *Manual of Clinical Periodontics*. Hudon, OH: Lexi-Comp, Inc., 2002, pp. 59–60.

Stamm JW, Banting DW, Imrey PB: Adult root caries survey of two similar communities with contrasting natural water levels. *Journal of the American Dental Association*, 120(2), 143–149, 1990.

Walker C: The supplemental use of antibiotics in periodontal therapy. *Compendium of Continuing Education in Dentistry*, 20(4) (Suppl.), 4–11, 1999.

Weinberg MA, Westphal C, Oakat M, Froum SJ: *Comprehensive Periodontics for the Dental Hygienist*, 2nd ed. Upper Saddle River, NJ: Prentice Hall, 2006, pp. 56–58, 157–158, 253, 265–266, 420–432.

Wilkins EM: *Clinical Practice of the Dental Hygienist*, 9th ed. Philadelphia: Lippincott Williams & Wilkins, 2006, pp. 7–12, 348–349, 473–474, 549, 561, 721–722, 726–741, 822–823, 841–847.

Wilson TG, Glover ME, Schoen J, Baus C, Jacobs T: Compliance with maintenance therapy in a private periodontal practice. *Journal of Periodontology*, 55, 468–473, 1984.

CASE E

Louis Riddick

SITUATION

Louis Riddick and his wife owned and managed their own business until their sons took over last year. Now enjoying early retirement, Louis is still very active in his community. An easy-going, confident man, he has a close circle of friends with whom he enjoys playing golf. Recently diagnosed with prehypertension, he is not overly concerned about his health. He is here today because his wife made the appointment for him after he mentioned that he thought his teeth might be getting loose.

LEARNING GOALS

Following integration of core scientific concepts and application of dental hygiene theory to the care of this patient, you will be able to

1. **Assess patient characteristics.**
   A. Classify occlusal relationships.
   B. Identify deviations in gingival appearance.
   C. Determine etiology of diastema.
   D. Apply appropriate terminology to identify white lesions.

2. **Obtain and interpret radiographs.**
   A. Differentiate between normal radiographic anatomy and pathosis.
   B. Utilize radiographs as an aid in identifying local contributing factors for periodontal disease.
   C. Apply radiographic interpretation to determine clinical findings.

3. **Plan and manage dental hygiene care.**
   A. Individualize treatment planning for the periodontally involved patient.
   B. Appropriately recommend a self-care product for the periodontally involved patient.

4. **Perform periodontal procedures.**
   A. Recognize periodontal disease's effect on the dentition.
   B. Utilize periodontal instruments effectively.
   C. Describe bone loss patterns associated with periodontal disease.

   D. Classify furcation involvement according to severity.
   E. Measure clinical attachment level.
   F. Identify the local contributing factor in the presence of a periodontal pocket.
   G. Identify periodontal disease risk factors.
   H. Predict outcomes of periodontal disease treatment interventions.
   I. Recommend appropriate maintenance interval for the periodontally involved patient.

5. **Use preventive agents.**
   A. Select an appropriate chemotherapeutic agent for patient self-care following nonsurgical periodontal therapy.

6. **Provide supportive treatment services.**
   A. Assist the patient in smoking cessation efforts.

7. **Demonstrate professional responsibility.**
   A. Identify effective communication that assists the patient in understanding treatment outcomes.
   B. Use communication that is appropriate for the dental hygiene professional.
   C. Identify communication that hinders patient motivation and compliance.

ADULT-PERIODONTAL PATIENT—*Louis Riddick*
PATIENT HISTORY SYNOPSIS

Age	*56 years*
Gender	*male*
Height	*5' 3"*
Weight	*150 lbs.*

VITAL STATISTICS

Blood Pressure	*139/89 mm Hg*
Pulse Rate	*70 bpm*
Respiration	*17 rpm*

1. Under care of physician
   Yes [X] No [ ]
   Condition: *blood pressure*
   smoking cessation
   _____

2. Hospitalized within the last 5 years
   Yes [ ] No [X]
   Reason: _____
   _____

3. Has or had the following conditions
   prehypertension
   _____
   _____

4. Current medications
   bupropion hydrochloride (Zyban)—antidepressant
   as aid in smoking cessation
   nicotine polacrilex (Nicorette)—nicotine
   replacement therapy

5. Smokes or uses tobacco products
   Yes [ ] No [X]

6. Is pregnant
   Yes [ ] No [ ] N/A [X]

MEDICAL HISTORY
This patient's prehypertension was diagnosed after he attended a blood pressure screening last month. At that time, he received a complete physical exam and was advised to quit smoking. He has not had a cigarette in 5 days.

DENTAL HISTORY
Patient reports that he had several teeth extracted "years ago," but that he gets along just fine without them. In fact, he jokes, "I now have less to brush." His last dental hygiene appointment was 12 months ago.

SOCIAL HISTORY
Patient considers his golf outings as exercise and important to his well-being. His relationship with his family is important to him and his wife's concern for his dental health is what got him here today.

CHIEF COMPLAINT
Patient reports mentioning to his wife last month that his teeth appeared to be getting loose. At first he dismissed this as a natural part of the aging process, until his wife expressed concern. He is here today to find out the cause.

CURRENT ORAL HYGIENE STATUS
Moderate subgingival plaque especially interproximal and generalized bleeding upon probing. He recently began using a power toothbrush.

SUPPLEMENTAL ORAL EXAMINATION FINDINGS
Slight tongue thrust
Generalized Class I mobility
Slight generalized calculus

ADULT CLINICAL EXAMINATION

	1	2	3	4	5	6	7	8	9	10	11	12	13	14	15	16
Probe 2	X	456	859	736	735	423	423	323	323	324	434	533	335	566	X	544
Probe 1	X	567	9610	847	846	534	534	434	434	435	545	644	446	677	X	655

F / **P**

	1	2	3	4	5	6	7	8	9	10	11	12	13	14	15	16
Probe 1	X	758	9711	745	446	534	434	434	434	434	335	645	656	757	X	656
Probe 2	X	647	8610	634	335	423	323	323	323	323	224	534	545	646	X	545

R   **L**

	32	31	30	29	28	27	26	25	24	23	22	21	20	19	18	17
Probe 2	444	X	X	434	433	323	322	222	222	222	323	334	434	X	X	555
Probe 1	655	X	X	545	544	424	423	222	223	323	323	324	435	X	X	666

L / **F**

	32	31	30	29	28	27	26	25	24	23	22	21	20	19	18	17
Probe 1	655	X	X	435	534	435	534	323	323	323	324	445	545	X	X	656
Probe 2	544	X	X	324	423	324	423	323	323	323	223	334	434	X	X	545

Legend:
- Clinically visible carious lesion
- X Clinically missing tooth
- △ Furcation
- ▲ "Through and through" furcation
- Probe 1: Initial probing depth
- Probe 2: Probing depth 6 weeks after periodontal therapy

L

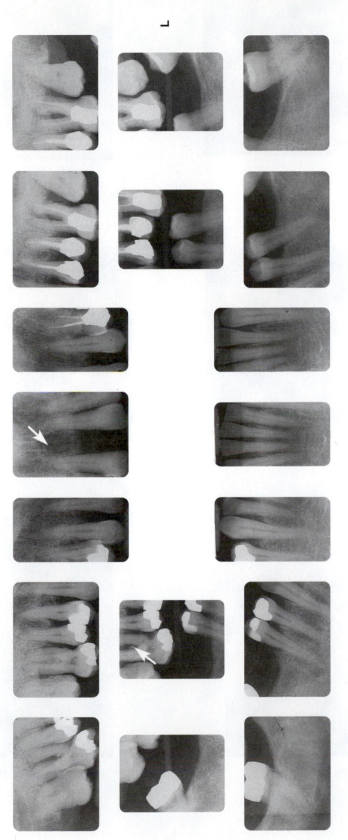

R

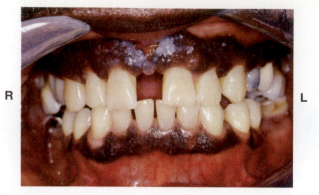

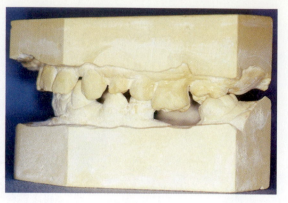

Left side

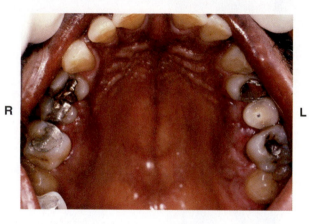

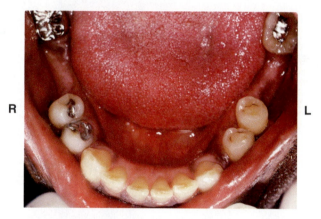

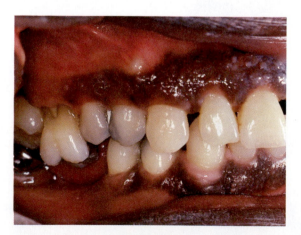

Right side

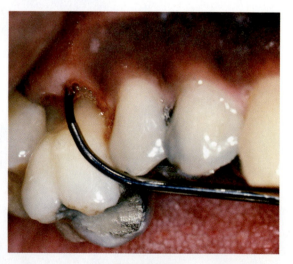

Right side

CASE QUESTIONS

ASSESSING PATIENT CHARACTERISTICS
Basic Level Questions

1. Which of the following is the best assessment of this patient's anterior occlusal relationship?
   A. Crossbite
   B. Edge-to-edge
   C. Open bite
   D. Overjet
   E. Underjet

2. The dark appearance of the facial gingiva most likely indicates
   A. Melanin pigmentation
   B. Smoking stains
   C. Lichen planus
   D. Contact stomatitis
   E. Discoid lupus erythematosus

Competency Level Questions

3. Which of the following is the most likely cause of this patient's maxillary central diastema?
   A. Tongue thrust
   B. Enlarged incisive papilla
   C. Periodontal involvement
   D. Developing radicular cyst
   E. Location of the frenal attachment

4. Which of the following is the most likely assessment of the white patch present on the soft tissue located near the maxillary central incisors that does not wipe off with gauze?
   A. Leukodema
   B. Leukoplakia
   C. Candidiasis
   D. Nicotinic stomatitis
   E. Fordyce's granules

OBTAINING AND INTERPRETING RADIOGRAPHS
Basic Level Questions

5. Which of the following is the most likely interpretation of the oval radiolucency between the maxillary central incisors (arrow)?
   A. Mental foramen
   B. Mandibular foramen
   C. Incisive foramen
   D. Lingual foramen
   E. Infraorbital foramen

Competency Level Questions

6. Which of the following is the most likely interpretation of the radiopaque finding between the roots of the maxillary right first molar (arrow)?
   A. Calculus
   B. Pulp stone
   C. Enamel pearl
   D. Hypercementosis
   E. Composite restoration

7. The gray hue exhibited by the maxillary left first premolar is
   A. An indication that this tooth is not vital
   B. The result of tetracycline staining
   C. A condition of dentinogenesis imperfecta
   D. Caused by the presence of metallic restorative materials
   E. Hypocalcified enamel

PLANNING AND MANAGING DENTAL HYGIENE CARE
Basic Level Questions

8. Which of the following would most likely be planned for this patient's first appointment?
   A. Application of desensitizing agents
   B. Instruction in oral self-care
   C. Extraction of the maxillary first molars
   D. Full-mouth periodontal scaling and root debridement
   E. Antifungal treatment of the white patches

Competency Level Questions

9. Which of the following would be the most beneficial oral self-care education for this patient?
   A. Recommend modified Bass toothbrushing.
   B. Suggest using the dental floss holder.
   C. Introduce the end-tuft brush.
   D. Provide a brochure on the interdental brush.
   E. Review patient skill with the power toothbrush.

PERFORMING PERIODONTAL PROCEDURES
Basic Level Questions

10. What factors contributed to the super eruption of the maxillary first molars?
    A. Furcation involvement
    B. Long junctional epithelium
    C. Absence of mandibular first molars
    D. Surgical intervention for periodontal disease
    E. Inadequate attached gingiva

11. The purpose of the instrument shown in the photograph of the maxillary right first molar is to
    A. Measure furcation involvement.
    B. Scale posterior teeth.
    C. Explore for calculus.
    D. Record pocket depths.
    E. Apply subgingival irrigation.

12. Which of the following instruments would be the best choice for removing calculus on the mesial of the mandibular right second molar?
    A. Gracey 1/2 curet—miniature working end
    B. Gracey 11/12 curet—rigid shank
    C. Gracey 13/14 curet—standard
    D. Universal sickle scaler
    E. Chisel scaler

13. Which of the following best describes the type of bone loss associated with the maxillary right first and second premolars?
    A. Angular
    B. Vertical
    C. Dehiscence
    D. Fenestration
    E. Horizontal

14. Which of the following is the correct classification of furcation involving the maxillary right first molar?
    A. Grade I
    B. Grade II
    C. Grade III
    D. Grade IV

Competency Level Questions

15. Using the furcation probe calibrated marking as a guide (pictured), the recession on the facial surface of the maxillary right first molar appears to be 4 mm. What is the measurement of the clinical attachment level at the reevaluation appointment?
    A. 10 mm
    B. 9 mm
    C. 8 mm
    D. 6 mm
    E. 5 mm

16. Which of the following may be a contributing etiologic factor to the periodontal defect present on the mesial surface of the maxillary left first premolar?
    A. Endodontic therapy
    B. Overhanging restoration
    C. Tooth root morphology
    D. Incipient carious lesion
    E. Occlusal trauma

17. Which of the following is the most likely cause of this patient's tooth mobility?
    A. Periodontal disease
    B. Untreated high blood pressure
    C. Medications
    D. Premature loss of permanent teeth
    E. Smoking history

18. Which of the following has been the greatest risk factor for this patient's periodontal disease?
    A. Brushing habits
    B. Medications
    C. Stress
    D. Prehypertension
    E. Smoking

19. Each of the following is a likely reason for the generalized reduction in pocket depths at the reevaluation appointment EXCEPT one. Which one is the EXCEPTION?
    A. Tissue shrinkage with a return to normal color, size, and contour
    B. Improved integrity of the clinical attachment
    C. Formation of a long junctional epithelial attachment
    D. Regeneration of new bone, cementum, and periodontal ligament
    E. Reformation of collagen that resists probing

20. Based on the oral conditions and patient self-care knowledge and effectiveness assessed at the initial appointment, and on the probing depths at the reevaluation appointment, when should this patient's next periodontal maintenance appointment be scheduled?
    A. 1 month
    B. 3 months
    C. 4 months
    D. 6 months
    E. 12 months

USING PREVENTIVE AGENTS
Competency Level Questions

21. Which of the following chemotherapeutic rinses would be the best recommendation for this patient to use following his initial appointment until he returns for the 6-week reevaluation appointment?
    A. Essential oils (Listerine®)
    B. Zinc chloride (Breathe Rx®)
    C. Cetylpyridinium chloride (Crest Pro Health®)
    D. Chlorhexidine gluconate (Peridex®)
    E. Hydrogen peroxide (Prevention Mouth Rinse®)

PROVIDING SUPPORTIVE TREATMENT SERVICES
Competency Level Questions

22. Which of the following should be included in this patient's smoking cessation follow-through from the dental hygienist?
    A. Instruct him to chew nicotine gum as one would conventional chewing gum.
    B. Provide positive reinforcement, emphasizing the benefits of stopping smoking.
    C. Warn the patient that a single slip, smoking one cigarette, will make him a user again.
    D. Inform the patient that nicotine withdrawal symptoms will subside in 5 to 7 days.
    E. Use photos of failed periodontal therapy as a scare tactic.

DEMONSTRATING PROFESSIONAL RESPONSIBILITY
Basic Level Questions

23. The dental hygienist is obligated to explain each of the following possible negative outcomes of periodontal therapy treatment to this patient EXCEPT one. Which one is the EXCEPTION?
    A. Appearance of long teeth
    B. Increased dentinal sensitivity
    C. Increased tooth mobility
    D. Statistics on success rates of treatment
    E. Blunting of papillae

Competency Level Questions

24. Which of the following statements is appropriate and legally within the scope of practice for a dental hygienist to make regarding this patient?
    A. "Following nonsurgical periodontal therapy the mobility should improve."
    B. "Both maxillary first molars should be extracted."
    C. "You will need a referral to be evaluated by a periodontist."
    D. "Your physician should have prescribed a blood pressure medication."
    E. "Implants can be used to replace your missing teeth."

25. Which of the following is the best initial response to this patient's comments reported in his dental history?
    A. "Although you may not realize it, you have the ability to achieve good dental health."
    B. "Why did you wait so long to come in for dental treatment?"
    C. "We are going to set you up with four appointments for deep scaling."
    D. "If you don't begin to take care of your teeth you will most likely be losing some more."
    E. "Great! Next, you'll be telling us that we should charge you less because you have less teeth to clean. Just kidding."

SETTING PATIENT GOALS

ESTABLISHING A DENTAL HYGIENE CARE PLAN

To assist this patient in meeting his needs, develop a dental hygiene care plan that establishes a framework within which to help him identify goals for obtaining oral health. In addition to the clinical assessment, a well-prepared dental hygiene care plan should take into account the patient's age, gender, lifestyle, culture, attitudes, health beliefs, and knowledge level. To help link this patient's needs for overall well-being with his oral conditions, and to provide motivation for achieving better health, the following is a partial list of possible deficits based on the Human Needs Conceptual Model to Dental Hygiene Practice. (See the appendix for an explanation of the Human Needs Conceptual Model to Dental Hygiene Practice to help you identify additional unmet needs.) Use this partial list of unmet needs or deficits as a guide in preparing a dental hygiene care plan for this patient. One set of goals and dental hygiene actions/implications has been completed as an example.

Deficit identified in Protection from Health Risks

Due to: smoking history
Evidenced by: self-report

Goals: _____

Dental hygiene actions/implications: _____

Deficit identified in Skin and Mucous Membrane Integrity of the Head and Neck

Due to: significant pocket depths
Evidenced by: the presence of gingival inflammation and bleeding

Goals: *maintain pocket depth reduction noted at reevaluation appointment; reduce pockets depths that remain unchanged.*

Dental hygiene actions/implications: *evaluate outcomes of periodontal debridement; assess patient understanding of the disease process and commitment to goals; determine the need for scaling residual calculus and reinstrumenting regions of unchanged pocket depths; perform periodontal debridement; refer to periodontist.*

Deficit identified in Biologically Sound Dentition

Due to: potential for tooth loss
Evidenced by: tooth mobility

Goals: _____

Dental hygiene actions/implications: _____

Deficit identified in Conceptualization and Problem Solving

Due to: misconceptions associated with oral health care
Evidenced by: lack of replacement of missing teeth

Goals: _____

Dental hygiene actions/implications: _____

Deficit identified in Responsibility for Oral Health

Due to: lack of regular oral care; neglecting the signs and symptoms of periodontal disease

Evidenced by: periodontal disease and caries; lack of awareness of the patient's role in his own oral health

Goals: _____

Dental hygiene actions/implications: _____

REFLECTIVE ACTIVITIES

1. **Investigate tips and techniques to alleviate nicotine withdrawal symptoms that can be shared with this patient.**

2. **Role-play a script between the dental hygienist and a patient who: (1) is not interested in quitting smoking; (2) thinks that switching from smoking cigarettes to using spit tobacco is a safe alternative; and (3) is interested in quitting, but does not know how to begin.**

3. **Initiate a smoking cessation program (Ask, Advise, Assist, Arrange) with one of your patients who uses tobacco.**

REFERENCES

Darby ML, Walsh MM: *Dental Hygiene Theory and Practice,* 2nd ed. St. Louis: Saunders (Elsevier), 2003, pp. 41–58, 222–223, 466–470.

eMedicine. Web MD. http://www.emedicine.com/derm/topic647.htm . Accessed October 23, 2006.

eMedicine. Web MD. http://www.emedicine.com/derm/topic663.htm . Accessed October 23, 2006.

Gage TW, Little JW: *Mosby's 2007 Dental Drug Consult.* St. Louis: Mosby (Elsevier), 2005, pp. 96–97.

Glickman I: *Clinical Periodontology.* Philadelphia: Saunders, 1953.

Guntsch A, Erier M, Preshaw PM, Sigusch BW, Klinger G, Glockman E: Effect of smoking on crevicular polymorphonuclear neutrophil function in periodontally healthy subjects. *Journal of Periodontal Research,* 41, 184–188, 2006.

Kaplowitz G: Essential elements of oral care. *RDH,* 26(9), 2006.

Lupus Foundation of America. http://www.lupus.org/education/topics/oral.html . Accessed October 23, 2006.

Mecklenburg RE, Christen AG, Gerbert B, Gift HC, Glynn TJ, Jones RB, Lindsay E, Manley MW, Severson H: *How to Help Your Patients Stop Using Tobacco. A National Cancer Institute Manual for the Oral Health Team.* U.S. Department of Health and Human Services, Public Health Service, National Institutes of Health, American Cancer Society, NIH Publication No. 98–3191, 1998.

Nield-Gehrig JS: *Fundamentals of Periodontal Instrumentation,* 5th ed. Baltimore: Lippincott Williams & Wilkins, 2004, pp. 338–341, 457–459.

Perry DA, Beemsterboer P, Taggart EJ: *Periodontology for the Dental Hygienist,* 3rd ed. St. Louis: Saunders (Elsevier), 2007, pp. 151–152, 175–177, 269–270.

Serio FG, Hawley CE: *Manual of Clinical Periodontics.* Hudon, OH: Lexi-Comp, Inc., 2002, pp. 32–34.

Weinberg MA, Westphal C, Froum SJ, Palat M: *Comprehensive Periodontics for the Dental Hygienist,* 2nd ed. Upper Saddle River, NJ: Prentice Hall, 2006, pp. 26, 56–58, 157–158, 253, 255–256, 383–389, 424, 441, 428–431, 553–556.

White SC, Pharoah MJ: *Oral Radiology Principles and Interpretation,* 5th ed. St. Louis: Mosby (Elsevier), 2004, pp. 345–347.

Wilkins EM: *Clinical Practice of the Dental Hygienist,* 9th ed. Philadelphia: Lippincott Williams & Wilkins, 2005, pp. 225–240, 500–518, 609–619, 679–680.

Wolf HF, Hassell TM: *Color Atlas of Dental Hygiene. Periodontology.* New York: Thieme, 2006, pp. 54, 165, 222, 303.

Wright R: *Tough Questions, Great Answers. Responding to Patient Concerns about Today's Dentistry.* Chicago: Quintessence Publishing Co., Inc., 1997, pp. 79–108.

CASE F

Banu Radpur-Ansari

SITUATION

Banu Radpur-Ansari is currently working as a graduate teaching assistant in the engineering department at the local university and completing her PhD in statistics and engineering. Dedication to her research and teaching responsibilities have left her little time for activities outside university life. Intelligent and motivated by her current oral conditions and the problems they pose, she is here today to make a commitment to improving her oral health.

LEARNING GOALS

Following integration of core scientific concepts and application of dental hygiene theory to the care of this patient, you will be able to

1. **Assess patient characteristics.**
   A. Recognize normal anatomic features of the hard palate.
   B. Identify occlusal disharmonies.
   C. Determine the cause of food impaction.

2. **Obtain and interpret radiographs.**
   A. Identify the presence of dental materials radiographically.
   B. Interpret suspected caries radiographically.
   C. Recognize situations that require alteration of radiographic techniques.
   D. Recognize the appearance of normal radiographic anatomy.

3. **Plan and manage dental hygiene care.**
   A. Determine the need for antibiotic premedication.
   B. Identify the prophylactic regimen for antibiotic premedication.
   C. Plan scaling and root planing sequence for the premedicated patient.
   D. Choose appropriate pain control methods.

4. **Perform periodontal procedures.**
   A. Identify risk factors for periodontal disease.
   B. Classify periodontal disease status.
   C. Identify mucogingival involvement.
   D. Assess treatment outcomes.
   E. Recognize the impact periodontal disease has on the patient's ability to maintain oral self-care.
   F. Determine the etiology of gingival swelling.

5. **Use preventive agents.**
   A. Recognize contraindications for the use of preventive agents.
   B. Identify the role antibiotic therapy plays in treating periodontal diseases.

6. **Provide supportive treatment services.**
   A. Make appropriate referrals in treating periodontal diseases.
   B. Recognize contraindications for the use of whitening products.

7. **Demonstrate professional responsibility.**
   A. Identify requirements for informed consent.
   B. Identify potential causes of patient dissatisfaction with treatment outcomes.

ADULT-PERIODONTAL PATIENT—*Banu Radpur-Ansari*
PATIENT HISTORY SYNOPSIS

Age __*35 years*__
Gender __*female*__
Height __*5' 8"*__
Weight __*125 lbs.*__

VITAL STATISTICS

Blood Pressure __*114/62 mm Hg*__
Pulse Rate __*72 bpm*__
Respiration __*18 rpm*__

---

1. Under care of physician
   Yes [X] No [ ]
   Condition: *hypothyroidism*
   (myxedema)

2. Hospitalized within the last 5 years
   Yes [X] No [ ]
   Reason: *infective endocarditis*

3. Has or had the following conditions
   Currently taking medication for a sinus infection

4. Current medications
   levothyroxine sodium (Synthroid)—thyroid hormone
   vitamin D (Drisdol Drops)—vitamin supplement
   amoxicillin (Amoxil)—antibiotic

5. Smokes or uses tobacco products
   Yes [ ] No [X]

6. Is pregnant
   Yes [ ] No [X] N/A [ ]

MEDICAL HISTORY
Last year she developed a high fever following a colonoscopy procedure. She was told that she had developed infective endocarditis and was admitted to the hospital where she was given intravenous antibiotics for 5 days.

DENTAL HISTORY
Has had sporadic dental care due to her busy schedule. Is currently using over-the-counter tooth whiteners. She does not remember when her last dental hygiene appointment was, but does recall being scheduled for multiple appointments that she was unable to keep.

SOCIAL HISTORY
Attended universities in Great Britain and the United States and moved permanently to the United States from Tehran when she was 25. She is married to a fellow researcher, has no children, and is dedicated to advancing her research at the local university where she is a doctoral student.

CHIEF COMPLAINT
Throbbing pain and bad taste coming from the maxillary left posterior region.
A few years ago, the maxillary right second and third molars became loose and were extracted. Before the pain started, she noticed that the left molars were beginning to feel like the extracted teeth did and she is worried that these too are destined for extraction. She is interested in professional tooth whitening.

ADULT CLINICAL EXAMINATION

Maxillary (R → L):

	1	2	3	4	5	6	7	8	9	10	11	12	13	14	15	16
Probe 2	X	X	346	753	212	212	212	212	212	212	212	222	224	567	758	1075
Probe 1	X	X	345	643	323	313	323	323	323	323	223	323	335	556	758	1086
Probe 1	X	X	346	533	323	212	222	222	222	222	323	323	424	435	637	846
Probe 2	X	X	336	523	313	212	212	212	212	212	212	313	313	426	638	945

Mandibular (R → L):

	32	31	30	29	28	27	26	25	24	23	22	21	20	19	18	17
Probe 2	434	423	323	312	212	213	312	212	213	312	213	213	323	333	444	434
Probe 1	545	534	434	433	333	324	423	323	325	523	324	324	434	434	554	445
Probe 1	423	414	414	323	313	214	423	322	224	423		223	223	346	655	525
Probe 2	423	313	314	312	212	213	312	217	213	312		212	213	335	544	424

R ... L

CURRENT ORAL HYGIENE STATUS
General moderate bleeding on probing. She brushes up and down three to four times per day. She uses a plastic toothpick product (Brush Picks®) after eating to remove food particles that get stuck in the embrasures of the posterior teeth.

SUPPLEMENTAL ORAL EXAMINATION FINDINGS
Exudate upon probing the maxillary left second and third molars.
Class I mobility noted for maxillary right first molar, maxillary left second molar, and mandibular left second and third molars. Class II mobility noted for the maxillary left third molar. Food impaction between the mandibular right first and second molars.
Heavy subgingival calculus in all four posterior quadrants and in the mandibular anterior region.

⊔ Clinically visible carious lesion

✗ Clinically missing tooth

△ Furcation

▲ "Through and through" furcation

Probe 1: Initial probing depth

Probe 2: Probing depth 6 weeks after periodontal therapy

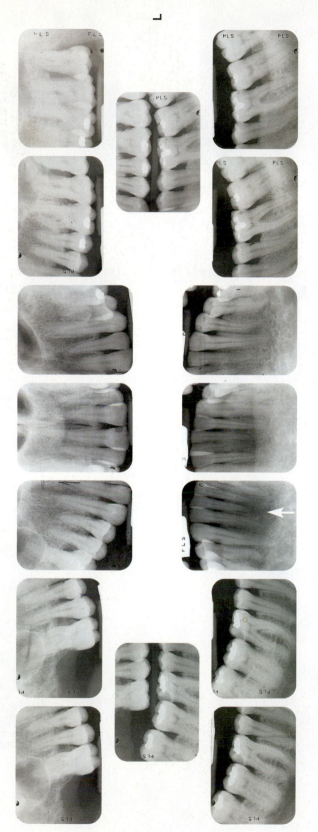

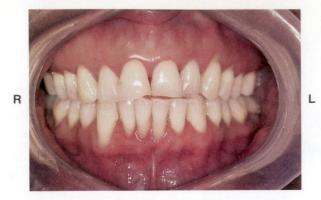

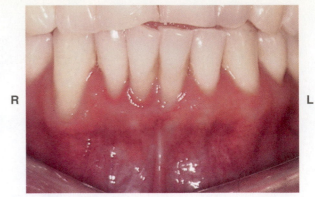

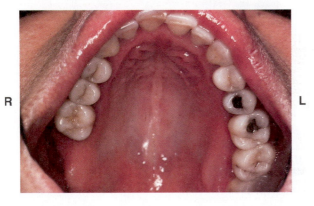

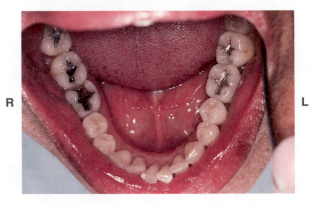

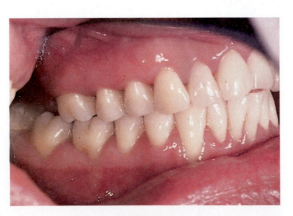

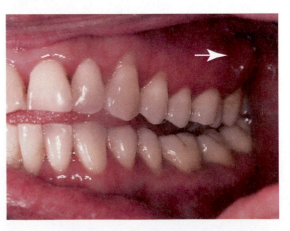

Right side

Left side

CASE QUESTIONS

ASSESSING PATIENT CHARACTERISTICS
Basic Level Questions

1. The pronounced, raised ridges evident on the anterior region of the hard palate is indicative of
   A. Torus palantinus
   B. Rugae
   C. Salivary duct openings
   D. Blisterform lesions
   E. Trauma

2. The appearance of the maxillary anterior teeth indicates
   A. Erosion
   B. Abrasion
   C. Attrition
   D. Caries
   E. Abfraction

Competency Level Questions

3. What is the potential risk associated with the mandibular right second and third molars?
   A. Extrusion
   B. Ankylosis
   C. Impaction
   D. Hypercementosis
   E. Fusion

4. What is the most likely reason for food impaction between the mandibular right first and second molars?
   A. Mobility
   B. Blunted papilla
   C. Recession
   D. Caries
   E. Diastema

OBTAINING AND INTERPRETING RADIOGRAPHS
Basic Level Questions

5. Which of the following teeth has been restored with a composite restoration?
   A. Maxillary right first molar
   B. Maxillary right central incisor
   C. Mandibular left first molar
   D. Mandibular left lateral incisor
   E. Mandibular right first molar

6. Caries is evident radiographically on which of the following teeth?
   A. Maxillary right central incisor
   B. Maxillary left second molar
   C. Mandibular left first molar
   D. Mandibular right canine
   E. Mandibular right second molar

Competency Level Questions

7. What radiographic technique was used to image the maxillary left third molar?
    A. Water's
    B. Posterior-anterior
    C. Occlusal
    D. Localization
    E. Disto-oblique

8. The most likely interpretation of the radiolucency at the apices of the mandibular anterior teeth (arrow) is
    A. The lingual foramen
    B. The mental fossa
    C. Periapical cemental dyplasia
    D. Signs of osteoporosis
    E. A periapical abscess

PLANNING AND MANAGING DENTAL HYGIENE CARE
Basic Level Questions

9. What is the reason that this patient must be premedicated before periodontal probing and subgingival debridement procedures?
    A. History of infective endocarditis
    B. Thyroid condition
    C. Sinus infection
    D. Foreign born
    E. Blood pressure

10. What is the recommended antibiotic premedication for this patient?
    A. 2 g amoxicillin orally 1 hour before treatment
    B. 2 g ampicillin IM 30 minutes before treatment
    C. 600 mg clindamycin orally 1 hour before treatment
    D. 1 g cefazolin IV 30 minutes before treatment

Competency Level Questions

11. Which of the following would be the most appropriate treatment plan for scaling and root planing for this patient?
    A. One quadrant each week
    B. One quandrant every 2 weeks
    C. Half mouth each week
    D. Half mouth every 2 weeks
    E. Complete mouth at one appointment

12. Which of the following pain control choices is required for debridement of the maxillary left quadrant?
    A. Nitrous oxide–oxygen analgesia
    B. Topical anesthetic benzocaine 20%
    C. Infiltration anesthesia prilocaine 4%
    D. Noninjectable anesthetic lidocaine 2.5% and prilocaine 2.5% gel
    E. Block anesthesia bupivacaine 0.5% with epinephrine

PERFORMING PERIODONTAL PROCEDURES
Basic Level Questions

13. Which of the following is a risk factor for this patient's periodontal disease?
    A. Endocrine
    B. Stress
    C. Hormones
    D. Age
    E. Race

14. What is the American Academy of Periodontology's classification of this patient's periodontal status?
    A. Chronic periodontitis
    B. Aggressive periodontitis
    C. Drug-induced gingival disease
    D. Periodontitis as a manifestation of systemic diseases
    E. Necrotizing periodontitis

15. Each of the following teeth appears to be at risk for mucogingival involvement EXCEPT one. Which one is the EXCEPTION?
    A. Maxillary left canine
    B. Maxillary left second molar
    C. Mandibular left central incisor
    D. Mandibular right canine
    E. Mandibular right second molar

16. At the reevaluation appointment, which of the following areas should be retreated and monitored closely for signs of further attachment loss?
    A. All four posterior quadrants
    B. Entire mandibular arch
    C. Maxillary right and left posterior regions
    D. Maxillary and mandibular anterior sextants
    E. Maxillary right posterior, maxillary left posterior, mandibular left central, and lateral incisor regions

Competency Level Questions

17. Which of the following is the most likely reason that this patient has chosen to use plastic picks to remove food from between her teeth?
    A. Too busy to floss
    B. Furcation involvement
    C. Gingival recession
    D. Blunted papillae
    E. Cultural influence

18. The extended and enlarged, bulbous area located on the attached gingiva apical to the maxillary left second and third molars (arrow) is most likely the result of
    A. A periodontal abscess
    B. Trauma from plastic picks
    C. Bone exostosis
    D. Occlusal disharmonies
    E. An impacted tooth

19. Based on probe readings at the reevaluation appointment, which of the following is the most accurate assessment of this patient's periodontal condition?
    A. Classified as recurrent periodontal disease and should reenter initial nonsurgical therapy
    B. Considered refractory periodontal disease and should reenter initial nonsurgical therapy
    C. Determined to be a potential candidate for periodontal surgery and should be referred to a periodontist
    D. Categorized as necrotizing ulcerative periodontitis and should be referred to a periodontist
    E. Suspected drug-influenced gingival enlargement and should be referred to a physician

USING PREVENTIVE AGENTS
Basic Level Questions

20. Which of the following would require contacting this patient's physician before recommending for at-home use?
    A. Rinsing with essential oils
    B. Oral irrigation with chlorhexidine gluconate
    C. Brushing with sodium fluoride
    D. Applying a whitening product
    E. Use of disclosing tablets

Competency Level Questions

21. Each of the following is a reason that the antibiotic this patient is currently taking for her sinus infection has failed to improve her periodontal abscess and generalized periodontal condition EXCEPT one. Which one is the EXCEPTION?
    A. Too low a concentration reaching the oral site
    B. Unfavorable local risk factors present
    C. Microorganisms are not susceptible to the antibiotic
    D. Inadequate or incorrect dose being taken
    E. Patient noncompliance

PROVIDING SUPPORTIVE TREATMENT SERVICES
Basic Level Questions

22. If painful symptoms do not subside after vigorous subgingival debridement of the maxillary left molar region, when should the patient be referred for emergency periodontal surgery to access the furcation area?
    A. Immediately following the scaling appointment
    B. When the anesthesia wears off
    C. After 24 hours
    D. Within 1 to 2 weeks
    E. At the next reevaluation appointment

Competency Level Questions

23. Each of the following is a potential contraindication of professional tooth whitening for this patient EXCEPT one. Which one is the EXCEPTION?
    A. Active pathological condition
    B. Periodontal status
    C. Anterior composite restoration
    D. Age
    E. Current shade of her teeth

DEMONSTRATING PROFESSIONAL RESPONSIBILITY
Basic Level Questions

24. Prior to proceeding with the dental hygiene care plan, this patient's signature must be obtained to
    A. Verify her vital signs.
    B. Give consent to treatment.
    C. Show legal status in the United States.
    D. Validate her commitment to self-care.
    E. Document when her last dental appointment was.

Competency Level Questions

25. This patient is unlikely to be satisfied with results obtained by in-office bleaching because it is likely that
    A. She has unrealistic expectations of the outcome.
    B. Tooth sensitivity will result.
    C. The composite restoration will no longer match her natural teeth shade.
    D. She will have an allergic reaction to the bleaching products.
    E. Soft tissue sensitivity will develop.

SETTING PATIENT GOALS

ESTABLISHING A DENTAL HYGIENE CARE PLAN

To assist this patient in meeting her needs, develop a dental hygiene care plan that establishes a framework within which to help her identify goals for obtaining oral health. In addition to the clinical assessment, a well-prepared dental hygiene care plan should take into account the patient's age, gender, lifestyle, culture, attitudes, health beliefs, and knowledge level. To help link this patient's needs for overall well-being with her oral conditions, and to provide motivation for achieving better health, the following is a partial list of possible deficits based on the Human Needs Conceptual Model to Dental Hygiene Practice. (See the appendix for an explanation of the Human Needs Conceptual Model to Dental Hygiene Practice to help you identify additional unmet needs.) Use this partial list of unmet needs or deficits as a guide in preparing a dental hygiene care plan for this patient. One set of goals and dental hygiene actions/implications has been completed as an example.

Deficit identified in Protection from Health Risks

Due to: potential to develop infective endocarditis
Evidenced by: self-reported past infective endocarditis

Goals: _____

Dental hygiene actions/implications: _____

Deficit identified in Freedom from Head and Neck Pain

Due to: periodontal abscess
Evidenced by: periodontal disease, lack of plaque control

Goals: *patient will seek regular professional care; periodontal disease will be brought under control.*

Dental hygiene actions/implications: *educate patient on disease process; plan number and length of appointments; discuss treatment plan and potential outcomes with patient; initiate nonsurgical periodontal treatment; make appropriate referral recommendations.*

Deficit identified in Skin and Mucous Membrane Integrity of the Head and Neck

Due to: bacterial plaque accumulation
Evidenced by: attachment loss and mucogingival involvement

Goals: _____

Dental hygiene actions/implications: _____

Deficit identified in Wholesome Facial Image

Due to: unrealistic expectations regarding tooth whitening
Evidenced by: request for professional whitening products

Goals: _____

Dental hygiene actions/implications: _____

REFLECTIVE ACTIVITIES

1. **To assist with answering patient questions regarding what whitening products to use, investigate a number of different whitening products currently marketed to the public. Use magazine or television ads, the Web, or products promoted by oral health care facilities in your area to make a list of at least five different products. Determine the active ingredients, instructions for use, cost, manufacturer's claims on efficacy, and availability of supportive research on efficacy; and list advantages and disadvantages of the various products.**

2. **Divide the class into two sides for a philosophical debate on tooth whitening's role in the oral health care practice. One team should prepare for the debate by taking the side that whitening procedures are cosmetic and should not play a serious role in treatment planning for the patient. The other side should champion whitening services as an integral component of total oral health care.**

REFERENCES

CRA Foundation: Non-injectable local anesthetic for periodontal administration. *CRA Newsletter*, 29(4), 3–4, 2005.

Darby ML, Walsh MM: Application of the human needs conceptual model to dental hygiene practice. *Journal of Dental Hygiene*, 74(3), 230–237, 2000.

Darby ML, Walsh MM: *Dental Hygiene Theory and Practice*, 2nd ed. St. Louis: Saunders (Elsevier), 2003, pp. 694–705.

Hatrick CD, Eakle WS, Bird WF: *Dental Materials. Clinical Applications for Dental Assistants and Dental Hygienists.* Philadelphia: Saunders (Elsevier), 2003, pp. 102–106.

Johnson ON, Thomson EM: *Essentials of Dental Radiography for Dental Assistants and Hygienists*, 8th ed. Upper Saddle River, NJ: Prentice Hall, 2007, pp. 201–204, 339–344, 374–376.

Little JW, Falce DA, Miller CS, Rhodus NL: *Dental Management of the Medically Compromised Patient*, 7th ed. St. Louis: Mosby (Elsevier), 2008, pp. 248, 259–260.

Pickett FA, Gurenlian JR: *The Medical History: Clinical Implications and Emergency Prevention in Dental Settings*, Philadelphia: Lippincott Williams & Wilkins, 2005, pp. 53–56.

Raposa K: The whitening generation: What you need to know to help your patients and your practice make the right decision about tooth whitening. *Access*, 20(8), 24–28, 2006.

Serio FG, Hawley CE: *Manual of Clinical Periodontics.* Hudon, OH: Lexi-Comp, Inc., 2002, pp. 58–60, 105–107.

Weinberg MA, Westphal C, Oakat M, Froum SJ: *Comprehensive Periodontics for the Dental Hygienist*, 2nd ed. Upper Saddle River, NJ: Prentice Hall, 2006, pp. 31–38, 93–102, 151.

White SC, Pharoah MJ: *Oral Radiology. Principles and Interpretation*, 5th ed. St. Louis: Mosby (Elsevier), 2004, pp. 492, 524.

Wilkins EM: *Clinical Practice of the Dental Hygienist*, 9th ed. Philadelphia: Lippincott Williams & Wilkins, 2005, pp. 122–125, 267–269, 448–449, 583–607, 1041–1043.

Wolf HF, Hassell TM: *Color Atlas of Dental Hygiene. Periodontology.* New York: Thieme, 2006, p. 217.

CASE **G**

Juan Hernandez

SITUATION

Juan Hernandez looks forward to coming to his regularly scheduled 6-month dental hygiene appointments. He is usually accompanied by his granddaughter, who he depends on for transportation. This patient is ambulatory, with the use of a cane.

LEARNING GOALS

Following integration of core scientific concepts and application of dental hygiene theory to the care of this patient, you will be able to

1. **Assess patient characteristics.**
   A. Recognize etiology of deviations in gingival appearance.
   B. Distinguish normal anatomic features from pathology.
   C. Assess occlusal relationships.
   D. Identify conditions that result in the need for Class V restorations.
   E. Determine the etiology of gingival recession.
   F. Identify the interrelationship of arthritis and oral function.

2. **Obtain and interpret radiographs.**
   A. Recognize dental materials radiographically.
   B. Apply appropriate techniques to correct radiographic errors.
   C. Appropriately recommend the use of vertical or horizontal bitewing radiographs.
   D. Differentiate between normal radiographic anatomy and pathology.

3. **Plan and manage dental hygiene care.**
   A. Identify possible effects of prescribed medications on dental hygiene treatment.
   B. Identify health risks that contraindicate dental hygiene treatment.
   C. Modify dental hygiene treatment when necessary for the medically compromised patient.
   D. Plan periodontal debridement sequence based on patient needs.

4. **Perform periodontal procedures.**
   A. Assess periodontal status.
   B. Identify oral conditions that hinder instrumentation.
   C. Provide appropriate follow-up care for the periodontally involved patient.
   D. Recommend periodontal maintenance schedule based on tissue response to nonsurgical periodontal treatment.

5. **Use preventive agents.**
   A. Determine the need for appropriate supplemental oral hygiene devices and agents.

6. **Provide supportive treatment services.**
   A. Recognize the appropriate method for margination of an overhang amalgam.
   B. Select appropriate treatment for temporomandibular disorder (TMD).

7. **Demonstrate professional responsibility.**
   A. Demonstrate effective communication techniques with the stroke victim.
   B. Determine the components of implied consent.
   C. Identify the role that characteristics of a geriatric patient play in ethical care planning.
   D. Determine the components of informed consent.

GERIATRIC PATIENT—*Juan Hernandez*
PATIENT HISTORY SYNOPSIS

VITAL STATISTICS

Age	_81 years_	Blood Pressure	_140/90 mm Hg_
Gender	_male_	Pulse Rate	_70 bpm_
Height	_5' 10"_	Respiration	_14 rpm_
Weight	_175 lbs._		

1. Under care of physician
   Yes [X]   No [ ]
   Condition: _hypertension_ _____
   _____
   _____

2. Hospitalized within the last 5 years
   Yes [X]   No [ ]
   Reason: _cerebrovascular_
   accident (CVA)

3. Has or had the following conditions
   atherosclerosis _____
   osteoarthritis _____
   _____

4. Current medications
   warfarin sodium (Coumadin)—anticoagulant
   chlorothiazide (Diuril)—diuretic
   atorvastatin (Lipitor)—antihyperlipidemic
   naproxen (Naproxsyn)—anti-inflammatory/antiarthritic

5. Smokes or uses tobacco products
   Yes [ ]   No [X]

6. Is pregnant
   Yes [ ]   No [ ]   N/A [X]

MEDICAL HISTORY
This patient has slightly limited use of his right side since his stroke, 5 years ago. He experiences morning stiffness especially in his hands, hips, and knees.

DENTAL HISTORY
Proud that he has all of his teeth and has not had to experience dentures. Attributes his oral condition to "the goodness of faith" and the good food of his culture. He brushes once per day using a horizontal scrubbing action and has had instruction in flossing, but his arthritic hands have not "had much luck" using floss.

SOCIAL HISTORY
Lives with the youngest of his six children. His extended family is close and he enjoys being the family patriarch. His wife of 58 years is deceased.

CHIEF COMPLAINT
Temporomandibular joint has become somewhat problematic with an increased stiffness and a crackling sensation that has manifested bilaterally.

ADULT CLINICAL EXAMINATION

	1	2	3	4	5	6	7	8	9	10	11	12	13	14	15	16
Probe 2	X	324	425	534	212	212	212	212	212	212	315	434	334	424	434	X
Probe 1	X	324	425	534	212	312	212	212	212	212	315	434	334	434	434	X

(F / P)

	1	2	3	4	5	6	7	8	9	10	11	12	13	14	15	16
Probe 1	X	466	435	523	323	313	212	212	212	212	214	414	424	523	465	X
Probe 2	X	466	435	523	322	212	212	212	212	212	213	314	424	523	444	X

R / L

	32	31	30	29	28	27	26	25	24	23	22	21	20	19	18	17
Probe 2	X	525	525	524	414	212	212	212	212	212	214	415	424	424	525	X
Probe 1	X	525	525	524	414	333	322	212	212	212	214	415	525	525	525	X

(L / F)

	32	31	30	29	28	27	26	25	24	23	22	21	20	19	18	17
Probe 1	X	425	526	524	412	212	212	212	212	212	212	214	412	424	433	X
Probe 2	X	424	526	524	412	212	212	212	212	212	212	214	312	324	423	X

CURRENT ORAL HYGIENE STATUS
Bleeding upon probing interproximally in posterior regions
Slight generalized calculus
Moderate generalized marginal plaque

SUPPLEMENTAL ORAL EXAMINATION FINDINGS
Moderate xerostomia
TMJ moderate crepitus bilaterally
Mandibular left premolars exhibit fremitus.

⊓ Clinically visible carious lesion

X Clinically missing tooth

△ Furcation

▲ "Through and through" furcation

Probe 1: Initial probing depth

Probe 2: Probing depth 6 weeks after periodontal therapy

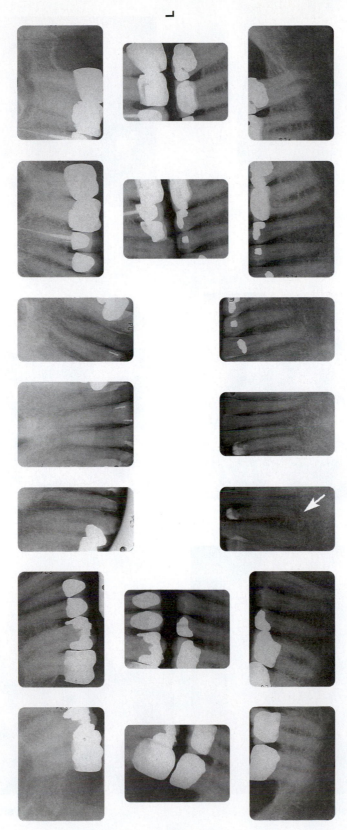

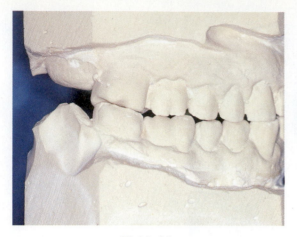

Right side

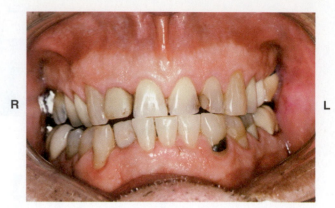

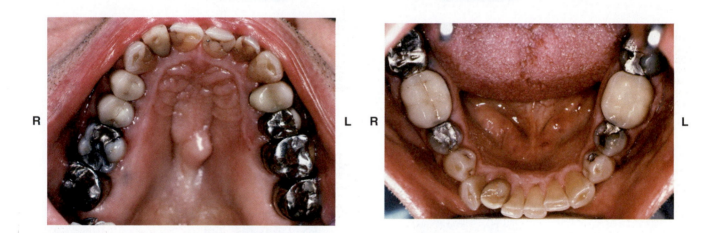

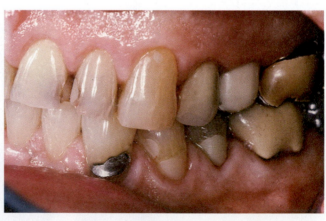

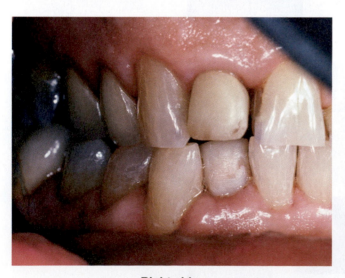

Right side   **Left side**

CASE QUESTIONS

ASSESSING PATIENT CHARACTERISTICS

Basic Level Questions

1. Which of the following best describes the bluish gingival tissue lingual to the maxillary right first molar?
   A. Necrosis
   B. Cyanosis
   C. Leukoplakia
   D. Exostosis
   E. Amalgam tattoo

2. Which of the following is the most likely assessment of this patient's palate?
   A. Granular tumor
   B. Pseudocyst
   C. Gingival fibromatosis
   D. Torus palantinus
   E. Hyperplastic salivary ducts

3. Which of the following correctly describes this patient's molar occlusal relationship on the right side?
   A. Open bite
   B. Edge-to-edge
   C. End-to-end
   D. Cross bite
   E. Protruded

Competency Level Questions

4. Each of the following may have contributed to the need for the Class V restorations placed on the mandibular left canine, first premolar, and second premolar EXCEPT one. Which one is the EXCEPTION?
   A. Cervical burnout
   B. Toothbrush abrasion
   C. Aggressive scaling
   D. Root caries
   E. Abfraction

5. Age and occlusal trauma are the cause of this patient's gingival recession.

   This patient's gingival recession has increased his risk of root caries.
   A. The first statement is true, the second statement is false.
   B. The first statement is false, the second statement is true.
   C. Both statements are true.
   D. Both statements are false.

6. Which of the following is the most likely contributing factor in this patient's temporo-mandibular joint disorder (TMD)?
   A. History of a stroke
   B. High blood pressure
   C. Osteoarthritis
   D. Age
   E. Attrition

OBTAINING AND INTERPRETING RADIOGRAPHS
Basic Level Questions

7. Radiographically, the maxillary left second premolar shows signs of
   A. Endodontic therapy
   B. Endosseous implant
   C. Internal root resorption
   D. Pulp stones
   E. Apicoectomy

Competency Level Questions

8. Which one of the following would correct the technique error evidenced in the maxillary right canine periapical radiograph?
   A. Move the film posteriorly.
   B. Move the film anteriorly.
   C. Decrease the vertical angulation.
   D. Increase the vertical angulation.
   E. Move the PID inferiorly.

9. Which of the following is the best reason for exposing vertical and not horizontal bitewing radiographs on this patient?
   A. Age
   B. Periodontal status
   C. Presence of maxillary torus
   D. Limited opening because of TMD
   E. Will eliminate the need for periapical radiographs

10. Which of the following is the most likely interpretation of the radiolucency observed near the mandibular right lateral incisor? (arrow)
    A. Genial tubercles
    B. Mental foramen
    C. Periapical abscess
    D. Film identification dot
    E. Mandibular torus

PLANNING AND MANAGING DENTAL HYGIENE CARE
Basic Level Questions

11. Which medication currently taken by this patient may contraindicate proceeding with treatment today?
    A. Diuril
    B. Lipitor
    C. Naprosyn
    D. Coumadin

12. Each of the following is important when planning oral health care appointments for this patient EXCEPT one. Which one is the EXCEPTION?
    A. Schedule treatment for early morning.
    B. Allow frequent position changes during treatment.
    C. Treatment chair should be comfortable.
    D. Provide physical supports such as pillows.
    E. Plan short treatment segments.

Competency Level Questions

13. Given that this patient has an acceptable prothrombin time and treatment may continue, which of the following would still be contraindicated?
    A. Subgingival instrumentation with hand instruments
    B. Air-powder polishing with sodium bicarbonate
    C. Ultrasonic instrumentation with narrow profile tip
    D. Nitrous oxide sedation
    E. Sodium fluoride varnish application

14. Which of the following would be the most appropriate treatment plan for this patient?
    A. One appointment for full-mouth oral prophylaxis, followed up with a 6-month recall appointment
    B. One appointment for full-mouth nonsurgical periodontal therapy, followed up with a 6-week reevaluation appointment
    C. One appointment for full-mouth disinfection, followed up with a 4-week reevaluation appointment
    D. Two appointments for half-mouth periodontal debridement, followed up with a 6-week reevaluation appointment
    E. Four appointments for quadrant scaling and root planing, followed up with a 4-week reevaluation appointment

PERFORMING PERIODONTAL PROCEDURES
Basic Level Questions

15. What is this patient's periodontal status?
    A. Aggressive periodontitis
    B. Slight chronic periodontitis
    C. Moderate chronic periodontitis
    D. Severe chronic periodontitis
    E. Refractory periodontitis

16. Each of the following may hinder periodontal debridement procedures for this patient EXCEPT one. Which one is the EXCEPTION?
    A. Furcation involvement
    B. Poorly contoured crown margins
    C. Cervical restorations
    D. Increased bleeding
    E. Cultural attitude toward treatment

Competency Level Questions

17. Based on this patient's probing depths at the reevaluation appointment, each of the following would be indicated EXCEPT one. Which one is the EXCEPTION?
    A. Prescribing oral antibiotic therapy
    B. Referral to a periodontist
    C. Instrumenting pockets and bleeding areas
    D. Oral irrigation with chemotherapeutic agents
    E. Using locally delivered drug therapy

18. Based on the probe readings at the reevaluation appointment, when should this patient's next periodontal maintenance appointment be scheduled?
    A. 1 month
    B. 3 months
    C. 6 months
    D. 12 months

USING PREVENTIVE AGENTS
Basic Level Questions

19. Each of the following would be an appropriate recommendation for this patient's oral self-care program EXCEPT one. Which one is the EXCEPTION?
    A. Automatic toothbrush
    B. Power-driven oral irrigation device
    C. Home fluoride rinse
    D. Interproximal brush
    E. Floss holder

PROVIDING SUPPORTIVE TREATMENT SERVICES
Competency Level Questions

20. To improve the restoration present on the mesial of the maxillary right first molar, the dentist would most likely
    A. Smooth the mesial overhang using fine diamond interproximal finishing strips.
    B. Remove the mesial overhang using a flame-shaped silicon carbide bur.
    C. Cut the mesial overhang by inserting a gold knife.
    D. Trim the mesial overhang using a fine-fluted, pointed tungsten carbide bur.

21. Which of the following should NOT be recommended for this patient's TMD?
    A. Soft diet
    B. Moist heat to face/jaw
    C. Acetaminophen (Tylenol Arthritis Extended Relief)
    D. Occlusal appliance
    E. Physician referral

DEMONSTRATING PROFESSIONAL RESPONSIBILITY
Basic Level Questions

22. Each of the following enhance effective communication with this patient EXCEPT one. Which one is the EXCEPTION?
    A. Remove face mask and face the patient when speaking.
    B. Give frequent and immediate feedback regarding demonstration of self-care techniques.
    C. Use simple drawings to explain dental procedures.
    D. When changing positions, move slowly around the patient.
    E. Allow the patient to get himself into position for treatment; provide assistance only when asked.

23. The implied consent given by this patient does NOT include
    A. Disclosing to determine the presence of biofilms
    B. Periodontal debridement of one quadrant
    C. Occlusal evaluation and test for fremitus
    D. Probing all four quadrants
    E. Physical extraoral palpation of TMJ function

Competency Level Questions

24. According to OSCAR (Oral, Systemic, Capability, Autonomy, Reality), a system developed by the American Academy of Oral Medicine to assist in care planning for geriatric and disabled patients, each of the following can play a role in treatment planning for this patient EXCEPT one. Which one is the EXCEPTION?
    A. Ethnicity and culture
    B. Decision-making ability
    C. Financial ability to pay for treatment
    D. Anticipated life span remaining
    E. Functional ability to perform self-care

25. Which of the following would NOT be a requirement for this patient's informed consent?
    A. Explanation of why periodontal debridement may not reduce pocket depths
    B. Warning that treatment may cause his gums to recede
    C. Listing of alternative treatments and their costs
    D. His granddaughter's presence when he signs the documents
    E. Caution that disease may progress with no treatment

SETTING PATIENT GOALS

ESTABLISHING A DENTAL HYGIENE CARE PLAN

To assist this patient in meeting his needs, develop a dental hygiene care plan that establishes a framework within which to help him identify goals for obtaining oral health. In addition to the clinical assessment, a well-prepared dental hygiene care plan should take into account the patient's age, gender, lifestyle, culture, attitudes, health beliefs, and knowledge level. To help link this patient's needs for overall well-being with his oral conditions, and to provide motivation for achieving better health, the following is a partial list of possible deficits based on the Human Needs Conceptual Model to Dental Hygiene Practice. (See the appendix for an explanation of the Human Needs Conceptual Model to Dental Hygiene Practice to help you identify additional unmet needs.) Use this partial list of unmet needs or deficits as a guide in preparing a dental hygiene care plan for this patient. One set of goals and dental hygiene actions/implications has been completed as an example.

Deficit identified in Protection from Health Risks

Due to: excessive bleeding during instrumentation
Evidenced by: medications reported on the health history

Goals: _____

Dental hygiene actions/implications: _____

Deficit identified in Skin and Mucous Membrane Integrity of the Head and Neck

Due to: presence of marginal plaque
Evidenced by: bleeding on probing and periodontal disease

Goals: _____

Dental hygiene actions/implications: _____

Deficit identified in Biologically Sound Dentition

Due to: future caries risk
Evidenced by: caries and xerostomia

Goals: *avoid future caries; improve oral conditions by supplementing salivary flow.*

Dental hygiene actions/implications: *perform comprehensive dental charting and interpretation of radiographs; refer to dentist for confirmation of the presence of caries and to determine which lesions need restoration and which may benefit from remineralization therapies; assess severity of diminished salivary flow; educate patient regarding the interrelationship between saliva and caries; determine the appropriate recommendation for reduced salivary flow; determine the need for fluoride therapies both professional and self-applied.*

Deficit identified in Conceptualization and Problem Solving

Due to: lack of awareness of effective brushing technique
Evidenced by: marginal plaque; self-report of scrub brushing technique

Goals: _____

Dental hygiene actions/implications: _____

Deficit identified in Responsibility for Oral Health

Due to: ineffective daily home care
Evidenced by: periodontal disease and caries

Goals: _____

Dental hygiene actions/implications: _____

REFLECTIVE ACTIVITIES

1. List ten physiologic age-related changes of the human body and discuss their impact on dental hygiene treatment.

2. To simulate decreased manual dexterity, often encountered in stroke survivors, brush your teeth using your nondominant hand. (If you are right-handed, brush your teeth with your left hand.) Disclose and evaluate your plaque removal ability. Write an essay on how you would assist a patient with reduced manual dexterity to perform oral self-care.

3. List a belief about health care from your own cultural background. How does this belief assist in helping and/or hindering access to health care for the people of your culture?

REFERENCES

Alvarez KH: *Williams & Wilkins' Dental Hygiene Handbook.* Baltimore: Lippincott Williams & Wilkins, 1998, pp. 326–333, 375–389.

Darby ML: *Mosby's Comprehensive Review of Dental Hygiene,* 6th ed. St. Louis: Mosby (Elsevier), 2006, pp. 586–590, 719.

Darby ML, Walsh MM: *Dental Hygiene Theory and Practice,* 2nd ed. Philadelphia: Saunders (Elsevier), 2003, pp. 219–220, 317, 553, 873–912, 960–985.

Gage TW, Little JW: *Mosby's 2007 Dental Drug Consult.* St. Louis: Mosby (Elsevier), 2007, pp. 102–103, 251–253, 855–857, 1298–1300.

Little JW, Falce DA, Miller CS, Rhodus NL: *Dental Management of the Medically Compromised Patient,* 7th ed. St. Louis: Mosby (Elsevier), 2008, pp. DM2–DM3, 35–48, 469–474.

Requa-Clark B: *Applied Pharmacology for the Dental Hygienist,* 4th ed. St. Louis: Mosby (Elsevier), 2000, pp. 321–364.

Ship JA, Mohammad AR (eds.): *The Clinician's Guide to Oral Health in Geriatric Patients.* Baltimore: American Academy of Oral Medicine, 1999.

Weinberg MA, Westphal C, Oakat M, Froum SJ: *Comprehensive Periodontics for the Dental Hygienist,* 2nd ed. Upper Saddle River, NJ: Prentice Hall, 2006, pp. 348–361, 555–l557.

Wilkins EM: *Clinical Practice of the Dental Hygienist,* 9th ed. Philadelphia: Lippincott Williams & Wilkins, 2005, pp. 254–272, 755–761.

CASE **H**

Virginia Carson

SITUATION

Virginia Carson appears to struggle into the operatory and to get situated in the treatment chair. She wheezes and appears out of breath with each movement. It has taken a lot of effort for her to get to this appointment today because she does not drive. She relies on the community's senior citizen transportation. This patient knows that she needs to be here, but does not like "going to the dentist."

LEARNING GOALS

Following integration of core scientific concepts and application of dental hygiene theory to the care of this patient, you will be able to

1. **Assess patient characteristics.**
   A. Categorize blood pressure readings.
   B. Classify furcation involvement.
   C. Determine preliminary diagnosis of oral conditions that deviate from normal.

2. **Obtain and interpret radiographs.**
   A. Differentiate between a variety of normal radiographic anatomical landmarks.
   B. Interpret radiolucencies and radiopacities observed on a periapical radiograph.

3. **Plan and manage dental hygiene care.**
   A. Recognize medical conditions that require antibiotic premedication.
   B. Identify appointment-planning considerations for the geriatric patient.
   C. Take steps to avoid a medical emergency.
   D. Select appropriate interdental devices based on patient needs.
   E. Identify risks to oral and general health.

4. **Perform periodontal procedures.**
   A. Identify types of periodontal pockets.
   B. Classify periodontal disease based on extent and severity.
   C. Select appropriate scaling instruments for effective and efficient calculus removal.
   D. Differentiate between the severity of periodontal conditions that affect prognosis.
   E. Identify periodontal risk indicators.

5. **Use preventive agents.**
   A. Select treatment recommendations following reevaluation of initial periodontal debridement.

6. **Provide supportive treatment services.**
   A. Recommend appropriate treatment interventions based on patient need.
   B. Differentiate between acrylic products used in dental appliances.
   C. Recommend appropriate denture care.

7. **Demonstrate professional responsibility.**
   A. Demonstrate effective communication strategies for the geriatric patient.
   B. Identify professional responsibility in maintaining an oral health care facility accessible to the geriatric patient.
   C. Recognize ethical treatment planning for the geriatric patient.
   D. Communicate appropriately with the medically compromised geriatric patient about the link between periodontal diseases and systemic health.

GERIATRIC PATIENT—*Virginia Carson*
PATIENT HISTORY SYNOPSIS

VITAL STATISTICS

Age	*66 years*	Blood Pressure	*142/94 mm Hg*
Gender	*female*	Pulse Rate	*69 bpm*
Height	*5' 3"*	Respiration	*14 rpm*
Weight	*165 lbs.*		

1. Under care of physician
   Yes [X]   No [ ]   Condition: *congestive heart failure* _____

2. Hospitalized within the last 5 years
   Yes [X]   No [ ]   Reason: *heart attack* _____

3. Has or had the following conditions
   hepatitis C
   bronchitis (COPD—chronic obstructive pulmonary disease)

4. Current medications
   atenolol (Tenormin)—beta¹-adrenergic blocker
   digoxin (Lanoxicaps)—cardiac glycoside
   enalapril maleate (Vasotec)—antihypertensive
   fluticasone propionate/salmeterol (Advair Diskus)—respiratory inhalant combination furosemide (Lasix)—diuretic
   multivitamin with iron (Stress Tabs)—over-the-counter dietary supplement

5. Smokes or uses tobacco products
   Yes [X]   No [ ]

6. Is pregnant
   Yes [ ]   No [X]   N/A [ ]

MEDICAL HISTORY
Although her physician has recommended smoking cessation, this patient still smokes a pack of cigarettes a day.

DENTAL HISTORY
Received a new, full maxillary denture last month. Although she has been back to the office several times for adjustments, she appears to be happy with the appliance.

SOCIAL HISTORY
A widow, she has lived alone since her husband passed away 9 years ago. Striving to live comfortably on a small pension, this patient takes advantage of senior citizen assistance available to her in the community. She recently moved to a senior citizen condominium where she is acquiring a new social life.

CHIEF COMPLAINT
Her immediate dental complaint has been addressed with a new full maxillary denture that replaces her chipped and ill-fitting 20-year-old appliance. She was referred for dental hygiene treatment and made this appointment out of respect for the dentist who made her denture. She promised him that she would return to the office to take care of her lower teeth after her denture was made.

ADULT CLINICAL EXAMINATION

	32	31	30	29	28	27	26	25	24	23	22	21	20	19	18	17
Probe 2		656	635	525	323	333	434	434	434	434	434	434	434	546	746	
Probe 1		657	635	525	333	434	434	434	434	434	434	434	434	546	756	
Probe 1		757	555	454	434	534	424	434	535	555	555	554	554	545	645	
Probe 2		757	555	454	434	534	424	424	424	444	445	555	554	545	635	

CURRENT ORAL HYGIENE STATUS
Poor oral hygiene with generalized heavy marginal plaque and calculus. She brushes once daily and has tried flossing, but her teeth are too tight and the floss does not fit in between them.

SUPPLEMENTAL ORAL EXAMINATION FINDINGS
Spontaneous bleeding

🦷 Clinically visible carious lesion
✗ Clinically missing tooth
△ Furcation
▲ "Through and through" furcation
Probe 1: Initial probing depth
Probe 2: Probing depth 6 weeks after periodontal therapy

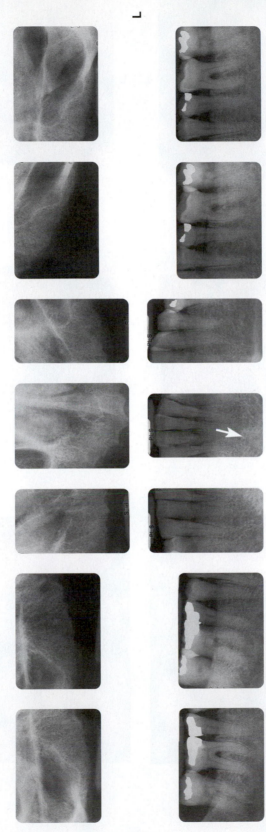

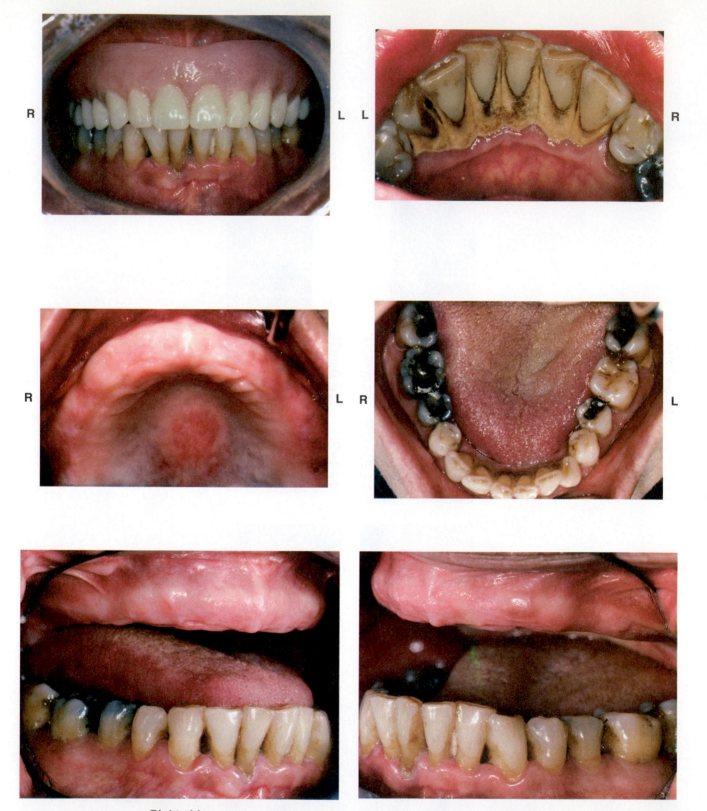

Right side

Left side

CASE QUESTIONS

ASSESSING PATIENT CHARACTERISTICS
Basic Level Questions

1. This patient's blood pressure category is
   A. Hypotension
   B. Normal
   C. Prehypertension
   D. Hypertension stage 1
   E. Hypertension stage 2

2. What is the classification of furcation involvement of the mandibular right first molar?
   A. Grade I
   B. Grade II
   C. Grade III
   D. Grade IV

Competency Level Questions

3. Which of the following is the most likely assessment of the condition seen on this patient's palate?
   A. Primary herpetic gingivostomatitis
   B. Chronic atrophic candidiasis
   C. Herpetiform aphthous ulcer
   D. Melanin pigmentation
   E. Torus palatinus

OBTAINING AND INTERPRETING RADIOGRAPHS
Basic Level Questions

4. What is the interpretation of the radiopaque circle, identified by the arrow, seen on the mandibular central incisor periapical radiograph?
   A. Genial tubercles
   B. Symphysis
   C. Mental foramen
   D. Retrocuspid papilla
   E. Trabeculae

5. What is the scalloped radiopaque line visible radiographically across the mandibular central incisors?
   A. Cementoenamel junction
   B. Dense enamel layer
   C. Calculus buildup
   D. Composite resin
   E. Cementicles

Competency Level Questions

6. Which of the following is the most likely reason for the radiopaque appearance of the nasal fossa?
   A. Soft tissue of the nose imaged
   B. Film fog artifact
   C. Sinus infection
   D. Deviated septum
   E. Conchae present

7. Which one of the following is the most likely interpretation of the radiolucency observed on the distal surface of the mandibular right first premolar?
   A. Toothbrush abrasion
   B. Cervical burnout
   C. Root fracture
   D. Abfraction lesion
   E. Caries

PLANNING AND MANAGING DENTAL HYGIENE CARE
Basic Level Questions

8. Which of the following medical conditions predisposes this patient for the need to premedicate with prophylactic antibiotic coverage?
   A. Bronchitis
   B. Hepatitis C
   C. Congestive heart failure
   D. Spontaneous gingival bleeding
   E. None of the above

9. The best time to schedule appointments for this patient is
   A. First appointment of the morning
   B. Early morning, 8:00 A.M. to 10:00 A.M.
   C. Midmorning to early afternoon, 11:00 A.M. to 2:00 P.M.
   D. Late afternoon, after 3:00 P.M.
   E. Last appointment of the day

Competency Level Questions

10. Each of the following will help avoid an emergency situation when treating this patient EXCEPT one. Which one is the EXCEPTION?
    A. Use anesthesia with vasoconstrictor.
    B. Avoid orthostatic hypotension.
    C. Use a semisupine or upright position for treatment.
    D. Follow stress reduction protocol.
    E. Monitor vital signs.

11. Which of the following interdental devices should NOT be recommended for this patient?
    A. Wooden interdental cleaner
    B. Tufted dental floss
    C. Interdental tip
    D. Saline irrigation
    E. Toothpick in holder

12. This patient is at increased risk for each of the following EXCEPT one. Which one is the EXCEPTION?
    A. Halitosis
    B. Nicotine stomatitis
    C. Periodontal disease
    D. Extrinsic tooth stains
    E. Oral cancer

PERFORMING PERIODONTAL PROCEDURES
Basic Level Questions

13. Which of the following best describes the type of periodontal pocketing found on the mesial aspect of the mandibular left second premolar?
    A. Gingival sulcus
    B. Gingival pocket
    C. Pseudopocket
    D. Periodontal intrabony pocket
    E. Periodontal suprabony pocket

14. Based on extent and severity, how would this patient's periodontal disease be classified?
    A. Localized moderate
    B. Localized advanced
    C. Generalized early
    D. Generalized moderate
    E. Generalized advanced

15. Which one of the following instruments should be selected to begin removal of supragingival calculus from the lingual surfaces of this patient's mandibular anterior teeth?
    A. Universal curette
    B. Area-specific curette
    C. Anterior sickle scaler
    D. Standard ultrasonic tip
    E. Periodontal ultrasonic tip

Competency Level Questions

16. Which of the following teeth presents with the poorest prognosis?
    A. Mandibular right second molar
    B. Mandibular right first premolar
    C. Mandibular right central incisor
    D. Mandibular left lateral incisor
    E. Mandibular left second premolar

17. This patient presents with each of the following risk indicators for periodontal disease EXCEPT one. Which one is the EXCEPTION?
    A. Age
    B. Gender
    C. Cigarette smoking
    D. Poor home care habits
    E. Socioeconomic status

USING PREVENTIVE AGENTS
Competency Level Questions

18. Following her 6-week reevaluation appointment, what should be scheduled next for this patient?
    A. Periodontist referral
    B. Pulp vitality testing
    C. Pit and fissure sealants
    D. Dental restorations
    E. Desensitization

PROVIDING SUPPORTIVE TREATMENT SERVICES
Basic Level Questions

19. Which one of the following interventions is most appropriate for this patient?
    A. Dietary counseling
    B. Oral cancer referral
    C. Dental implant evaluation
    D. Tobacco cessation program
    E. Advanced infection control procedures

20. Considering the clinical appearance of the maxillary denture, what dental material was used to manufacture it?
    A. Bis-phenol A-glycidal methacrylate (bis-GMA)
    B. Urethane dimethacrylate (UEDMA)
    C. Poly methyl methacrylate (MMA) resin
    D. Hydroxyethyl methacrylate (HEMA)
    E. Dipentaerythiol penta-acrylate monophosphate (PENTA-P)

21. To prevent stain accumulation on her new denture, which of the following home care regimens should be recommended?
    A. Soak weekly in mouthwash.
    B. Brush daily with dentifrice using a denture brush.
    C. Immerse in sodium hypochlorite overnight.
    D. Brush once a month using a household scouring powder.
    E. Clean by placing in the dishwasher once every 6 months.

DEMONSTRATING PROFESSIONAL RESPONSIBILITY
Basic Level Questions

22. Each of the following will help to improve communication with this patient EXCEPT one. Which one is the EXCEPTION?
    A. Face the patient, make eye contact, and speak clearly.
    B. Be nonjudgmental in recommending that she take steps to improve her health.
    C. Eliminate distracting background noise and music.
    D. Repeat self-care instructions and give her written take-home instructions.
    E. Use endearing terms such as "Honey" and "Dear" to address her in an accepting manner.

23. A throw rug and reduced hallway lighting can be physical barriers and potential hazards for the older adult patient with impaired vision or motor control.

    Altering the oral health care treatment facility for the older adult patient may be viewed as discriminatory.
    A. The first statement is true, the second statement is false.
    B. The first statement is false, the second statement is true.
    C. Both statements are true and related.
    D. Both statements are true but not related.
    E. Both statements are false.

Competency Level Questions

24. Dental hygiene care for this patient should be based on palliative treatment.

    Long-term periodontal health maintenance is important for the medically compromised older adult.
    A. The first statement is true, the second statement is false.
    B. The first statement is false, the second statement is true.
    C. Both statements are true.
    D. Both statements are false.

25. Each of the following is applicable and appropriate to approach a discussion with this patient EXCEPT one. Which one is the EXCEPTION?
    A. "Periodontal disease and cardiovascular disease share the same risk factors."
    B. "Patients with periodontal disease have higher levels of cardiovascular disease."
    C. "Poor oral health, periodontitis, and oral infections increase the odds of myocardial infarction."
    D. "Periodontal disease causes coronary heart disease and chronic obstructive pulmonary disease."
    E. "An association has been established between periodontitis and chronic obstructive pulmonary disease."

SETTING PATIENT GOALS

ESTABLISHING A DENTAL HYGIENE CARE PLAN

To assist this patient in meeting her needs, develop a dental hygiene care plan that establishes a framework within which to help her identify goals for obtaining oral health. In addition to the clinical assessment, a well-prepared dental hygiene care plan should take into account the patient's age, gender, lifestyle, culture, attitudes, health beliefs, and knowledge level. To help link this patient's needs for overall well-being with her oral conditions, and to provide motivation for achieving better health, the following is a partial list of possible deficits based on the Human Needs Conceptual Model to Dental Hygiene Practice. (See the appendix for an explanation of the Human Needs Conceptual Model to Dental Hygiene Practice to help you identify additional unmet needs.) Use this partial list of unmet needs or deficits as a guide in preparing a dental hygiene care plan for this patient. One set of goals and dental hygiene actions/implications has been completed as an example.

Deficit identified in Protection from Health Risks

Due to: tobacco usage
Evidenced by: periodontal disease diminished response to treatment

Goals: _____

Dental hygiene actions/implications: _____

Deficit identified in Freedom from Stress

Due to: uneasiness regarding dental hygiene appointments
Evidenced by: lack of motivation and commitment to regular professional care

Goals: _____

Dental hygiene actions/implications: _____

Deficit identified in Skin and Mucous Membrane Integrity of the Head and Neck

Due to: bacterial plaque and inadequate oral health behaviors
Evidenced by: the presence of gingival inflammation, pockets, and bleeding

Goals: _____

Dental hygiene actions/implications: _____

Due to: chronic infection
Evidenced by: degree of periodontal involvement

Goals: _____

Dental hygiene actions/implications: _____

Deficit identified in Conceptualization and Problem Solving

Due to: misconceptions associated with oral health care
Evidenced by: lack of concern regarding condition of mandibular teeth

Goals: _____

Dental hygiene actions/implications: _____

Deficit identified in Responsibility for Oral Health

Due to: irregular dental hygiene visits
Evidenced by: heavy calculus deposits

Goals: *schedule and keep regular periodontal maintenance appointments during this next year.*

Dental hygiene actions/implications: *help patient identify roadblocks to achieving this goal; help patient to rate her desire for oral health in relation to these roadblocks; encourage patient to participate in developing solutions that will help her get to the oral health care facility.*

REFLECTIVE ACTIVITIES

1. Make a list of possible barriers to receiving regular professional oral health care faced by the geriatric patient. Together with your class, brainstorm possible solutions for overcoming these barriers.

2. Based on the needs of this patient, establish priorities in the dental and dental hygiene care plan. Keep in mind the following, which will most likely influence the establishment of these priorities: attitude of the patient toward dental and dental hygiene treatment; physical abilities or disabilities; philosophy and attitude of the health care provider.

3. Develop a table or chart that lists the oral manifestations of aging that can be used as an aid in performing an intraoral and extraoral examination of the geriatric patient. Include age-related changes likely to present in the soft tissues of the head and neck region, including the salivary glands, the lips, oral mucosa, and tongue; changes in the teeth that include color, evidence of wear, types of caries, and radiographic findings; and changes in the periodontal tissues including the supporting bone.

REFERENCES

Anusavice KJ (ed.): *Phillips' Science of Dental Materials*, 11th ed. Philadelphia: Saunders (Elsevier), 2003, pp. 721–757.

Darby ML: *Mosby's Comprehensive Review of Dental Hygiene*, 6th ed. St. Louis: Mosby (Elsevier), 2006, pp. 570–571, 585–586.

Fried JL: *The Dental Hygienist's Role in Tobacco Use, Prevention and Cessation*. Chicago: ADHA Self Study Course, 1995.

Gage TW, Little JW: *Mosby's 2007 Dental Drug Consult*. St. Louis: Mosby (Elsevier), 2005, pp. 98–100, 369–371, 422–424, 540–542.

Glickman I: *Clinical Periodontology*. Philadelphia: Saunders, 1953.

Ibsen OAC, Phelan JA: *Oral Pathology for the Dental Hygienist*, 4th ed. Philadelphia: Saunders (Elsevier), 2004, pp. 48–49, 135–136.

Johnson ON, Thomson EM: *Essentials of Dental Radiography for Dental Assistants and Hygienists*, 8th ed. Upper Saddle River, NJ: Prentice Hall, 2007, pp. 127–131, 249–265, 329.

Little JW, Falce DA, Miller CS, Rhodus NL: *Dental Management of the Medically Compromised Patient*, 7th ed. St. Louis: Mosby (Elsevier), 2008, pp. 92–97, 140–151, 534–550.

Perry DA, Beemsterboer P, Taggart EJ: *Periodontology for the Dental Hygienist*, 2nd ed. Philadelphia: Saunders (Elsevier), 2001, pp. 107–130.

Pickett FA, Terezhamlmy GT: *Lippincott Williams & Wilkins' Dental Drug Reference with Clinical Implications*. Baltimore: Lippincott Williams & Wilkins, 2006, pp. 424–425.

Weinberg, MA, Westphal C, Pilat M, Froum SJ: *Comprehensive Periodontics for the Dental Hygienist*, 2nd ed. Upper Saddle River, NJ: Prentice Hall, 2006, pp. 31–38, 154–161, 245–253, 426, 438–440.

Wilkins EM: *Clinical Practice of the Dental Hygienist*, 9th ed. Philadelphia: Lippincott Williams & Wilkins, 2005, pp. 17–33, 36, 123, 246–259, 426–438, 477–480, 596, 663.

CASE I

Eleanor Gray

SITUATION

Eleanor Gray is a great-grandmother who recently moved to the area with her husband to be closer to their daughters and their families. Diagnosed with Alzheimer's disease (AD), she and her husband agreed that being nearer to their children may help to lighten the burden of coping with the disease progression. Additionally, the local medical community is known for its resources for patients with AD and their families. Eleanor plans to enroll in an AD clinical trial ongoing at the medical center.

LEARNING GOALS

Following integration of core scientific concepts and application of dental hygiene theory to the care of this patient, you will be able to

1. **Assess patient characteristics.**
   A. Distinguish pathology from common oral conditions.
   B. Identify the cause of tooth staining.
   C. Recognize normal and abnormal conditions of the roots of the teeth.
   D. Identify dental materials.

2. **Obtain and interpret radiographs.**
   A. Determine the need for vertical bitewing radiographs.
   B. Identify radiographic anatomy and landmarks.
   C. Identify film size used for adult periapical radiographs.
   D. Identify the cause of radiographic error.

3. **Plan and manage dental hygiene care.**
   A. Link medications with adverse oral side effects.
   B. Recognize the interrelationship of self-care of natural teeth and of the dental materials used to restore function to the dentition.
   C. Recommend appropriate oral hygiene aids for the patient with a removable partial denture.
   D. Establish the appropriate setting for oral self-care instructions for the geriatric patient with AD.
   E. Identify contraindications for treatment of the geriatric patient with AD.

4. **Perform periodontal procedures.**
   A. Calculate total loss of attachment from patient assessment data.
   B. Identify the effect of periodontal intervention on tooth mobility.
   C. Recognize possible adverse effects of non-surgical periodontal procedures.
   D. Determine the role of secondary dentin.

5. **Use preventive agents.**
   A. Determine the appropriate fluoride therapy based on patient assessment data.

6. **Provide supportive treatment services.**
   A. Instruct patient in the appropriate care of a removable partial denture.
   B. Counsel the geriatric patient with AD and her family on the interrelationship of oral health, medications, AD, and osteoporosis.

7. **Demonstrate professional responsibility.**
   A. Recognize terms used to describe the demographics of the elderly population.
   B. Design a treatment plan based on risk and benefits for the geriatric patient with AD.

GERIATRIC PATIENT—*Eleanor Gray*
PATIENT HISTORY SYNOPSIS

VITAL STATISTICS

Age	*75 years*	Blood Pressure	*122/82 mm Hg*
Gender	*female*	Pulse Rate	*68 bpm*
Height	*5′ 4″*	Respiration	*18 rpm*
Weight	*135 lbs.*		

1. Under care of physician
   Yes [X] No [ ]
   Condition: *mild late-onset Alzheimer's disease*
   osteoporosis
2. Hospitalized within the last 5 years
   Yes [ ] No [X]
   Reason: ______
3. Has or had the following conditions
   knee arthroplasty (total replacement surgery - left knee) 7 years ago
   no complications and no subsequent infections
4. Current medications
   donepezil (Aricept)—reversible cholinesterase inhibitor
   risperidone (Risperdal)—antipsychotic
   alendronate sodium (Fosamax)—bisphosphonate
   calcium carbonate supplement (Caltrate)—over-the-counter supplement
5. Smokes or uses tobacco products
   Yes [ ] No [X]
6. Is pregnant
   Yes [ ] No [X] N/A [ ]

MEDICAL HISTORY
Over the last year began to exhibit the following symptoms: short-term memory loss, difficulty performing familiar tasks, disorientation of time and place, all of which have contributed to the diagnosis of AD. She is being screened to participate in a clinical trial on the effects of antioxidants such as vitamin E and C on the progression of AD at the local research institute.

DENTAL HISTORY
Has undergone extensive dental treatment including orthodontia, endodontic therapy, prosthedontics, and periodontal surgeries. She has been on a periodontal maintenance schedule for several years, alternating 3-month appointments with a general practicioner and a periodontist.
A defective, loose cantilever fixed bridge was removed 18 months ago and replaced with a removable partial denture.

SOCIAL HISTORY
A weekly golfer in the senior ladies league at her club until knee surgery. She and her husband recently moved into a senior community with optional assisted living services near their children and grandchildren. Her husband and daughter report that she has recently begun to be fearful and easily agitated.

CHIEF COMPLAINT
Her family wants to reestablish the periodontal maintenance schedule she was on before moving. However, during her last visit the patient became disruptive and refused treatment.

ADULT CLINICAL EXAMINATION

	1	2	3	4	5	6	7	8	9	10	11	12	13	14	15	16
Probe 2	X	223	322	212	212	212	212	213	312	212	212	212	212	212	412	X
Probe 1	X	223	323	212	212	212	212	212	212	212	212	212	224	433	433	X

F

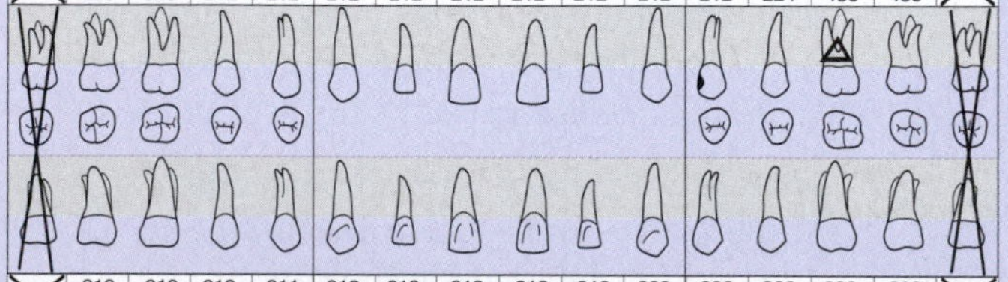

P

	1	2	3	4	5	6	7	8	9	10	11	12	13	14	15	16
Probe 1	X	213	212	212	211	212	212	212	212	212	323	323	322	323	333	X
Probe 2	X	212	313	212	211	212	212	212	212	212	213	322	222	212	312	X

R L

	32	31	30	29	28	27	26	25	24	23	22	21	20	19	18	17
Probe 2	X	X	X	112	113	212	111	112	112	111	212	212	212	X	X	212
Probe 1	X	X	X	112	212	212	212	212	112	111	212	222	222	X	X	212

L

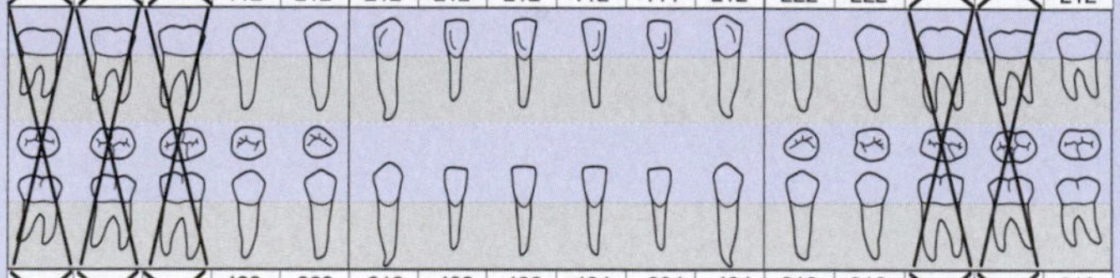

F

	32	31	30	29	28	27	26	25	24	23	22	21	20	19	18	17
Probe 1	X	X	X	423	323	313	423	423	424	324	424	212	312	X	X	313
Probe 2	X	X	X	323	323	212	313	313	313	313	313	212	213	X	X	313

CURRENT ORAL HYGIENE STATUS
Generalized slight bleeding on probing
Uses a water pick.

SUPPLEMENTAL ORAL EXAMINATION FINDINGS
Family has expressed doubt that she will maintain care of the removable partial denture and has expressed interest in a permanent bridge with implant

Clinically visible carious lesion
Clinically missing tooth
△ Furcation
▲ "Through and through" furcation
Probe 1: Initial probing depth
Probe 2: Probing depth 6 weeks after periodontal therapy

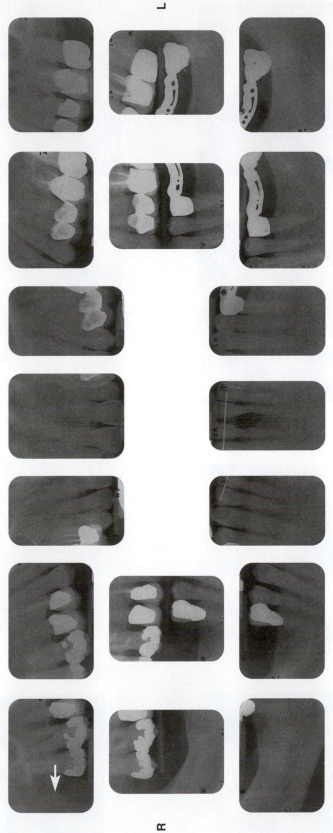

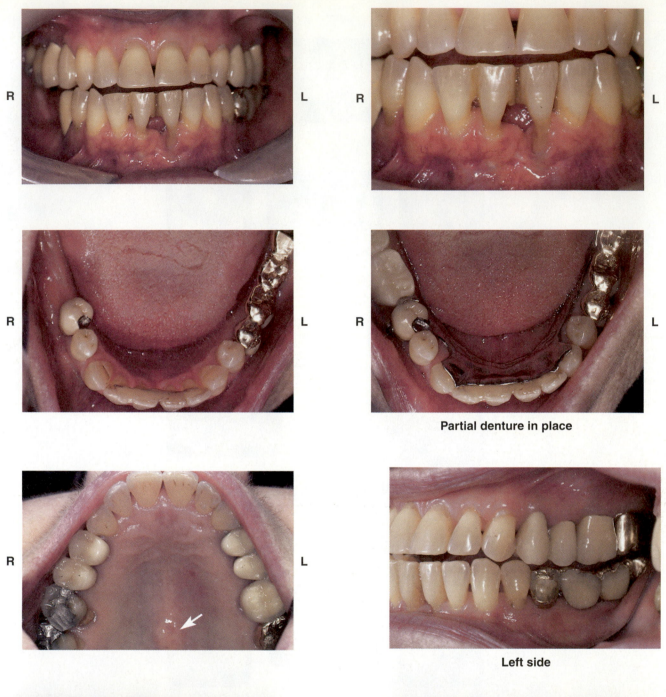

Partial denture in place

Left side

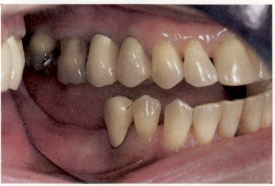

Right side

Right side
Partial denture in place

CASE QUESTIONS

ASSESSING PATIENT CHARACTERISTICS
Basic Level Questions

1. The raised, hard nodule observed in the midline of the palate (arrow) is most likely
   A. Denture stomatitis
   B. A torus palatinus
   C. Herpangina
   D. The median palatine suture
   E. A traumatic ulcer

2. Which of the following can be observed on the lingual surfaces of the maxillary anterior teeth?
   A. Green stain resulting from poor oral hygiene
   B. Orange stain resulting from chromogenic bacteria
   C. Black line stain that often manifests in clean mouths
   D. Brown stain resulting from foodstuffs such as coffee or tea
   E. Yellow stain associated with the presence of biofilm

3. Which of the following is the likely explanation for the darker yellow color of the facial aspect of the anterior teeth at the gingival margin?
   A. Accumulation of biofilm
   B. Intrinsic, endogenous staining
   C. Exposed root surfaces
   D. Effect of medications
   E. Enamel hypoplasia

4. The mandibular left second premolar is restored with a
   A. Porcelain-fused-to-metal crown
   B. Full-coverage cast gold crown
   C. MODBL amalgam
   D. Porcelain veneer
   E. Gold onlay

5. Which of the following mandibular teeth serve(s) as abutments?
   A. Right second premolar
   B. Each of the remaining mandibular teeth
   C. Left central incisor and right central incisor
   D. Left lateral incisor and right lateral incisor
   E. Left second premolar and left third molar

6. The missing teeth on the mandibular left have been restored with a
   A. Cantilever bridge
   B. Maryland bridge
   C. Fixed partial denture
   D. Removable partial denture
   E. Resin-bonded cast metal bridge

Competency Level Questions

7. The metal appearance on the mesial occlusal of the mandibular right premolar indicates
   A. A post-and-core buildup for support of the crown
   B. A depression in the crown surface that has picked up stain
   C. An amalgam restoration present on this portion of the crown
   D. That occlusal forces have worn through the porcelain exposing the metal
   E. Where the rest of the partial denture connects with the crown

OBTAINING AND INTERPRETING RADIOGRAPHS
Basic Level Questions

8. Which of the following is the most likely reason vertical bitewings were exposed on this patient?
   A. To adapt to the presence of tori
   B. To image more of the alveolar bone
   C. To assist with managing a gag reflex
   D. To provide increased comfort during film packet placement
   E. Usually recommended for the geriatric patient

9. The arrow drawn on the maxillary right molar radiograph is pointing to the
   A. Coronoid process of the mandible
   B. Maxillary tuberosity
   C. Lateral pterygoid plate
   D. Patient's finger
   E. Condyle

10. What film size was used to expose the maxillary central incisor periapical radiograph?
    A. Size no. 0
    B. Size no. 1
    C. Size no. 2
    D. Size no. 3
    E. Size no. 4

Competency Level Questions

11. Which of the following is the cause of the lack of image contrast of this patient's full mouth series of radiographs?
    A. The PID was not aligned perpendicular to the film packet.
    B. The bisecting technique was used.
    C. The open end of the PID was positioned an increased distance from the patient.
    D. The partial denture was not removed before exposure.
    E. The film packets were not properly stored away from stray radiation.

PLANNING AND MANAGING DENTAL HYGIENE CARE
Basic Level Questions

12. Which of this patient's medications puts her at risk for osteonecrosis of the jaws?
    A. Donepezil (Aricept)
    B. Risperidone (Risperdal)
    C. Alendronate sodium (Fosamax)
    D. Calcium carbonate (Caltrate)

13. This patient must regularly clean the partial denture to maintain the health status of the mandibular right second premolar.

    The longevity of the partial denture depends on the health of the mandibular right second premolar.
    A. The first statement is true, the second statement is false.
    B. The first statement is false, the second statement is true.
    C. Both statements are true.
    D. Both statements are false.

14. Which of the following brushes should be recommended to help this patient care for her partial denture?
    A. Clasp brush
    B. Toothbrush used for natural teeth
    C. Power toothbrush
    D. Interproximal brush
    E. End-tuft brush

Competency Level Questions

15. Each of the following should be considered when giving instructions for oral self-care to this patient EXCEPT one. Which one is the EXCEPTION?
    A. Ask permission to include her caregiver in the education process.
    B. Request that she put on her glasses during instruction and at home during self-care.
    C. Eliminate distracting background noise and sit facing the patient when speaking.
    D. Introduce a new oral hygiene aid to augment her use of the oral irrigator.
    E. Encourage implementation of oral self-care at the same times each day.

16. Each of the following is contraindicated for this patient EXCEPT one. Which one is the EXCEPTION?
    A. Air polishing
    B. Antibiotic premedication
    C. Implant surgery
    D. Supine position in the treatment chair
    E. Short-acting antianxiety medication before appointments

PERFORMING PERIODONTAL PROCEDURES
Basic Level Questions

17. At the reevaluation appointment, the measurement of recession on the facial surface of the mandibular left central incisor is 6 mm. What is the total loss of attachment in this region?
    A. 5 mm
    B. 6 mm
    C. 7 mm
    D. 8 mm

Competency Level Questions

18. Which of the following is the reason the mandibular central incisors do not exhibit mobility?
    A. Periodontal splint
    B. Medication for osteoporosis
    C. Effective oral self-care
    D. Surgical intervention
    E. Regular maintenance appointments

19. The hourglass shape exhibited by the mandibular anterior incisors is most likely caused by
    A. Scrub-method brushing technique
    B. Years of scaling and root planing
    C. The use of course grit polishing agents
    D. Congenital defect
    E. Chemical erosion

20. Scaling is not likely to elicit hypersensitivity of this patient's root surfaces because of the presence of significant secondary dentin.

    Secondary dentin is helping to protect this patient's root surfaces from decay.
    A. The first statement is true, the second statement is false
    B. The first statement is false, the second statement is true.
    C. Both statements are true.
    D. Both statements are false.

USING PREVENTIVE AGENTS
Competency Level Questions

21. Which of the following would be contraindicated for this patient?
    A. 0.05% sodium fluoride rinse
    B. 2% sodium fluoride gel
    C. 5% sodium fluoride varnish
    D. 1.23% acidulated phosphate fluoride foam
    E. 0.76% sodium monofluorophosphate dentifrice

PROVIDING SUPPORTIVE TREATMENT SERVICES
Basic Level Questions

22. Which of the following agents should be recommended for at-home cleaning of this patient's partial denture?
    A. Bleach (sodium hypochloride)
    B. Vinegar (acetic acid)
    C. Hot water
    D. Hydrogen peroxide
    E. Household scouring abrasive

Competency Level Questions

23. This patient and her family may benefit from counseling regarding each of the following EXCEPT one. Which one is the EXCEPTION?
    A. The link between nutrition and root caries
    B. The link between osteoporosis and periodontal disease
    C. The link between joint replacement and prophylactic premedication
    D. The link between bisphosphonate therapy and osteonecrosis of the jaws
    E. The link between the caregiver's active participation in the patient's oral self-care and oral health

DEMONSTRATING PROFESSIONAL RESPONSIBILITY
Basic Level Questions

24. Classifying this patient as "aged" is a form of ageism.

    This patient is considered functionally dependent.
    A. The first statement is true, the second statement is false.
    B. The first statement is false, the second statement is true.
    C. Both statements are true.
    D. Both statements are false.

Competency Level Questions

25. Which of the following is the best course of action considering the defective restorative treatment of the mandibular left second premolar?
    A. Application of composite material to the facial surface
    B. Metal bonding of composite veneer to the facial surface
    C. Removing the defective crown and replacing with a new fixed bridge
    D. Removing the defective crown and replacing with a partial denture similar to the one recently applied to the mandibular right side
    E. No restorative action required at this time

SETTING PATIENT GOALS

ESTABLISHING A DENTAL HYGIENE CARE PLAN

To assist this patient in meeting her needs, develop a dental hygiene care plan that establishes a framework within which to help her and her potential caregivers identify goals for obtaining oral health. In addition to the clinical assessment, a well-prepared dental hygiene care plan should take into account the patient's age, gender, lifestyle, culture, attitudes, health beliefs, and knowledge level. To help link this patient's needs for overall well-being with her oral conditions, and to provide motivation for achieving better health, the following is a partial list of possible deficits based on the Human Needs Conceptual Model to Dental Hygiene Practice. (See the appendix for an explanation of the Human Needs Conceptual Model to Dental Hygiene Practice to help you identify additional unmet needs.) Use this partial list of unmet needs or deficits as a guide in preparing a dental hygiene care plan for this patient. One set of goals and dental hygiene actions/implications has been completed as an example.

Deficit identified in Protection from Health Risks

Due to: risk of osteonecrosis of the jaws
Evidenced by: medication

Goals: _____

Dental hygiene actions/implications: _____

Deficit identified in Freedom from Stress

Due to: disorientation and confusion resulting from the progression of Alzheimer's disease
Evidenced by: anxiety and disruption caused at previous dental hygiene appointment

Goals: *establish a 3-month periodontal maintenance schedule for the purpose of achieving maximum beneficial care comfortably.*

Dental hygiene actions/implications: *consult with the caregiver to determine the best time of day for appointments; schedule short appointments; schedule appointments when the office is least busy; eliminate distracting background noise, such as music, ultrasonic scaling, or dental hard piece in adjacent treatment rooms; schedule treatment with the same dental hygienist and same dental hygiene assistant, and in the same treatment room each time; allow her caregiver to remain in the treatment room to assist with verbal communication and with interpreting the patient's body language as needed; maintain a warm, caring attitude; smile and use comforting touch if it does not frighten the patient; consult with physician and dentist regarding the use of antianxiety medication before appointments.*

Deficit identified in Conceptualization and Problem Solving

Due to: lack of understanding of the interrelationship of medical conditions and medications and periodontal disease and oral health
Evidenced by: request for dental implant

Goals: _____

Dental hygiene actions/implications: _____

Deficit identified in Responsibility for Oral Health

Due to: progression of Alzheimer's disease
Evidenced by: gingivitis

Goals: _____

Dental hygiene actions/implications: _____

REFLECTIVE ACTIVITIES

1. Develop a self-care instructional manual for caregivers of a patient with Alzheimer's disease. Using a digital camera, produce images that will supplement your manual or that can be used as pull-out sheets that the caregiver can tape to the bathroom mirror to aid the patient in performing the skills needed to maintain oral health.

2. Develop reference sheets with tips and strategies that the dental hygienist can use when treating the patient with mild, moderate, and severe stages Alzheimer's disease.

3. Develop a comprehensive three-part self-care program for the patient preparing for oral rehabilitation and the placement of multiple, complex restorative treatments. Part 1 should instruct and evaluate the patient's ability to effectively remove biofilm; part 2 should include instruction in methods of self-care while temporary restorations are in place; and part 3 should focus on self-care techniques that meet the needs of the rehabilitated mouth.

REFERENCES

Alzheimer's Disease Education and Referral (ADEAR) Center: *Can Alzheimer's Disease Be Prevented?* Silver Spring, MD: U.S. Department of Health and Human Services National Institutes of Health and National Institute on Aging, NIH Publication No. 05-5503, 2005.

American Association of Oral and Maxillofacial Surgeons: Bisphosphonate therapy and osteonecrosis of the jaws. *Contemporary Oral Hygiene*, 6(12), 36–37, 2006.

Ashcroft D: The dental hygiene ramifications of bisphosphonate therapy. *Access*, 21(2), 20–24, 2007.

Darby M: *Mosby's Comprehensive Review of Dental Hygiene*, 6th ed. St. Louis: Mosby (Elsevier), 2006, p. 291.

DeDiase CB, Austin SL: Oral health and older adults. *Journal of Dental Hygiene*, 77(11), 125–143, 2003.

Gage TW, Little JW: *Mosby's 2007 Dental Drug Consult*. St. Louis: Mosby (Elsevier), 2007, pp. 32–33, 392–394, 1097–1099.

Gladwin M, Bagby M: *Clinical Aspects of Dental Materials. Theory, Practice, and Cases,* 2nd ed. Philadelphia: Lippincott Williams & Wilkins, 2004, pp. 137–140, 159.

Hatrick CD, Eakle WS, Bird WF: *Dental Materials. Clinical Applications for Dental Assistants and Dental Hygienists*. Philadelphia: Saunders (Elsevier), 2003, pp. 49, 77, 164.

Johnson ON, Thomson EM: *Essentials of Dental Radiography for Dental Assistants and Hygienists*, 8th ed. Upper Saddle River, NJ: Prentice Hall, 2007, pp. 39–42, 81, 217–221, 225–226.

Little JW, Falce DA, Miller CS, Rhodus NL: *Dental Management of the Medically Compromised Patient*, 7th ed. St. Louis: Mosby (Elsevier), 2008, pp. 478–481, 534–551.

Nield-Gehrig JS: *Fundamentals of Periodontal Instrumentation and Advanced Root Instrumentation*, 5th ed. Philadelphia: Lippincott Williams & Wilkins, 2004, p. 278.

Perry DA, Beemsterboer P, Taggart EJ: *Periodontology for the Dental Hygienist*, 3rd ed. St. Louis: Saunders (Elsevier), 2007, pp. 266–267.

Pickett FA, Gurenlian JR: *The Medical History: Clinical Implications and Emergency Prevention in Dental Settings*. Philadelphia: Lippincott Williams & Wilkins, 2005, pp. 83–86.

Prajer R, Kacerik M: Treating patients with Alzheimer's disease. *Dimensions of Dental Hygiene*, 4(9), 24–26, 2006.

Ship JA: *Clinician's Guide. Oral Health in Geriatric Patients*, 2nd ed. Hamilton, Ontario: BC Decker Inc., 2006, pp. 71–76.

Stein PS, Scheff S, Dawson DR: Alzheimer's disease and periodontal disease: Mechanisms underlying a potential bi-directional relationship. *Grand Rounds in Oral-Systemic Medicine*, 1(3), 14–24, 2006.

Stefanac SJ, Nesbit SP: *Treatment Planning in Dentistry*, 2nd ed. St. Louis: Mosby (Elsevier), 2007, p. 415.

Tolle SL: Treating patient's with Alzheimer's disease: Considerations for dental hygienists. *Journal of Practical Hygiene*, 14(9), 9–13, 2005.

Wactawski-Wende J: Oral disease and osteoporosis. *Oral and Whole Body Health*. New York: Scientific American, Inc., 2006, p. 33.

Weinberg MA, Westphal C, Oakat M, Froum SJ: *Comprehensive Periodontics for the Dental Hygienist*, 2nd ed. Upper Saddle River, NJ: Prentice Hall, 2006, p. 191.

Wilkins EM: *Clinical Practice of the Dental Hygienist*, 9th ed. Philadelphia: Lippincott Williams & Wilkins, 2005, pp. 183, 314–322, 469–491, 552–561, 825–837.

CASE J

Thoroughgood Epps

SITUATION

Thoroughgood Epps recently retired as an officer in the armed services. He is currently attending college to train for a new career since leaving the army. He is still being treated at a local veteran's hospital for osteoarthritis and became a dental implant candidate after a car accident 3 years ago.

LEARNING GOALS

Following integration of core scientific concepts and application of dental hygiene theory to the care of this patient, you will be able to

1. **Assess patient characteristics.**
   A. Identify dental materials.
   B. Classify restorations.

2. **Obtain and interpret radiographs.**
   A. Interpret a panoramic radiograph.
   B. Utilize radiographs to determine characteristics of dental implants.
   C. Interpret deviations from normal appearance of structures noted on radiographs.

3. **Plan and manage dental hygiene care.**
   A. Identify possible adverse oral effects of medications.
   B. Introduce appropriate oral self-care devices for the patient with dental implants and fixed bridges.
   C. Apply appropriate dental hygiene treatment alterations for the patient with degenerative joint disease.
   D. Select a dental hygiene care plan for periodontal debridement based on patient needs.

4. **Perform periodontal procedures.**
   A. Select appropriate debridement instruments based on the patient's oral conditions.
   B. Determine periodontal maintenance intervals for the patient with dental implants.

   C. Identify the effect of untreated caries on periodontal tissue healing.
   D. Select appropriate assessment parameters for evaluating the success of dental implants.

5. **Use preventive agents.**
   A. Select appropriate preventive agents based on patient needs.
   B. Identify contraindications for using preventative agents/procedures given patient characteristics.

6. **Provide supportive treatment services.**
   A. Select the appropriate extrinsic stain removal procedure based on conditions the patient presents.

7. **Demonstrate professional responsibility.**
   A. Identify the role the patient plays in maintaining oral health.
   B. Determine the appropriate radiographic assessment of need based on the conditions the patient presents.
   C. Identify dental implant candidate assessment criteria.
   D. Evaluate the quality of dental restorations.

SPECIAL NEEDS PATIENT—*Thoroughgood Epps*
PATIENT HISTORY SYNOPSIS

Age	*43 years*
Gender	*male*
Height	*6' 0"*
Weight	*210 lbs.*

VITAL STATISTICS

Blood Pressure	*120/82 mm Hg*
Pulse Rate	*63 bpm*
Respiration	*14 rpm*

1. Under care of physician
   Yes [X]   No [ ]
   Condition: *osteoarthritis (degenerative joint disease)*

2. Hospitalized within the last 5 years
   Yes [X]   No [ ]
   Reason: *car accident*

3. Has or had the following conditions
   Received steroid injections for acute flare-ups of pain.
   Currently taking Toradol for acute pain

4. Current medications
   ketorolac (Toradol)—nonsteroidal anti-inflammatory drug
   acetaminophen (Tylenol)—nonnarcotic analgesic
   trolamine salicylate (Aspercreme)—analgesic topical ointment

5. Smokes or uses tobacco products
   Yes [ ]   No [X]

6. Is pregnant
   Yes [ ]   No [ ]   N/A [X]

MEDICAL HISTORY
His physician recently prescribed Toradol for 5 days to help manage acute pain associated with C3–C7 of the cervical spine. He has had numerous x-ray examinations of his neck, back, and chest in the past 3 years.

DENTAL HISTORY
Traumatic injury to his back and mandible following a car accident 3 years ago

SOCIAL HISTORY
Single and enjoying a new life since retiring from active military duty

CHIEF COMPLAINT
Seeking to maintain his oral health since leaving the military

CURRENT ORAL HYGIENE STATUS
Light subgingival calculus interproximally in the posterior regions
Generalized moderate interproximal plaque accumulation with moderate bleeding on probing localized in the maxillary posterior regions

SUPPLEMENTAL ORAL EXAMINATION FINDINGS
In addition to brushing, he uses waxed dental floss several times a week and toothpicks after lunch every day. He was given floss threaders to clean the mandibular anterior region, but he reports that he hasn't had much success at using them.

🦷 Clinically visible carious lesion

✕ Clinically missing tooth

△ Furcation
▲ "Through and through" furcation
Probe 1: Initial probing depth
Probe 2: Probing depth 6 weeks after peridontal therapy

ADULT CLINICAL EXAMINATION

Maxillary (teeth 1–16):

	1	2	3	4	5	6	7	8	9	10	11	12	13	14	15	16
Probe 2	X	222	313	313	312	212	312	211	212	211	112	112	313	X	323	X
Probe 1	X	222	224	423	323	313	312	212	212	212	212	212	313	X	425	X

(F / P)

	1	2	3	4	5	6	7	8	9	10	11	12	13	14	15	16
Probe 1	X	324	413	313	312	222	222	223	312	212	212	223	324	X	524	X
Probe 2	X	213	213	312	212	211	112	212	212	212	112	112	213	X	312	X

Mandibular (teeth 32–17):

	32	31	30	29	28	27	26	25	24	23	22	21	20	19	18	17
Probe 2	322	X	223	312	212	212	X	X	X	X	X	X	214	413		424
Probe 1	435	X	534	322	322	212	X	X	X	X	X	X	224	334		534

(L / F)

	32	31	30	29	28	27	26	25	24	23	22	21	20	19	18	17
Probe 1	435	X	434	423	423	323	X	X	X	X	X	X	334	435		534
Probe 2	424	X	324	412	212	213	X	X	X	X	X	X	325	523		424

R / L

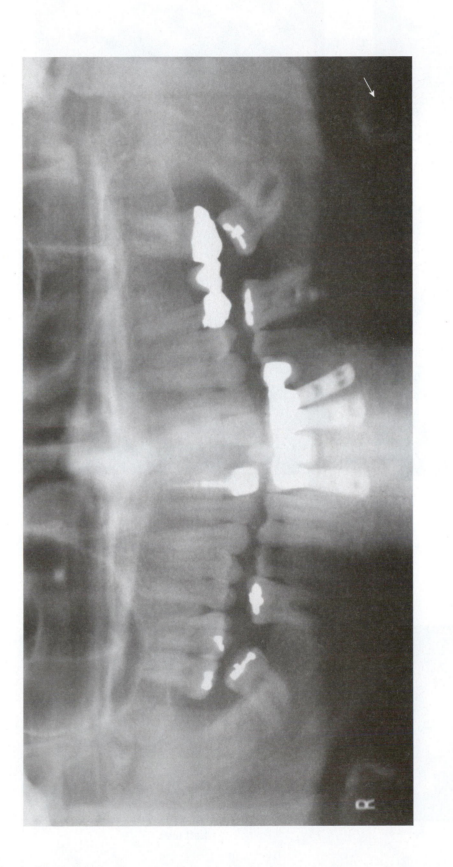

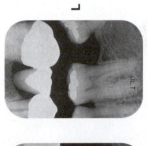

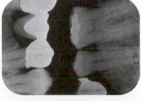

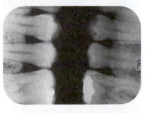

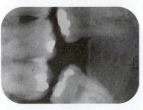

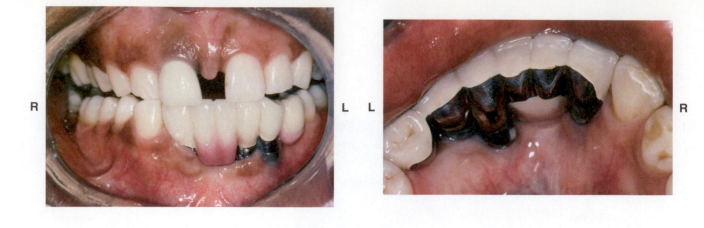

R   L   L   R

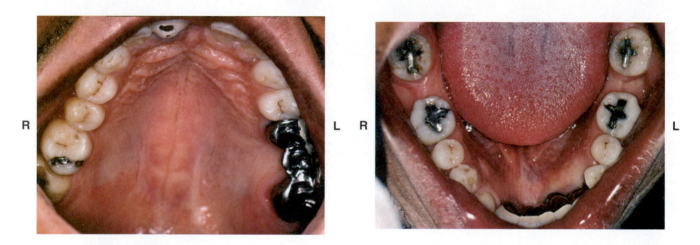

R   L   R   L

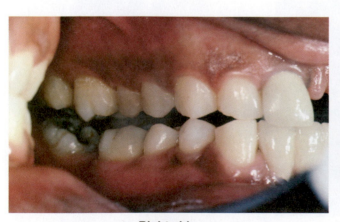

Right side

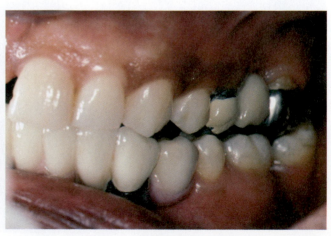

Left side

CASE QUESTIONS

ASSESSING PATIENT CHARACTERISTICS
Basic Level Questions

1. The restorative treatment of the mandibular anterior teeth is a(n)
   A. Removable partial denture
   B. Metal framework and overdenture
   C. Implant-retained prosthesis
   D. Periodontal splint
   E. Lingual retainer

2. Which of the following terms applies to the maxillary left second molar?
   A. Abutment
   B. Pontic
   C. Retainer
   D. Cantilever
   E. Rest

3. What classification is the restoration on the mandibular left first molar?
   A. Class I
   B. Class II
   C. Class III
   D. Class IV
   E. Class V

Competency Level Questions

4. Why does the left side of the mandibular anterior restorative treatment appear not to be attached to the adjacent natural tooth?
   A. The implant has failed.
   B. This is a cantilever pontic.
   C. The tooth root has resorbed.
   D. There is a clasp missing from the bridge.
   E. This portion of the restoration is temporary.

OBTAINING AND INTERPRETING RADIOGRAPHS
Basic Level Questions

5. The arrow drawn on the lower corner of the panoramic radiograph is pointing to
   A. The shadow of the lead-equivalent thyroid collar
   B. A calcification of the carotid artery
   C. C-3 of the spinal column
   D. The chin rest of the x-ray unit
   E. An image of the hyoid bone

6. With what type of implant does this patient present?
   A. Endodontic
   B. Subperiosteal
   C. Transosteal
   D. Endosteal
   E. Post and core

7. Which of the following describes the implant?
   A. Blade
   B. Cylinder
   C. Staple
   D. Plate form
   E. Screw

Competency Level Questions

8. Which of the following explains the bilateral increased radiolucencies in the regions of the submandibular fossae?
   A. Pathologic bone resorption or unexplained bone loss
   B. Superimposition of several structures imaged in the same place
   C. Negative shadows representing areas of decreased density
   D. Radiographic error that resulted in black artifacts
   E. Accidental exposure of the film to white light

9. Which of the following is observed in the pulp chamber of the mandibular right first molar?
   A. Secondary dentin
   B. Enamel pearl
   C. Condensing osteitis
   D. Hypercementosis
   E. Dens invaginatus

PLANNING AND MANAGING DENTAL HYGIENE CARE
Basic Level Questions

10. This patient's medications put him at risk for developing which of the following?
    A. Glossitis
    B. Angular cheilitis
    C. Gingival hyperplasia
    D. Xerostomia
    E. Black hairy tongue

11. Which one of these oral hygiene aids might be contraindicated for this patient?
    A. Wooden wedges
    B. Holder for toothpick
    C. End-tuft brush
    D. Interproximal brush
    E. Tufted floss

Competency Level Questions

12. Each of the following is recommended for managing this patient's treatment EXCEPT one. Which one is the EXCEPTION?
    A. Use a semisupine position.
    B. Use physical supports such as a neck pillow.
    C. Allow for frequent position changes.
    D. Schedule short appointments.
    E. Schedule morning appointments.

13. Which of the following is the most appropriate dental hygiene care plan for this patient?
    A. One 1-hour appointment for oral prophylaxis; followed by a maintenance appointment in 3 to 4 months
    B. One 90-minute appointment for full-mouth disinfection and one 1-hour appointment 24 hours later to evaluate tissue response and perform a second full-mouth disinfection if inflammation persists; followed by a reevaluation appointment in 4 to 6 weeks

C. One 1-hour appointment for full-mouth debridement and one 45-minute appointment 7 to 10 days later to evaluate tissue response and to instrument if inflammation persists; followed by a reevaluation appointment in 4 to 6 weeks

D. One 90-minute appointment for half-mouth periodontal debridement and one 90-minute appointment 7 to 10 days later for half-mouth periodontal debridement of the other side; followed by a reevaluation appointment in 4 to 6 weeks

E. Four 1-hour appointments scheduled 7 to 10 days apart for periodontal debridement by quadrant; followed by a reevaluation appointment in 4 to 6 weeks

PERFORMING PERIODONTAL PROCEDURES
Basic Level Questions

14. Which of the following hand-activated instruments would be the best choice to effectively and efficiently debride all natural teeth?
   A. Area-specific curets
   B. Universal curets
   C. Extended-shank curets
   D. Sickle scalers
   E. Periodontal files

15. Instruments made of each of the following types of materials may be used to scale subgingival deposits in the mandibular anterior region of this patient EXCEPT one. Which one is the EXCEPTION?
   A. Metal
   B. Plastic
   C. Gold tipped
   D. Nylon
   E. Graphite

Competency Level Questions

16. What is the appropriate length of time between periodontal maintenance appointments for this patient's recall?
   A. 1-month intervals
   B. 6-week intervals
   C. 3-month intervals
   D. 6-month intervals
   E. Dictated by patient needs

17. Which of the following may have contributed to the lack of tissue response in the interproximal region of the mandibular left second premolar and first molar at the 6-week reevaluation appointment?
   A. Inappropriate time interval for tissue response
   B. Bacterial seeding from dental caries
   C. History of repeated radiation exposure
   D. Undetected systemic conditions
   E. Inappropriate use of toothpicks

18. Which of the following is the most reliable indicator of this patient's implant success?
   A. Gingival color
   B. Papillary shape
   C. Lack of mobility
   D. Pocket depths
   E. Amount of bleeding on probing

USING PREVENTIVE AGENTS
Competency Level Questions

19. Which of the following will benefit this patient the most?
    A. Pit and fissure sealants
    B. Professional fluoride varnish
    C. Direct, local application of chlorhexidine
    D. Oral irrigation with essential oils
    E. Administration of potassium oxalate

20. Which of the following would be contraindicated for this patient?
    A. Mouth rinses containing alcohol
    B. Acidulated phosphate fluoride
    C. Tartar control dentifrice
    D. Disclosing solution
    E. Periapical radiographs

PROVIDING SUPPORTIVE TREATMENT SERVICES
Basic Level Questions

21. If necessary, each of the following may be used to remove stains from the implant superstructure EXCEPT one. Which one is the EXCEPTION?
    A. Ultrasonic scaling with a slim-diameter tip
    B. Light, sweeping motion with the air polisher
    C. Rotary rubber cup with tin oxide
    D. Sonic scaling with a specially designed plastic tip sleeve
    E. Nonabrasive paste applied with dental tape

DEMONSTRATING PROFESSIONAL RESPONSIBILITY
Basic Level Questions

22. Who is responsible for maintaining this patient's oral health?
    A. The dentist
    B. The dental hygienist
    C. The dentist and dental hygienist
    D. The patient
    E. The patient, dentist, and dental hygienist

23. How often should radiographs be taken of the mandibular anterior region?
    A. Every 3 months
    B. Every 6 months
    C. Once a year
    D. Once every 24 to 36 months
    E. Depends on the signs and symptoms at the time of assessment

Competency Level Questions

24. Each of the following played a role in determining that this patient was a good candidate for dental implants EXCEPT one. Which one is the EXCEPTION?
    A. Medical condition
    B. Attitude and emotional health
    C. Tobacco use
    D. Periodontal condition
    E. Genetic testing

25. Each of the following is a poor design characteristic of the restorative treatment of the mandibular anterior region EXCEPT one. Which one is the EXCEPTION?
    A. Acrylic that contacts the gingival surface
    B. Left pontic not attached to adjacent natural tooth
    C. Widely shaped pontics
    D. Overcontoured crowns
    E. Narrowed embrasures

SETTING PATIENT GOALS

ESTABLISHING A DENTAL HYGIENE CARE PLAN

To assist this patient in meeting his needs, develop a dental hygiene care plan that establishes a framework within which to help him identify goals for obtaining oral health. In addition to the clinical assessment, a well-prepared dental hygiene care plan should take into account the patient's age, gender, lifestyle, culture, attitudes, health beliefs, and knowledge level. To help link this patient's needs for overall well-being with his oral conditions, and to provide motivation for achieving better health, the following is a partial list of possible deficits based on the Human Needs Conceptual Model to Dental Hygiene Practice. (See the appendix for an explanation of the Human Needs Conceptual Model to Dental Hygiene Practice to help you identify additional unmet needs.) Use this partial list of unmet needs or deficits as a guide in preparing a dental hygiene care plan for this patient. One set of goals and dental hygiene actions/implications has been completed as an example.

Deficit identified in Protection from Health Risks

Due to: risk for prolonged bleeding during scaling
Evidenced by: use of nonsteroidal anti-inflammatory drugs (NSAIDs)

Goals: _____

Dental hygiene actions/implications: _____

Deficit identified in Freedom from Head and Neck Pain

Due to: risk for aggravating osteoarthritis during dental hygiene treatment
Evidenced by: previous neck injury, recent acute pain

Goals: _____

Dental hygiene actions/implications: _____

Deficit identified in Skin and Mucous Membrane Integrity of the Head and Neck

Due to: insufficient biofilm control
Evidenced by: 4 to 5 mm probing depths and localized moderate bleeding on probing

Goals: _____

Dental hygiene actions/implications: _____

Deficit identified in Biologically Sound Dentition

Due to: oral conditions conducive to caries
Evidenced by: two-surface carious lesion

Goals: *referral for restoration; eliminate conditions conducive to caries; prevent future occurrences*

Dental hygiene actions/implications: *evaluate cause: presence of cariogenic bacteria, supply of substrate for acid production, and/or host susceptibility; implement strategies based on cause(s); educate patient regarding the caries process; plan a self-care regimen for biofilm control; recommend appropriate oral self-care aids.*

Deficit identified in Responsibility for Oral Health

Due to: lack of appropriate oral self-care
Evidenced by: generalized interproximal and subgingival plaque

Goals: _____

Dental hygiene actions/implications: _____

REFLECTIVE ACTIVITIES

1. **Describe implant instrument design and stroke application used for**
   a. Assessment of the periodontal tissues
   b. Debridement of the apical region of the prosthetic framework
   c. Debridement of the abutment posts
   d. Subgingival debridement

2. **Update this patient's dental charting to reflect the restorations present. Copy and enlarge the Adult Clinical Examination chart page from this case and use appropriately colored pencils to draw in all the dental materials observed on the photographs and radiographs.**

REFERENCES

American Dental Association and the U.S. Department of Health and Human Services: *The selection of patients for x-ray examinations.* Rockville, MD: ADA, DHHS-FDA 88-8273, revised 2004.

Anusavice KJ: Efficacy of non-surgical management of the initial caries lesion. *Journal of Dental Education,* 61, 895–905, 1997.

Anusavice KJ: *Phillips' Science of Dental Materials,* 11th ed. Philadelphia: Saunders (Elsevier), 2003, pp. 257–260, 263–267.

Blackwell RE: *GV Black's Operative Dentistry,* Vol. II, 9th ed. Milwaukee: Medico Dental Publishing, 1955, pp. 1–4.

Ciancio SG: Recommending mouthrinses. *Dimensions of Dental Hygiene,* 3(11), 24–25, 2005.

Darby ML: *Mosby's Comprehensive Review of Dental Hygiene,* 6th ed. St. Louis: Mosby (Elsevier), 2006, p. 393.

Darby ML, Walsh MM: *Dental Hygiene Theory and Practice,* 2nd ed. St. Louis: Saunders (Elsevier), 2003, pp. 241–242, 342–343, 359–360, 494–495, 642.

Gage TW, Little JW: *Mosby's 2007 Dental Drug Consult.* St. Louis: Mosby (Elsevier), 2007, pp. 669–672.

Gladwin M, Bagby M: *Clinical Aspects of Dental Materials. Theory, Practice, and Cases,* 2nd ed. Philadelphia: Lippincott Williams & Wilkins, 2004, pp. 14–15.

Kuskins H: Panoramic radiography: Screening for carotid calcifications. *Access,* 2(18), 32–34, 2004.

Little JW, Falace DA, Miller CS, Rhodus NL: *Dental Management of the Medically Compromised Patient,* 7th ed. St. Louis: Mosby (Elsevier), 2008, pp. 326–329.

Merrifield S: Maintaining today's esthetic restorations responsibly. *Contemporary Oral Hygiene,* 7(1), 18–22, 2007.

Nield-Gehrig JS: *Fundamentals of Periodontal Instrumentation,* 5th ed. Philadelphia: Lippincott Williams & Wilkins, 2004, pp. 307–322, 387, 592.

Phinney DJ, Halstead JH: *Essential Skills and Procedures for Chairside Dental Assisting.* Albany, NY: Delmar, 2002, p. 55.

Sison SG: Implant maintenance and the dental hygienist. *Access,* 1 (Suppl.), 1–12, 2003.

Sonis ST: *Dental Secrets,* 2nd ed. Philadelphia: Hanley and Belfus, Inc., 1999, pp. 198–200, 284.

Stefanac SJ, Nesbit SP: *Treatment Planning in Dentistry,* 2nd ed. St. Louis: Mosby (Elsevier), 2007, pp. 204–207.

Weinberg MA, Westphal C, Oakat M, Froum SJ: *Comprehensive Periodontics for the Dental Hygienist,* 2nd ed. Upper Saddle River, NJ: Prentice Hall, 2006, pp. 421–431, 487–510.

Wilkins EM: *Clinical Practice of the Dental Hygienist,* 9th ed. Philadelphia: Lippincott Williams & Wilkins, 2005, pp. 200–204, 432–433, 470–497, 648–650.

CASE **K**

Johnnie Johnson

SITUATION

Johnnie Johnson works as a disk jockey in dance clubs and for hire at other functions and parties. He admits to heavy drinking and "a lot of partying." His alcohol consumption appears to be affecting his physical appearance. His hands tremor slightly and he speaks rapidly and nervously. He does not appear to be intoxicated at this time, however, his breath indicates recent alcohol consumption.

LEARNING GOALS

Following integration of core scientific concepts and application of dental hygiene theory to the care of this patient, you will be able to

1. **Assess patient characteristics.**
   A. Determine the etiology of oral findings.
   B. Distinguish anatomic characteristics of the periodontium.
   C. Identify materials used for dental restorations.
   D. Identify the risk factors for oral cancer.
   E. Recognize oral conditions resulting from excessive alcohol intake.

2. **Obtain and interpret radiographs.**
   A. Interpret radiographic deviation from normal anatomic conditions.
   B. Identify suspected carious lesions radiographically.

3. **Plan and manage dental hygiene care.**
   A. Provide the appropriate preprocedural rinse for the alcohol-dependent patient.
   B. Counsel the patient who presents with oral manifestations of a vitamin deficiency.
   C. Identify barriers to professional care for the alcohol-dependent patient.
   D. Predict possible medical emergencies when treating the alcohol-dependent patient.

4. **Perform periodontal procedures.**
   A. Apply standard and advanced fulcruming techniques.
   B. Sequence periodontal intervention procedures.

5. **Use preventive agents.**
   A. Recommend appropriate self-care agents for the patient with high caries activity.

6. **Provide supportive treatment services.**
   A. Select the appropriate polishing agent when restorations are present.
   B. Recommend supportive treatments and referrals for the patient with special needs.

7. **Demonstrate professional responsibility.**
   A. Utilize appropriate interview questions to provide follow-up to the patient's health history.
   B. Recognize the ethical concept of self-determination.
   C. Make an informed decision regarding safe treatment of the alcohol-dependent patient.

SPECIAL NEEDS PATIENT—*Johnnie Johnson*
PATIENT HISTORY SYNOPSIS

Age	*38 years*
Gender	*male*
Height	*5' 10"*
Weight	*160 lbs.*

VITAL STATISTICS

Blood Pressure	*118/76 mm Hg*
Pulse Rate	*90 bpm*
Respiration	*24 rpm*

1. Under care of physician
   Yes ☐   No ☒   Condition: _____
   _____
   _____

2. Hospitalized within the last 5 years
   Yes ☐   No ☒   Reason: _____
   _____

3. Has or had the following conditions
   suspected stomach ulcers
   _____
   _____

4. Current medications
   calcium carbonate, magnesium hydroxide (Mylanta)—
   gastrointestinal agent/antacid
   famotidine (Pepcid Chewables)—gastrointestinal
   agent/antacid
   ibuprofen (Advil)—analgesic/nonsteroidal
   anti-inflammatory drug
   magnesium hydroxide, aluminum hydroxide,
   simethicone (Maalox)—gastrointestinal agent/antacid

5. Smokes or uses tobacco products
   Yes ☒   No ☐

6. Is pregnant
   Yes ☐   No ☐   N/A ☒

MEDICAL HISTORY

Unremarkable medical history. Anecdotal information indicates need for a medical examination. Patient has not had a physical exam in several years and although he is experiencing stomach problems, he has chosen not to see a physician. His current over-the-counter medications are self-prescribed.

DENTAL HISTORY

Extensive dental restorative work as a child and a teenager. Has received only sporadic and emergency professional oral health care in the past 10 years. He often schedules appointments that he ends up canceling or he does not show up.

SOCIAL HISTORY

Somewhat of a loner, his lifestyle in which he sleeps during the day and works in nightclubs and after-hours bars at night, prevents him from developing long-term friendships. He states that he often does not know the real names of many of the people he encounters. Likewise, "Johnnie" is the working, or stage name, he uses for his job. He recently moved in with his girlfriend in her mobile home.

CHIEF COMPLAINT

Not happy with the appearance of his teeth, but states that he does not have a lot of money for dental treatment. He made this appointment at the urging of his new girlfriend. Additionally, he thinks that the appearance of his front teeth may be causing him not to get the better DJ opportunities. He aspires to perform disk jockeying services at more upscale dance clubs and parties such as wedding receptions.

CURRENT ORAL HYGIENE STATUS

Moderate subgingival calculus in the posterior regions. Performs oral hygiene self-care reasonably well and consistently. Slight papillary bleeding on probing.

SUPPLEMENTAL ORAL EXAMINATION FINDINGS

Moderate xerostomia
Bilateral parotid gland enlargement

ADULT CLINICAL EXAMINATION

	1	2	3	4	5	6	7	8	9	10	11	12	13	14	15	16
Probe 2	535	534	422	323	313	313	313	312	212	213	213	313	323	436	X	636
Probe 1	645	535	544	434	423	323	323	313	313	313	313	423	324	536	X	635

(F / P)

	1	2	3	4	5	6	7	8	9	10	11	12	13	14	15	16
Probe 1	534	424	434	323	313	313	323	323	323	313	323	424	424	434	X	524
Probe 2	433	323	323	313	313	212	213	313	313	313	213	313	423	424	X	424

R / L

	32	31	30	29	28	27	26	25	24	23	22	21	20	19	18	17
Probe 2	534	434	433	323	313	313	313	313	313	313	313	323	434		X	535
Probe 1	635	534	433	323	323	323	313	313	313	313	413	424	425	535	X	535

(L / F)

	32	31	30	29	28	27	26	25	24	23	22	21	20	19	18	17
Probe 1	535	635	434	423	323	313	423	423	424	324	424	424	435	635	X	536
Probe 2	534	534	423	323	323	212	313	313	313	313	313	324	434		X	525

Clinically visible carious lesion
Clinically missing tooth
△ Furcation
▲ "Through and through" furcation
Probe 1: Initial probing depth
Probe 2: Probing depth 6 weeks after periodontal therapy

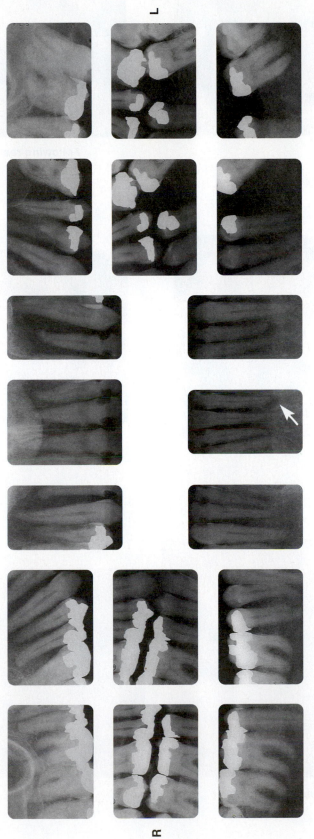

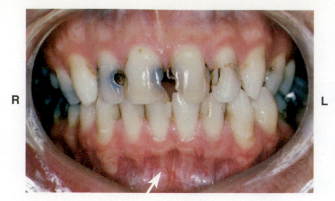

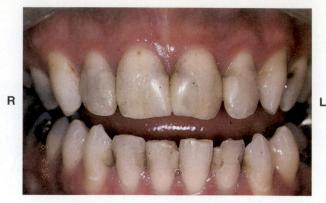

Following restorative appointment

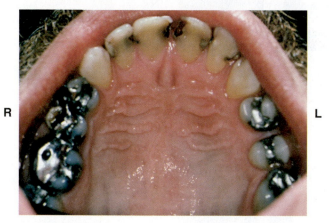

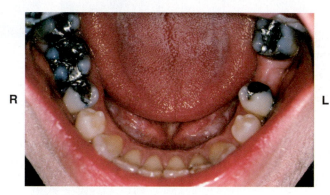

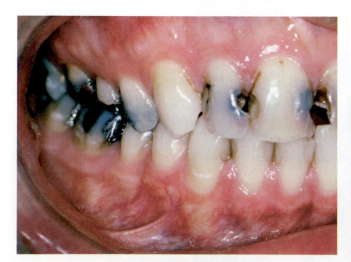

Right side

Left side

CASE QUESTIONS

ASSESSING PATIENT CHARACTERISTICS
Basic Level Questions

1. The small diffuse red dots on this patient's palate are indicative of
   A. Nicotine stomatitis
   B. Hyperkeratosis
   C. Pyogenic granuloma
   D. Kaposi's sarcoma
   E. Trauma from hot food

2. The deeper red tissue on the facial aspect of the mandibular anterior region (arrow) is called
   A. Free gingiva
   B. Attached gingiva
   C. Masticatory mucosa
   D. Alveolar mucosa
   E. Junctional epithelium

Competency Level Questions

3. What restorative dental materials were used to treat the caries observed in this patient's anterior teeth after the completion of initial therapy?
   A. Glass ionomers
   B. Acrylic resins
   C. Porcelain bonding
   D. Dental ceramics
   E. Multipurpose composites

4. Which of the following contributes to this patient's increased risk for oral cancer?
   A. Use of multiple antacids
   B. Alcohol use and smoking
   C. Xerostomia conditions
   D. High pulse and respiration rates
   E. Rampant caries with abscesses

5. This patient exhibits each of the following that may indicate heavy alcohol use and alcohol withdrawal syndrome EXCEPT one. Which one is the EXCEPTION?
   A. Hand tremors
   B. Rapid pulse
   C. Xerostomia
   D. Craving antacids
   E. Swollen glands

6. Painless, benign, bilateral parotid swellings frequently accompany chronic alcohol use.

   Reduced salivary output has allowed this patient's dental caries to spread between adjacent teeth.
   A. The first statement is true, the second statement is false.
   B. The first statement is false, the second statement is true.
   C. Both statements are true and related.
   D. Both statements are true, but not related.
   E. Both statements are false.

7. The reddening of the tip of this patient's tongue and the burning sensation is most likely the result of
   A. Cigarette smoking
   B. Use of antacids
   C. Folic acid deficiency
   D. Excessive alcohol intake
   E. Geographic tongue

OBTAINING AND INTERPRETING RADIOGRAPHS
Competency Level Questions

8. The radiolucency observed at the apex of the mandibular left lateral incisor (arrow) is most likely
   A. A periapical abscess
   B. Condensing osteitis
   C. A residual cyst
   D. The lingual foramen
   E. The mental foramen

9. Each of the following teeth exhibits caries at the initial appointment, before the patient has his teeth restored, EXCEPT one. Which one is the EXCEPTION?
   A. Maxillary right lateral incisor
   B. Maxillary right central incisor
   C. Maxillary left central incisor
   D. Mandibular left central incisor
   E. Mandibular left lateral incisor

PLANNING AND MANAGING DENTAL HYGIENE CARE
Basic Level Questions

10. A nonalcohol preprocedural rinse is indicated because of this patient's alcohol use pattern.
    A. The statement is true, the reason is false.
    B. The statement is false, the reason is true.
    C. Both the statement and reason are true and related.
    D. Both the statement and reason are true, but not related.
    E. Both the statements are false.

11. Which of the following can be added to this patient's diet to address his vitamin deficiency related to his burning tongue symptom?
    A. Sunlight exposure
    B. Liver meats
    C. Green vegetables
    D. Multiple vitamins
    E. Folate supplements

Competency Level Questions

12. Each of the following is a potential barrier to care planning for this patient EXCEPT one. Which one is the EXCEPTION?
    A. Limited finances
    B. Ability to keep appointments and follow through with treatment
    C. Aerosols and allergens present in the facility
    D. Liver impairment and bleeding potential
    E. Emotional stability during appointments

13. Which of the following is the leading cause of this patient's multiple carious lesions?
    A. Alcohol consumption
    B. Xerostomia
    C. Lack of professional care
    D. Tobacco use
    E. Poor oral self-care

14. Which of the following possible medical emergencies should be considered when treating this patient?
    A. Alcohol withdrawal syndrome
    B. Airway obstruction
    C. Adrenal crisis
    D. Anaphylaxis
    E. Asthma

15. Which of the following is the most likely reason this patient has difficulty keeping his scheduled dental hygiene appointments?
    A. Lack of knowledge regarding the importance of oral health
    B. Embarrassment about the condition of his smile
    C. Negative dental experiences as a child
    D. Preoccupation with drinking
    E. Fear of being in pain

PERFORMING PERIODONTAL PROCEDURES
Basic Level Questions

16. When scaling the maxillary left posterior buccal aspects, the dental hygienist should refrain from fulcruming
    A. In the maxillary left canine/premolar area
    B. With the palm of the hand on the patient's chin
    C. On the maxillary left incisors
    D. With the ring finger resting on the index finger of the nondominate hand

Competency Level Questions

17. Following the preliminary prephase of periodontal procedure sequencing where periapical emergencies are treated, this patient will enter which of the following treatment phases?
    A. Phase I Non-Surgical Initial Therapy
    B. Phase II Surgical and Corrective Therapy
    C. Phase III Restorative Care
    D. Phase IV Maintenance Therapy

USING PREVENTIVE AGENTS
Basic Level Questions

18. Which of the following self-care agents should be recommended for this patient?
    A. Peridex (chlorhexidine)
    B. Viadent (sanguinarine)
    C. Listerine (essential oils)
    D. Scope (cetylpyridinium chloride)
    E. Gel-Kam (stannous fluoride)

Competency Level Questions

19. Which of the following should be recommended for this patient?
    A. Tartar control dentifrice
    B. Fluoride varnish
    C. Sealants
    D. Locally delivered antimicrobial therapy
    E. Antifungal palliative care for the tongue

PROVIDING SUPPORTIVE TREATMENT SERVICES
Basic Level Questions

20. If stains are present on this patient's new anterior restorations at the next recall appointment, they can be removed with a(n)
    A. Ultrasonic scaler at high power
    B. Sonic scaler at low power
    C. Rubber cup and fine-grit abrasive
    D. Toothbrush and tartar control dentifrice
    E. Air polisher and sodium bicarbonate

Competency Level Questions

21. Which of the following should NOT be recommended for this patient?
    A. Fluoride supplementation
    B. Reduced alcohol consumption
    C. Tobacco cessation program
    D. Tooth-whitening procedures
    E. Nutritional counseling

22. Which of the following should be this patient's first referral?
    A. Physician
    B. Dietician
    C. Endodontist
    D. Alcoholism recovery group
    E. Smoking cessation classes

DEMONSTRATING PROFESSIONAL RESPONSIBILITY
Basic Level Questions

23. Because alcohol use can affect oral conditions and impact oral hygiene treatment, this patient's health history should be followed up with each of the following questions EXCEPT one. Which one is the EXCEPTION?
    A. "When was your last drink?"
    B. "How often do you drink?"
    C. "How much do you drink?"
    D. "What types of alcohol do you consume?"
    E. "What is your pattern of alcohol consumption?"

Competency Level Questions

24. Which of the following is the most likely reason this patient did not have his anterior teeth restored with porcelain veneer crowns or full porcelain-fused-to-metal crowns?
    A. The dentist and oral health care team knew that the patient could not afford crowns, so they did not waste time telling him about this treatment option.
    B. The patient was willing to forego the best dental treatment (crowns) to use his financial resources on some other nondental needs.
    C. Because this patient is at risk for keeping appointments, the dental hygienist recommended that he not put himself through the process of multiple appointments for fabricating the crowns.
    D. Composite restorative dental materials currently on the market make this the better choice over crowns for these carious anterior teeth.
    E. This patient is not capable of understanding the need for comprehensive restoration of these badly decayed teeth.

25. Although the patient has arrived for his dental appointment smelling of alcohol, his speech is not slurred and his gait is steady. The dental hygienist has chosen to continue with nonsurgical periodontal debridement treatment procedures. What is the basis for this decision?
    A. This patient should not be treated today.
    B. This patient has chosen to reveal his alcohol problem.
    C. The dental hygienist is covered by malpractice insurance.
    D. The dental hygienist is using the right of therapeutic privilege.
    E. This patient has decision-making capacity.

SETTING PATIENT GOALS

ESTABLISHING A DENTAL HYGIENE CARE PLAN

To assist this patient in meeting his needs, develop a dental hygiene care plan that establishes a framework within which to help him identify goals for obtaining oral health. In addition to the clinical assessment, a well-prepared dental hygiene care plan should take into account the patient's age, gender, lifestyle, culture, attitudes, health beliefs, and knowledge level. To help link this patient's needs for overall well-being with his oral conditions, and to provide motivation for achieving better health, the following is a partial list of possible deficits based on the Human Needs Conceptual Model to Dental Hygiene Practice. (See the appendix for an explanation of the Human Needs Conceptual Model to Dental Hygiene Practice to help you identify additional unmet needs.) Use this partial list of unmet needs or deficits as a guide in preparing a dental hygiene care plan for this patient. One set of goals and dental hygiene actions/implications has been completed as an example.

Deficit identified in Protection from Health Risks

Due to: alcohol and tobacco use
Evidenced by: effects on the oral cavity

Goals: *patient will demonstrate an understanding of the interrelationship of alcohol and tobacco use and oral health; patient will take steps to alter behaviors that pose a health risk.*

Dental hygiene actions/implications: *educate the patient on the risks to health of the combined use of tobacco and excessive alcohol; provide a demonstration, with the patient observing in a handheld mirror, of the oral effects of smoking (stains, periodontal disease) and excessive alcohol use (swollen parotid glands, condition of the tongue, dry mouth conditions); teach patient how to perform a self-screening for oral cancer; communicate that resources are available should he decide to moderate unhealthy behavior; provide resources as requested; encourage patient to make and keep appointments for dental treatment and regular dental hygiene care.*

Deficit identified in Skin and Mucous Membrane Integrity of the Head and Neck

Due to: xerostomia
Evidenced by: oral conditions, burning tongue, and parotid gland enlargement

Goals: _____

Dental hygiene actions/implications: _____

Deficit identified in Biologically Sound and Functional Dentition

Due to: lack of professional oral care
Evidenced by: multiple dental caries and defective restorations

Goals: _____

Dental hygiene actions/implications: _____

Deficit identified in Wholesome Facial Image

Due to: self-consciousness of appearance; dissatisfaction with smile
Evidenced by: severe rampant caries of anterior teeth; lack of regular dental care

Goals: _____

Dental hygiene actions/implications: _____

REFLECTIVE ACTIVITIES

1. Individuals who smoke and use excessive amounts of alcohol have a significantly increased risk of oral cancer. Determine how you would approach this patient regarding moderation of alcohol use and smoking cessation. Explain how counseling can contribute to his knowledge, attitudes, and practices regarding his unhealthy behavior.

2. Alcohol abuse and alcoholism often result in poor nutrition. Write a detailed treatment plan to assess this patient's diet and provide nutritional counseling. Include a description of the tools you will use to help provide an accurate survey of his eating habits.

3. In a small group activity, brainstorm several possible reasons why this patient has difficulty making and keeping dental and dental hygiene appointments. Use this list as a basis for role-playing how the dental hygienist might address each of the reasons.

REFERENCES

Alvarez K: *Dental Hygiene Handbook.* Baltimore: Williams and Wilkins, 1998, pp. 419–421.

Darby ML: *Mosby's Comprehensive Review of Dental Hygiene*, 6th ed. St. Louis: Mosby (Elsevier), 2006, pp. 586–590, 810.

Ibsen OAC, Phelan J: *Oral Pathology for the Dental Hygienist*, 4th ed. St. Louis: Saunders (Elsevier), 2004, pp. 56–57, 62, 67–68.

Langlais RP, Miller CS: *Color Atlas of Common Oral Disease*, 2nd ed. Philadelphia: Williams and Wilkins, 1998, pp. 48–51, 72–73, 76, 86–87, 164.

Medical Economics: *Physicians Desk Reference for Nonprescription Drugs and Dietary Supplements*, 60th ed. Montvale, NJ: Thomson Healthcare, 2006, p. 3392.

Miller RL, Gould AR, Bernstein ML, Read CJ: *General Pathology for the Dental Hygienist.* St. Louis: Mosby, 1995, pp. 200–201, 254–260.

Rule JT, Veatch RM: *Ethical Questions in Dentistry*, 2nd ed. Chicago: Quintessence Publishing Co. Inc., 2004, pp. 85–102.

Stegeman CA, Davis JR: *The Dental Hygienist's Guide to Nutritional Care*, 2nd ed. St. Louis: Saunders (Elsevier), 2005, pp. 130, 218–220.

Weinberg MA, Westphal C, Pilat M, Froum SJ: *Comprehensive Periodontics for the Dental Hygienist*, 2nd ed. Upper Saddle River, NJ: Prentice Hall, 2006, pp. 310–325.

Weinstein B: *Dental Ethics.* Philadelphia: Lea & Febiger, 1993, p. 69.

Wilkins E: *Clinical Practice of the Dental Hygienist*, 9th ed. Philadelphia: Lippincott Williams & Wilkins, 2005, pp. 1010–1020.

CASE **L**

Thomas Small

SITUATION

Thomas Small has presented for his dental hygiene appointment today with an eager seriousness. Although his mother is his legal guardian, his social services case worker has brought him in today. She explains that Thomas likes to have all procedures explained in detail before agreeing to treatment.

LEARNING GOALS

Following integration of core scientific concepts and application of dental hygiene theory to the care of this patient, you will be able to

1. **Assess patient characteristics.**
   A. Identify variations of normal head and neck anatomy.
   B. Recognize factors that contribute to the creation of nonpathologic oral deviations from normal.
   C. Determine the etiology of gingival inflammation.
   D. Identify the risk associated with opercula.

2. **Obtain and interpret radiographs.**
   A. Identify normal radiographic anatomy.
   B. Recognize radiographic artifacts.
   C. Recognize anatomic anomalies observed in radiographs.

3. **Plan and manage dental hygiene care.**
   A. Prepare appropriately for a possible medical emergency during dental hygiene treatment.
   B. Execute appropriate response to a medical emergency during dental hygiene treatment.
   C. Select appropriate treatment regimens for the patient with a seizure disorder.
   D. Recommend oral self-care strategies for the patient exhibiting mental retardation.
   E. Perform dental hygiene treatment for the patient with a seizure disorder.

4. **Perform periodontal procedures.**
   A. Utilize standard indices for assessing periodontal health.
   B. Identify microorganisms present in plaque biofilm.

   C. Select the appropriate calculus removal method.
   D. Select the appropriate instrument for removing calculus.
   E. Determine possible outcomes of oral health care instruction and nonsurgical periodontal therapy.

5. **Use preventive agents.**
   A. Select the appropriate fluoride treatment based on patient assessment data.

6. **Provide supportive treatment services.**
   A. Determine contraindications to treatment based on gingival conditions.
   B. Determine when medical emergency assistance should be initiated in response to an epileptic seizure.

7. **Demonstrate professional responsibility.**
   A. Identify professional obligation in determining the need for information regarding a patient's history of seizures.
   B. Classify mental retardation adaptive functioning.
   C. Identify the person legally responsible for providing informed consent for a patient under the care of another.
   D. Determine the competency of the patient to give informed consent.

SPECIAL NEEDS PATIENT—*Thomas Small*
PATIENT HISTORY SYNOPSIS

VITAL STATISTICS

Age	*32 years*
Gender	*male*
Height	*5' 7"*
Weight	*185 lbs.*

Blood Pressure	*135/89 mm Hg*
Pulse Rate	*88 bpm*
Respiration	*14 rpm*

1. Under care of physician
   Yes [X]   No [ ]   Condition: *seizure disorder* _____
   _____
   _____

2. Hospitalized within the last 5 years
   Yes [ ]   No [X]   Reason: _____
   _____

3. Has or had the following conditions
   epilepsy _____
   _____
   _____

4. Current medications
   carbamazepine (Tegretol)—anticonvulsant
   phenytoin (Dilantin)—anticonvulsant
   topiramate (Topamax)—anticonvulsant
   _____

5. Smokes or uses tobacco products
   Yes [ ]   No [X]

6. Is pregnant
   Yes [ ]   No [ ]   N/A [X]

MEDICAL HISTORY
Mental retardation. Epileptic seizures responding well to current medications and appear to be controlled. Last episode was 8 months ago; appear to be precipitated by monotonous sounds, music, and loud noises.

DENTAL HISTORY
Professional oral health has been sporadic. His last recall appointment was 18 months ago.

SOCIAL HISTORY
Patient enjoys his job at the supermarket, and is especially proud that he is learning where items are located in each aisle. He lives in an independent living group home.

CHIEF COMPLAINT
Thomas expresses frustration when asked about his oral hygiene practices. He explains that he hasn't been brushing, because he thinks one of the other men living at his group home keeps stealing his toothbrush.

ADULT CLINICAL EXAMINATION

	1	2	3	4	5	6	7	8	9	10	11	12	13	14	15	16
Probe 2																
Probe 1	544	445	324	314	414	323	323	436	634	434	433	333	333	334	444	444

	1	2	3	4	5	6	7	8	9	10	11	12	13	14	15	16
Probe 1	444	444	323	323	312	313	212	212	212	212	212	213	313	313	315	544
Probe 2																

R / L

	32	31	30	29	28	27	26	25	24	23	22	21	20	19	18	17
Probe 2																
Probe 1	X	534	323	313	313	424	212	222	222	222	222	223	324	426	428	X

	32	31	30	29	28	27	26	25	24	23	22	21	20	19	18	17
Probe 1	X	645	433	323	323	324	424	424	424	425	524	223	323	323	456	X
Probe 2																

CURRENT ORAL HYGIENE STATUS
Spontaneous marginal bleeding on probing
Generalized moderate subgingival calculus

SUPPLEMENTA ORAL EXAMINATION FINDINGS
The partially erupted mandibular third molars present with opercula
Lips parted in occlusion
Evidence of mouth breathing
Licks and sucks on lips excessively

⌒ Clinically visible carious lesion

✕ Clinically missing tooth

△ Furcation

▲ "Through and through" furcation

Probe 1: Initial probing depth

Probe 2: Probing depth 6 weeks after periodontal therapy

L

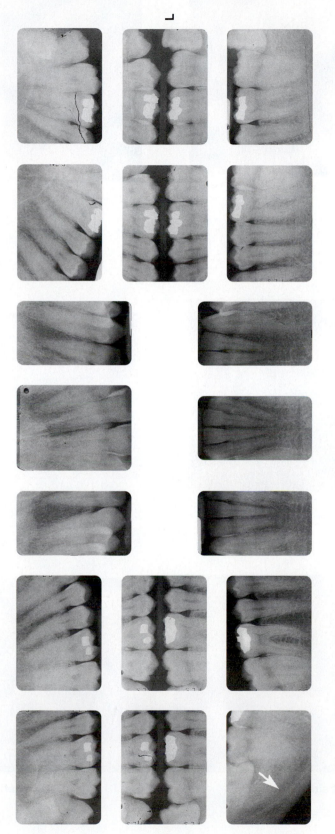

R

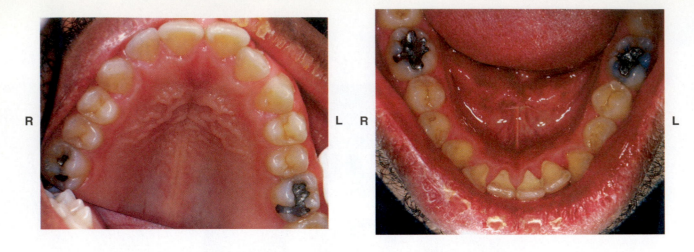

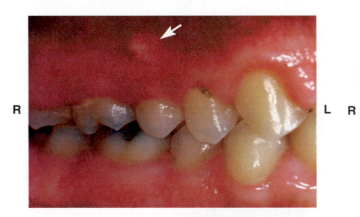

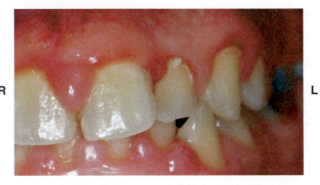

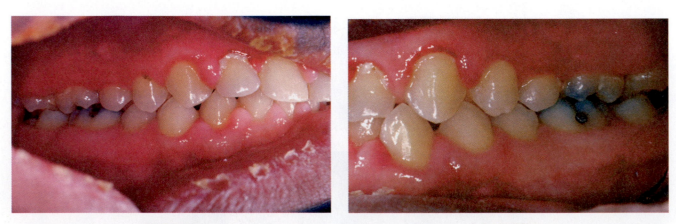

Right side

Left side

CASE QUESTIONS

ASSESSING PATIENT CHARACTERISTICS
Basic Level Questions

1. Which of the following is the most likely assessment of the hard nodulelike finding observed on the facial gingiva, adjacent to the maxillary right second premolar (arrow)?
   A. Papilloma
   B. Neurofibroma
   C. Exostosis
   D. Hyperkeratosis
   E. Lipoma

Competency Level Questions

2. Each of the following may be contributing to this patient's excessively dry lips EXCEPT one. Which one is the EXCEPTION?
   A. His medications
   B. Mouth breathing
   C. Evaporation of excessive moisture on the lips
   D. Seizure disorder
   E. Habit of sucking on the lips

3. Which of the following best applies to the enlarged gingiva in the anterior region?
   A. Linear gingival erythema
   B. Phenytoin-influenced gingival enlargement
   C. Hereditary gingival fibromatosis
   D. Necrotizing ulcerative gingivitis
   E. Acute herpetic gingivostomatitis

4. The mandibular third molars are at risk for developing which of the following?
   A. Pericoronitis
   B. Osteomyelitis
   C. Melanosis
   D. Mucocele
   E. Taurodontism

OBTAINING AND INTERPRETING RADIOGRAPHS
Basic Level Questions

5. Which of the following is the most likely interpretation of the long tubelike radiolucency (arrow) observed in the mandibular right molar periapical radiograph?
   A. Compound fracture
   B. Nutrient canal
   C. Oblique ridge
   D. Mylohyoid line
   E. Mandibular canal

6. Which of the following is the most likely assessment of the black line observed on the maxillary left molar periapical radiograph?
   A. Lint that stuck to the film while wet
   B. Static electricity that created an artifact
   C. Roller mark from the automatic processor
   D. Accidental chemical splash prior to processing
   E. Fingernail scratching the film emulsion

Competency Level Questions

7. Which of the following is the most likely interpretation of the anomalies observed in the maxillary molar periapical radiographs?
   A. Bony exostoses
   B. Dens invaginatus
   C. Enamel pearls
   D. Supernumerary teeth
   E. Impacted third molars

PLANNING AND MANAGING DENTAL HYGIENE CARE
Basic Level Questions

8. Each of the following should be considered when treating this patient, EXCEPT one. Which one is the EXCEPTION?
   A. Include a mouth prop in the treatment armamentarium
   B. Schedule appointments within the first few hours of daily medications
   C. Ask the patient to report aura sensation immediately upon sensing
   D. Ready life support oxygen for respiratory support
   E. Prepare to administer a bronchodilator

9. If this patient has a seizure in the dental chair, the primary task of management must be to protect him from injury to himself.

   At the start of a seizure, an attempt should be made to move this patient out of the treatment chair and onto the floor.
   A. The first statement is true, the second statement is false.
   B. The first statement is false, the second statement is true.
   C. Both statements are true and related.
   D. Both statements are true but not related.
   E. Both statements are false.

10. Each of the following should be executed if this patient begins to exhibit uncontrolled muscle motor movements EXCEPT one. Which one is the EXCEPTION?
    A. Monitor vital signs.
    B. Provide aggressive restraints.
    C. Place in a supine position.
    D. Remove instruments from the area.
    E. Maintain an open airway.

Competency Level Questions

11. Which of the following treatment regimens may pose the greatest risk for potentially exacerbating this patient's risk of a seizure?
    A. Coronal polishing
    B. Subgingival irrigation
    C. Ultrasonic scaling
    D. Root planing
    E. Toothbrush deplaquing

12. Which of the following oral hygiene care strategies should be implemented first to increase this patient's motivation to improve his oral self-care habits?
    A. Disclose and show plaque accumulation using a hand mirror.
    B. Provide a brochure with large pictures demonstrating brushing technique.
    C. Give him a new toothbrush with his name on it.
    D. Include the social services case worker in oral self-care instructions.
    E. Use a digital intraoral camera that images the oral cavity on a monitor.

13. Which of the following should be considered before subgingival debridement?
    A. Premedicate with appropriate antibiotics.
    B. Determine pretreatment bleeding time.
    C. Offer acetaminophen to manage discomfort.
    D. Rinse with an alcohol-containing mouth rinse.
    E. Irrigate pockets with saline.

PERFORMING PERIODONTAL PROCEDURES
Basic Level Questions

14. According to the Plaque Index of Silness and Löe, which of the following scores would be applied to this patient's maxillary anterior teeth?
    A. 0
    B. 1
    C. 2
    D. 3

15. Which of the following statements regarding the bacteria present in the plaque biofilm adjacent to the maxillary left lateral incisor and maxillary left canine is most accurate?
    A. Primarily gram-positive cocci and epithelial cells
    B. Increased numbers of gram-positive filamentous forms and short rods
    C. Mixed flora of rods, filamentous forms, and fusobacteria
    D. Gram-negative and anaerobic organisms that have begun to appear
    E. Vibrios and spirochetes that are prevalent

16. Which of the following is indicated for the brown spot on the maxillary right first premolar?
    A. Subgingivally irrigating with an antimicrobial agent
    B. Polishing with a medium-grit abrasive
    C. Toothbrushing with a fluoridated dentifrice
    D. Scaling with a universal curet
    E. Burnishing with fluoride

17. Which of the following instruments would be the best choice to remove the supragingival calculus observed on the lingual surfaces of this patient's mandibular anterior teeth?
    A. Curved scaler
    B. File scaler
    C. Hoe scaler
    D. Chisel scaler

Competency Level Questions

18. Following debridement and instruction in oral self-care, what reduction in probing depths can be expected at the 6-week reevaluation appointment?
    A. 0 to 1 mm
    B. 2 to 3 mm
    C. 4 to 5 mm
    D. Increased probing depths likely

USING PREVENTIVE AGENTS
Competency Level Questions

19. Which of the following self-applied fluorides would be the best recommendation for this patient?
    A. Low-potency sodium fluoride mouth rinse
    B. Acidulated phosphate fluoride custom tray application
    C. Stannous fluoride brush-on gel
    D. Extra-strength sodium monofluorophate dentifrice
    E. Dietary sodium fluoride tablet supplement

PROVIDING SUPPORTIVE TREATMENT SERVICES
Basic Level Questions

20. Which of the following will most likely be postponed until a later appointment?
    A. Fluoride varnish
    B. Polishing
    C. Root planing
    D. Scaling
    E. Probing

21. Should a seizure occur while treating this patient, emergency medical assistance must be summoned if the seizure lasts longer than
    A. 5 minutes
    B. 10 minutes
    C. 15 minutes
    D. 20 minutes
    E. 30 minutes

DEMONSTRATING PROFESSIONAL RESPONSIBILITY
Basic Level Questions

22. Each of the following must be identified before treating this patient EXCEPT one. Which one is the EXCEPTION?
    A. Type of seizure
    B. Frequency of seizure episodes
    C. Degree of control
    D. Known precipitating factors
    E. Change in mental status

23. This patient's mental retardation is considered
    A. Mild
    B. Moderate
    C. Severe
    D. Profound

24. Who must sign the informed consent document prior to treating this patient?
    A. The patient
    B. His case worker
    C. His mother
    D. The group home director
    E. The dentist

Competency Level Questions

25. With regard to the ability to give informed consent for dental hygiene treatment, this patient is
    A. Legally competent with decision-making capacity
    B. Legally competent with impaired decision-making capacity
    C. Legally incompetent with decision-making capacity
    D. Legally incompetent with impaired or no decision-making capacity

SETTING PATIENT GOALS

ESTABLISHING A DENTAL HYGIENE CARE PLAN

To assist this patient in meeting his needs, develop a dental hygiene care plan that establishes a framework within which to help him and his caregivers identify goals for obtaining oral health. In addition to the clinical assessment, a well-prepared dental hygiene care plan should take into account the patient's age, gender, lifestyle, culture, attitudes, health beliefs, and knowledge level. To help link this patient's needs for overall well-being with his oral conditions, and to provide motivation for achieving better health, the following is a partial list of possible deficits based on the Human Needs Conceptual Model to Dental Hygiene Practice. (See the appendix for an explanation of the Human Needs Conceptual Model to Dental Hygiene Practice to help you identify additional unmet needs.) Use this partial list of unmet needs or deficits as a guide in preparing a dental hygiene care plan for this patient. One set of goals and dental hygiene actions/implications has been completed as an example.

Deficit identified in Protection from Health Risks

Due to: potential for epileptic seizure during treatment
Evidenced by: medical history

Goals: _____

Dental hygiene actions/implications: _____

Deficit identified in Skin and Mucous Membrane Integrity of the Head and Neck

Due to: gingival inflammation
Evidenced by: spontaneous bleeding

Goals: _____

Dental hygiene actions/implications: _____

Deficit identified in Conceptualization and Problem Solving

Due to: mental retardation
Evidenced by: not taking alternative action to compensate for missing toothbrush

Goals: _____

Dental hygiene actions/implications: _____

Deficit identified in Responsibility for Oral Health

Due to: inadequate toothbrushing
Evidenced by: lack of a toothbrush

Goals: *assist patient with maintaining the self-care tools he needs to improve his oral health; increase toothbrushing frequency.*

Dental hygiene actions/implications: *provide the patient with a new toothbrush; allow the patient to choose his own brush from a selection of colors and types appropriate for his needs; personalize the brush with his name; assist the patient with determining how best to protect his brush and keep it safe so that he can use it often.*

REFLECTIVE ACTIVITIES

1. Consider a case in which a legally competent person's decision-making skills are questionable. Discuss how you would determine the following: whether the patient shows evidence of understanding the proposed treatment; whether the patient understands the risks and benefits of the treatment and the consequences of nontreatment; and whether the patient shows evidence of rationality in weighing the treatment options presented. What role would the patient's immediate family, friends, or others play in this scenario? Discuss how you would approach this situation.

2. Develop a seizure disorder supplement to a standard medical history with questions pertaining to seizures that the dental hygiene professional can use before treating the patient with a seizure disorder.

3. Develop a medical emergency sheet describing the steps the oral health care team would take to manage a seizure that occurred during treatment. Role-play an emergency scenario.

4. Role-play the dental hygienist meeting this patient for the first time. Demonstrate the establishment of a professional relationship. Use strategies that develop a rapport; gain patient confidence and interest; explain procedures and answer patient questions; and obtain legal consent for treatment.

REFERENCES

Alvarez K: *Dental Hygiene Handbook.* Philadelphia: Lippincott Williams & Wilkins, 1999, pp. 396–398.

Braun RJ, Cutilli BJ: *Manual of Emergency Medical Treatment for the Dental Team.* Philadelphia: Williams & Wilkins, 1999, pp. 92–94.

Darby ML: *Mosby's Comprehensive Review of Dental Hygiene,* 6th ed. St. Louis: Mosby (Elsevier), 2006, pp. 588, 591–592.

Darby ML, Walsh MM: *Dental Hygiene Theory and Practice,* 2nd ed. St. Louis: Saunders (Elsevier), 2003, pp. 816–833.

Davis JA: *Legal and Ethical Considerations for Dental Hygienists and Assistants.* St. Louis: Mosby, 2000, pp. 58–63.

Gage TW, Little JW: *Mosby's 2007 Dental Drug Consult.* St. Louis: Mosby (Elsevier), 2007, pp. 189–191, 543–544, 1225–1227.

Haveles, EB: *Applied Pharmacology for the Dental Hygienist.* 5th ed. St. Louis: Mosby (Elsevier). 2007, pp. 314–325.

Ibsen OAC, Phelan J: *Oral Pathology for the Dental Hygienist,* 4th ed. St. Louis: Saunders (Elsevier), 2004, pp. 55, 59, 133, 173–177, 190, 258, 279, 284.

Little JW, Falce DA, Miller CS, Rhodus NL: *Dental Management of the Medically Compromised Patient,* 7th ed. St. Louis: Mosby (Elsevier), 2008, pp. DM52–53, 464–469.

Löe H: The gingival index, the plaque index, and the retention index systems. *Journal of Periodontology,* 38, 610–611, 1967.

Nield-Gehrig JS, Willmann DE: *Foundations of Periodontics for the Dental Hygienists,* 2nd ed. Philadelphia: Lippincott Williams & Wilkins, 2008, pp. 74–77.

Perry DA, Beemsterboer PL: *Periodontology for the Dental Hygienist,* 3rd ed. St. Louis: Saunders (Elsevier), 2007, pp. 270, 358, 360, 379, 386–387, 403.

Pickett FA, Gurenlian JR: *The Medical History: Clinical Implications and Emergency Prevention in Dental Settings.* Philadelphia: Lippincott Williams & Wilkins, 2005, pp. 157–161.

Pickett FA, Terezhamlmy GT: *Lippincott Williams & Wilkins' Dental Drug Reference with Clinical Implications.* Philadelphia: Lippincott Williams & Wilkins, 2006, pp. 271–272, 625–626, 730–731.

Rule JT, Veatch RM: *Ethical Questions in Dentistry,* 2nd ed. Chicago: Quintessence Publishing Co., Inc., 2004, pp. 154–165.

Stefanac SJ, Nesbit SP: *Treatment Planning in Dentistry,* 2nd ed. St. Louis: Mosby (Elsevier), 2007, pp. 81–83, 256–257.

Wilkins EM: *Clinical Practice of the Dental Hygienist,* 9th ed. Philadelphia: Lippincott Williams & Wilkins, 2005, pp. 294–295, 551–561, 616–619, 690, 728–730, 882–911, 968–979.

CASE **M**

Nancy Foster

SITUATION

Nancy Foster is a senior in college and lives at home with her parents. She works part time as a waitress. Nancy is outgoing and has plans to further her education by attending graduate school. Diagnosed with diabetes at age 15, keeping her diabetes under control is a constant concern. She recently began using an insulin pump. She has presented today for her regular 6-month examination and prophylaxis.

LEARNING GOALS

Following integration of core scientific concepts and application of dental hygiene theory to the care of this patient, you will be able to

1. **Assess patient characteristics.**
   A. Identify the classifications of diabetes using current medical terminology.
   B. Determine the etiology of diabetes based on patient health history information.
   C. Classify fluorosis.
   D. Recognize diabetes effects on the oral cavity.
   E. Relate pathophysiology of diabetes with clinical symptoms.

2. **Obtain and interpret radiographs.**
   A. Identify common radiographic artifacts.
   B. Identify the cause of errors that diminish the quality of radiographs.
   C. Apply the appropriate corrective action to radiographic error.
   D. Identify normal radiographic landmarks.
   E. Use radiographs to classify carious lesions according to G. V. Black's method of classification.
   F. Interpret deviations from normal radiographic anatomy.

3. **Plan and manage dental hygiene care.**
   A. Recognize and manage a medical emergency during dental hygiene treatment.

4. **Perform periodontal procedures.**
   A. Classify the patient's periodontal condition using the American Academy of Periodontology classification system.
   B. Identify the causes of change in gingival tissues.
   C. Identify risk factors for periodontal disease.
   D. Assess outcomes of nonsurgical periodontal therapy.
   E. Appropriately recommend recare appointment time intervals.

5. **Use preventive agents.**
   A. Select appropriate teeth for pit and fissure sealant application.
   B. Select preventive agents based on patient needs.

6. **Provide supportive treatment services.**
   A. Recognize conditions that decrease the effectiveness of tooth whitening.

7. **Demonstrate professional responsibility.**
   A. Use health history follow-up questions to open communication with the patient for the purpose of avoiding the occurrence of a medical emergency during treatment.

MEDICALLY COMPROMISED PATIENT—*Nancy Foster*
PATIENT HISTORY SYNOPSIS

VITAL STATISTICS

Age	*21 years*
Gender	*female*
Height	*5' 3"*
Weight	*106 lbs.*

Blood Pressure	*90/60 mm Hg*
Pulse Rate	*96 bpm*
Respiration	*14 rpm*

1. Under care of physician
   Yes ☒   No ☐   Condition: *glycated hemoglobin test every 3 months* _____

2. Hospitalized within the last 5 years
   Yes ☐   No ☒   Reason: _____

3. Has or had the following conditions
   diabetes mellitus (DM) _____

4. Current medications
   regular (Humulin R) - insulin
   neutral protamine hagedorn (NPH)
   (Humulin N) - insulin

5. Smokes or uses tobacco products
   Yes ☐   No ☒

6. Is pregnant
   Yes ☐   No ☒   N/A ☐

MEDICAL HISTORY
Has experienced a recent weight loss of 7 lbs.

DENTAL HISTORY
Receives regular dental hygiene care at 6-month intervals; orthodontic treatment in her early teens.

SOCIAL HISTORY
A busy full-time college student with a part-time job, patient admits to less than ideal eating habits. Has a habit of biting her fingernails.

CHIEF COMPLAINT
Recently noticed that her gums look different and that they are sore and bleed. Interested in tooth whitening.

ADULT CLINICAL EXAMINATION

	1	2	3	4	5	6	7	8	9	10	11	12	13	14	15	16
Probe 2	X	213	313	313	X	212	212	111	111	111	111	X	212	212	212	X
Probe 1		324	524	323		322	212	212	212	212	223		323	323	323	

	1	2	3	4	5	6	7	8	9	10	11	12	13	14	15	16
Probe 1	X	323	523	323	X	322	212	212	212	212	212	X	325	323	323	X
Probe 2		313	312	212		211	111	111	111	111	111		212	212	212	

	32	31	30	29	28	27	26	25	24	23	22	21	20	19	18	17
Probe 2	X	313	413	313	X	212	111	111	111	111	111	X	212	323	323	X
Probe 1		334	534	323		323	212	212	111	111	212		323	434	433	

	32	31	30	29	28	27	26	25	24	23	22	21	20	19	18	17
Probe 1	X	323	323	212	X	212	211	111	111	111	112	X	212	313	323	X
Probe 2		313	312	212		212	111	111	111	111	111		112	313	323	

CURRENT ORAL HYGIENE STATUS
Slight, localized calculus in the mandibular anterior region.
Slight, generalized plaque biofilm.

SUPPLEMENTAL ORAL EXAMINATION FINDINGS
Moderate, generalized bleeding upon probing
Moderate xerostomia

⊌ Clinically visible carious lesion
☒ Clinically missing tooth
△ Furcation
▲ "Through and through" furcation
Probe 1: Initial probing depth
Probe 2: Probing depth 6 weeks after
   periodontal therapy

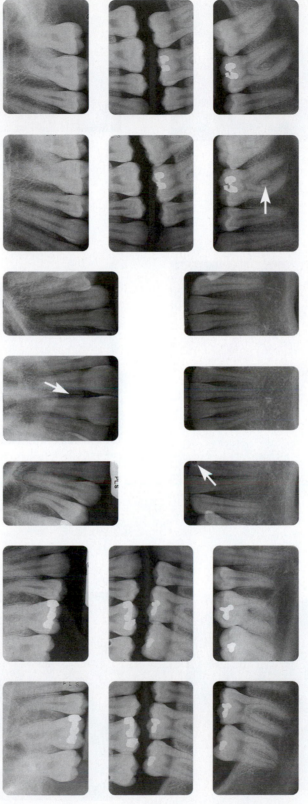

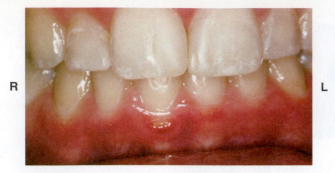

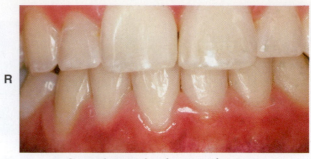

6–week reevaluation appointment

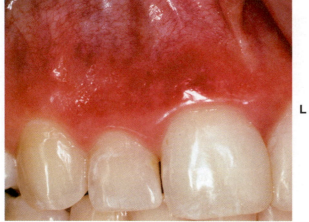

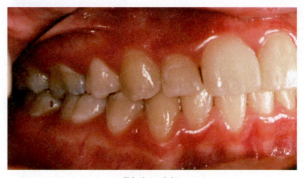

Right side

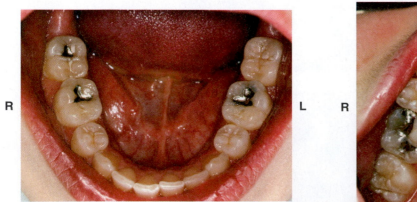

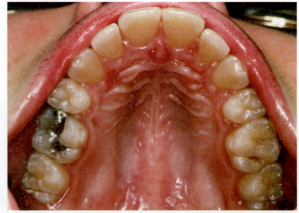

CASE QUESTIONS

ASSESSING PATIENT CHARACTERISTICS
Basic Level Questions

1. Based on the current American Diabetes Association classification system, this patient has which of the following?
   A. Type 1 diabetes
   B. Type 2 diabetes
   C. Gestational diabetes
   D. Drug-induced diabetes

2. Which of the following was the most likely etiology in the development of this patient's diabetes?
   A. Insulin resistance
   B. Inadequate insulin secretion
   C. Autoimmune destruction of beta cells
   D. Poor weight management
   E. Sucrose consumption

3. Based on the Tooth Surface Index of Fluorosis (TSIF) classification system, what is this patient's numerical score?
   A. 0
   B. 1
   C. 2
   D. 3
   E. 4

Competency Level Questions

4. What is the most likely cause of this patient's xerostomia?
   A. Periodontal disease
   B. Medication use
   C. Renal function
   D. Frequent meals
   E. Oral hygiene

5. Which of the following would NOT be related to poor glycemic control?
   A. Dental caries
   B. Weight loss
   C. Increased pulse rate
   D. Congenitally missing teeth
   E. Low blood pressure

6. This patient's medical condition has the potential to increase her risk for each of the following oral manifestations EXCEPT one. Which one is the EXCEPTION?
   A. Gingivitis
   B. Periodontitis
   C. Burning mouth syndrome
   D. Oral mucosal diseases
   E. Dentin hypersensitivity

OBTAINING AND INTERPRETING RADIOGRAPHS
Basic Level Questions

7. Which of the following is the most likely interpretation of the round radiolucency at the incisal edge of the mandibular right central incisor observed in the mandibular right lateral canine periapical radiograph (arrow)?
   A. Film identification dot
   B. Composite restoration
   C. Attrition
   D. Calculus deposit
   E. Caries

8. Which of the following has rendered the maxillary right premolar periapical radiograph undiagnostic?
   A. Interproximal spaces overlapped
   B. Root apices not visible
   C. Cone cutting present
   D. Herringbone effect
   E. Film holder imaged

Competency Level Questions

9. What corrective action is required when retaking the undiagnostic maxillary right premolar periapical radiograph?
   A. Decrease the vertical angulation.
   B. Shift the horizontal angulation to the mesial.
   C. Ensure that the patient bites down on the film holder.
   D. Reverse the film packet when placing into the oral cavity.
   E. Center the film within the x-ray beam.

10. Which of the following is the most likely interpretation of the radiolucent vertical line between the maxillary central incisors (arrow)?
    A. Nasal septum
    B. Nutrient canal
    C. Vertical bone loss
    D. Palatal fracture
    E. Midpalatine suture

11. The radiographs reveal which G. V. Black's classification of caries on the maxillary left first molar?
    A. II
    B. III
    C. IV
    D. V
    E. VI

12. Which of the following is the most likely interpretation of the radiopaque anomaly near the roots of the mandibular left first molar (arrow)?
    A. Microdont
    B. Mesiodens
    C. Secondary dentin
    D. Enamel pearl
    E. Pulp stone

13. Which of the following teeth presents with root dilaceration?
    A. Maxillary right second premolar
    B. Maxillary left first molar
    C. Mandibular left canine
    D. Mandibular right central incisor
    E. Mandibular right second molar

PLANNING AND MANAGING DENTAL HYGIENE CARE
Basic Level Questions

14. Which of the following would be considered the most likely medical emergency that may occur with this patient during treatment?
    A. Hyperglycemia
    B. Hypoglycemia
    C. Diabetic coma
    D. Ketoacidosis

15. Each of the following indicates that this patient is experiencing a medical emergency EXCEPT one. Which one is the EXCEPTION?
    A. Excessive perspiration
    B. Bounding pulse
    C. Slight paresthesia
    D. Increased anxiety
    E. Argumentative mood

Competency Level Questions

16. Which of the following will assist in managing a possible emergency medical situation regarding this patient?
    A. Premedicate with oral antibiotics.
    B. Place ammonia capsule on the bracket table for ready use.
    C. Request that the patient disconnect the insulin pump during treatment.
    D. Use a semisupine chair position.
    E. Have a source of oral sugar (e.g., orange juice) available.

PERFORMING PERIODONTAL PROCEDURES
Basic Level Questions

17. Based on the American Academy of Periodontology classification system, what is this patient's periodontal classification?
    A. Gingivitis associated with dental plaque only
    B. Nonplaque-induced gingival disease
    C. Gingival disease modified by medications
    D. Gingival disease modified by systemic factors
    E. Gingival manifestations of systemic conditions

Competency Level Questions

18. On a histologic level, each of the following is responsible for the color change of the gingiva observed at the initial appointment in the facial region of the maxillary right central incisor EXCEPT one. Which one is the EXCEPTION?
    A. Blood flow to this area has increased.
    B. Many dead and dying phagocytes are present.
    C. Osteoclast activity is being stimulated by prostaglandins.
    D. Leukocytes are invading the bacteria present at this site.
    E. Plasma proteins are leaking from the blood vessels in the tissue.

19. Periodontal disease may be considered a complication of diabetes.

    If this patient maintains control over her blood glucose levels, her risk for periodontal disease is likely to be no greater than that of nondiabetics.
    A. Both sentences are true.
    B. Both sentences are false.
    C. The first sentence is true, the second sentence is false.
    D. The first sentence is false, the second sentence is true.

20. What is the reason for the change in appearance of the facial gingiva in the region of the mandibular right central incisor at the 6-week reevaluation appointment?
    A. Weight gain of lost pounds
    B. Cessation of nail biting habit
    C. Change in method of insulin delivery
    D. Initiation of use of whitening products
    E. Periodontal debridement and improved self-care

21. Which of the following recare appointment intervals would benefit this patient?
    A. 1 month
    B. 3 months
    C. 6 months
    D. 9 months
    E. 12 months

USING PREVENTIVE AGENTS
Basic Level Questions

22. Which of the following should be indicated for placement of a sealant?
    A. Maxillary right second molar
    B. Maxillary right first molar
    C. Maxillary left first molar
    D. Mandibular left first molar
    E. Mandibular right first molar

Competency Level Questions

23. Which of the following would benefit this patient the most?
    A. End-tuft brush
    B. Tooth whitening product
    C. Dietary assessment
    D. Self-applied fluoride
    E. Disclosing tablets

PROVIDING SUPPORTIVE TREATMENT SERVICES
Competency Level Questions

24. Which of the following can be expected to minimize tooth whitening results for this patient?
    A. Gingival inflammation
    B. Nail biting habit
    C. Fluorosis
    D. Diabetes
    E. Sealants

DEMONSTRATING PROFESSIONAL RESPONSIBILITY
Basic Level Questions

25. Each of the following is a recommended health history interview question to determine the safe treatment of this patient today EXCEPT one. Which one is the EXCEPTION?
    A. "Did you take your usual dose of insulin today?"
    B. "How often do you have insulin reactions?"
    C. "What was your blood glucose level at the last test?"
    D. "Have you eaten your normal meals and snacks today?"
    E. "How much do you weigh?"

SETTING PATIENT GOALS

ESTABLISHING A DENTAL HYGIENE CARE PLAN

To assist this patient in meeting her needs, develop a dental hygiene care plan that establishes a framework within which to help her identify goals for obtaining oral health. In addition to the clinical assessment, a well-prepared dental hygiene care plan should take into account the patient's age, gender, lifestyle, culture, attitudes, health beliefs, and knowledge level. To help link this patient's needs for overall well-being with her oral conditions, and to provide motivation for achieving better health, the following is a partial list of possible deficits based on the Human Needs Conceptual Model to Dental Hygiene Practice. (See the appendix for an explanation of the Human Needs Conceptual Model to Dental Hygiene Practice to help you identify additional unmet needs.) Use this partial list of unmet needs or deficits as a guide in preparing a dental hygiene care plan for this patient. One set of goals and dental hygiene actions/implications has been completed as an example.

Deficit identified in Protection from Health Risks

Due to: inadequate nutrition
Evidenced by: self-report

Goals: _____

Dental hygiene actions/implications: _____

Deficit identified in Skin and Mucous Membrane Integrity of the Head and Neck

Due to: presence of generalized plaque
Evidenced by: gingival inflammation and bleeding

Goals: _____

Dental hygiene actions/implications: _____

Deficit identified in Biologically Sound and Functional Dentition

Due to: xerostomia
Evidenced by: caries

Goals: _____

Dental hygiene actions/implications: _____

Deficit identified in Conceptualization and Problem Solving

Due to: lack of awareness of interrelationship between diabetes and oral health
Evidenced by: focus of interest on teeth whitening instead of on signs and symptoms of gingival disease

Goals: _____

Dental hygiene actions/implications: _____

Deficit identified in Wholesome Facial Image

Due to: color of teeth
Evidenced by: request for whitening products

Goals: *assist patient with decision to use whitening product.*

Dental hygiene actions/implications: *perform a thorough exam to determine contraindications for the use of whitening products; take a whitening "history" on the patient to determine past use; determine patient satisfaction/dissatisfaction with past outcomes; determine patient expectations of future outcomes by allowing the patient to pick shades from a shade guide and then comparing shades with the patient's natural teeth; use co-discovery with the patient to determine realistic expectations; determine the patient knowledge level of products and educate the patient on product types, benefits, risks, compliance requirements, and lifestyle changes required, such as elimination of foods and beverages that stain the teeth.*

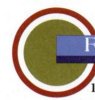

REFLECTIVE ACTIVITIES

1. Develop a list of healthy foods and snacks that would assist a busy college student in maintaining a healthy lifestyle.

2. Prepare a patient brochure on tooth whitening. Include information such as types of products and application methods; compliance requirements and lifestyle changes needed to ensure optimal outcomes; include contraindications and risks that will help answer patient questions regarding the whitening procedure.

REFERENCES

Blackwell RE: *G. V. Black's Operative Dentistry*, vol. II, 9th ed. Milwaukee: Medico-Dental Publishing, 1955, pp. 1–4.

Darby ML, Walsh MM (eds.): *Dental Hygiene Theory and Practice*, 2nd ed. St. Louis: Saunders (Elsevier), 2003, pp. 855–869.

Gage TW, Little JW: *Mosby's 2007 Dental Drug Consult*. St. Louis: Mosby (Elsevier), 2007, pp. 634–636.

Ibsen OAC, Phelan J: *Oral Pathology for the Dental Hygienist*, 4th ed. St. Louis: Saunders (Elsevier), 2004, pp. 38–39, 184–186, 277–278.

Little JW, Falce DA, Miller CS, Rhodus NL: *Dental Management of the Medically Compromised Patient*, 7th ed. St. Louis: Mosby (Elsevier), 2008, pp. 212–213.

Lyle DM: Diabetes mellitus. *RDH*, 23(3), 54–56, 88, 2003.

Marks RA: Tooth whitening and total patient care. *RDH*, 23(6), 46–52, 2003.

Mealey BL: The diabetic in the dental chair. *Scientific American Presents Oral and Whole Body Health*. New York: Scientific American, Inc. custom publication produced in collaboration with Crest and Oral-B, 2006, p. 21.

Mealey BL, Rose LF: Periodontal inflammation and diabetes mellitus. Recognizing the relationship. *Contemporary Oral Hygiene*, 7(1), 23–29, 2007.

Meiller TF, Wynn RL, McMullin AM, Biron C, Crossley HL: *Dental Office Emergencies. A Manual of Office Response Protocols*. Hudson, OH: Lexi-Comp, Inc., 2000, pp. 15, 19, 23.

Nield-Gehrig JS, Willmann DE: *Foundations of Periodontics for the Dental Hygienist*, 2nd ed. Philadelphia: Lippincott Williams & Wilkins, 2008, pp. 140–141, 150–160.

Ryan ME, Carnu O, Tenzler R: The impact of periodontitis on metabolic control and risk for diabetic complications. *Grand Rounds in Oral-Systemic Medicine*, 1(2), 24–34, 2006.

White SC, Pharoah MJ: *Oral Radiology. Principles and Interpretation*, 5th ed. St. Louis: Mosby (Elsevier), 2004, pp. 349–351.

Wilkins EM: *Clinical Practice of the Dental Hygienist*, 9th ed. Philadelphia: Lippincott Williams & Wilkins, 2005, pp. 264, 549, 571–572, 1072–1089.

Wolfe FD: Diabetes. Anyone. Any time. *RDH*, 27(3), 58–64, 116, 2007.

CASE N

Brian Bartlett

SITUATION

Until a toothache motivated him to make an appointment with the dentist last week, Brian Bartlett has not had regular professional oral hygiene care in over 2 years. He presents today on the recommendation of his physician and confirmed by the dentist. Recently diagnosed with diabetes and secondary high blood pressure, Brian's physician has prescribed medication, weight loss, and lifestyle changes to help him get his medical conditions under control. He seems serious about taking steps to improve his health.

LEARNING GOALS

Following integration of core scientific concepts and application of dental hygiene theory to the care of this patient, you will be able to

1. **Assess patient characteristics.**
   A. Determine the etiologic classification of diabetes based on patient health history information.
   B. Classify blood pressure readings with stages of hypertension.
   C. Identify the risks associated with an unhealthy body mass index (BMI).
   D. Identify adverse effects of medications taken by the medically compromised patient.
   E. Use appropriate terminology to describe gingival conditions.
   F. Identify a temporary restoration.
   G. Identify potential causes of recession.
   H. Assess potential risks of recession.

2. **Obtain and interpret radiographs.**
   A. Identify the cause of radiographic errors.
   B. Interpret caries radiographically.

3. **Plan and manage dental hygiene care.**
   A. Apply the appropriate technique for pain control for scaling procedures.
   B. Recognize potential adverse effects for medications and respond appropriately to prevent occurrence of a medical emergency.
   C. Select the appropriate anesthetic for pain control for scaling procedures.

4. **Perform periodontal procedures.**
   A. Classify a patient's periodontal status.
   B. Select the appropriate handheld instrument for scaling a region.
   C. Determine the total loss of attachment.

5. **Use preventive agents.**
   A. Recommend the appropriate preventive agents based on oral assessment.

6. **Provide supportive treatment services.**
   A. Identify reasons for selective polishing.
   B. Recognize dietary recommendations for medically compromised individuals.
   C. Recommend therapies for managing xerostomia.

7. **Demonstrate professional responsibility.**
   A. Communicate appropriately with the medically compromised patient about the link between periodontal diseases and systemic health.
   B. Recognize the link between periodontal diseases and diabetes.
   C. Obtain patient's written consent to treatment.

MEDICALLY COMPROMISED PATIENT—*Brian Bartlett*
PATIENT HISTORY SYNOPSIS

VITAL STATISTICS

Age	*40 years*
Gender	*male*
Height	*5' 11"*
Weight	*218 lbs.*

Blood Pressure	*144/96 mm Hg*
Pulse Rate	*96 bpm*
Respiration	*14 rpm*

1. Under care of physician
Yes [X]   No [ ]
Condition: *monitor glycemic control*
monitor blood pressure
monitor blood lipoproteins

2. Hospitalized within the last 5 years
Yes [ ]   No [X]   Reason: _____

3. Has or had the following conditions
diabetes mellitus (DM)
secondary hypertension

4. Current medications
metformin and rosiglitazone (Avandamet)—
antidiabetic combination
irbesartan (Avapro)—antihypertensive, angiotensin-II
antagonist
metolazone (Zaroxolyn)—thiazide-like diuretic
simvastatin (Zocor)—antihyperlipidemic

5. Smokes or uses tobacco products
Yes [ ]   No [X]

6. Is pregnant
Yes [ ]   No [ ]   N/A [X]

MEDICAL HISTORY
Current health problems have only recently been diagnosed. His physician is monitoring the efficacy of the medications he has recently started taking and his efforts at implementing dietary and lifestyle changes. He has met with a dietitian.

DENTAL HISTORY
Until a recent toothache prompted him to make an appointment with the dentist last week, he has not had professional dental hygiene care in over 2 years. Seems unaware of his oral condition, even though his physician has prescribed periodontal assessment and treatment in conjunction with other methods of restoring his overall health.

SOCIAL HISTORY
Lives with his girlfriend and her two children in the house he owns. Works as a computer technician in an electronics store and considers himself a devoted gamer. His goal is to produce his own line of video games.

CHIEF COMPLAINT
Had a temporary restoration placed last week and has scheduled today's appointment as directed by the dentist and his physician. Appears to have a low tolerance to probing subgingivally and once scaling started, he requested local anesthesia.

CURRENT ORAL HYGIENE STATUS
Moderate, generalized calculus
Heavy, generalized plaque biofilm

SUPPLEMENTAL ORAL EXAMINATION FINDINGS
Moderate, generalized bleeding upon probing
Edematous, spongy, sensitive gingival tissues
Right mandibular central incisor exhibits Class I mobility

ADULT CLINICAL EXAMINATION

	1	2	3	4	5	6	7	8	9	10	11	12	13	14	15	16
Probe 2	X															X
Probe 1		324	525	522	224	225	524	323	323	423	325	534	536	735	575	
Probe 1		428	755	665	525	424	423	323	222	522	223	445	525	537	545	
Probe 2	X															X

R / L

	32	31	30	29	28	27	26	25	24	23	22	21	20	19	18	17
Probe 2	X															X
Probe 1		766	635	524	323	323	116	222	312	223	112	213	324	536	656	
Probe 1		644	425	313	212	223	333	322	222	225	211	213	324	424	535	
Probe 2	X															X

Clinically visible carious lesion

Clinically missing tooth

△ Furcation
▲ "Through and through" furcation
Probe 1: Initial probing depth
Probe 2: Probing depth 6 weeks after periodontal therapy

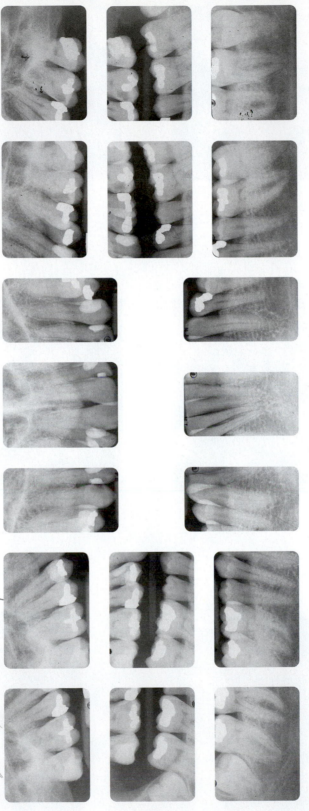

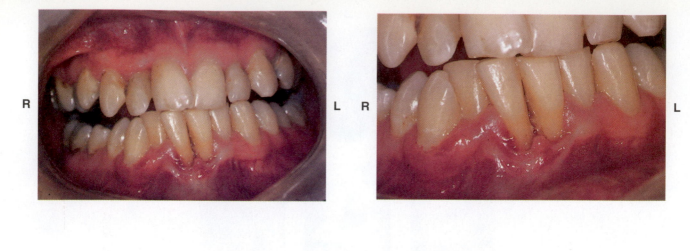

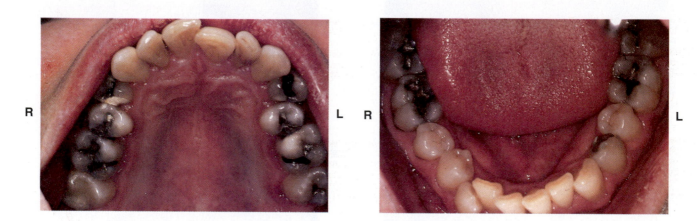

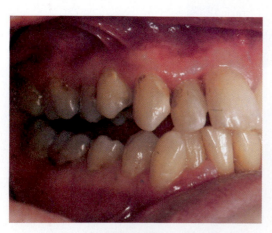

Right side

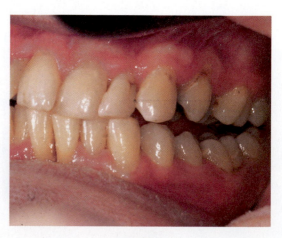

Left side

CASE QUESTIONS

ASSESSING PATIENT CHARACTERISTICS
Basic Level Questions

1. Based on the current American Diabetes Association classification system, this patient has Type 1 diabetes.

   Insulin resistance in the presence of normal insulin production is typical of patients with Type 1 diabetes.
   A. The first statement is true, the second statement is false.
   B. The first statement is false, the second statement is true.
   C. Both statements are true.
   D. Both statements are false.

2. This patient's blood pressure reading at today's appointment indicates
   A. A reading within normal limits
   B. A prehypertensive reading
   C. Stage 1 hypertension
   D. Stage 2 hypertension

3. This patient's body mass index (BMI) puts him at risk for each of the following EXCEPT one. Which one is the EXCEPTION?
   A. Diabetes
   B. Hypertension
   C. Dyslipidemia
   D. Decreased pain threshold
   E. Coronary artery disease

4. Which one of the medications taken by this patient does NOT put him at risk for dry mouth and/or taste disturbances?
   A. Avandamet
   B. Avapro
   C. Zaroxolyn
   D. Zocor

5. Which of the following terms is best applied to the location of the gingival margin in the region of the mandibular central incisors?
   A. Enlarged
   B. Recession
   C. Cratering
   D. Clefting
   E. Hyperplastic

6. Which of the following teeth presents with a temporary restoration?
   A. Maxillary right second molar
   B. Maxillary right first premolar
   C. Maxillary right canine
   D. Maxillary left lateral incisor
   E. Maxillary left canine

Competency Level Questions

7. Each of the following may be considered a contributing etiologic factor for the condition of the gingiva in the region of the mandibular anterior central incisors EXCEPT one. Which one is the EXCEPTION?

    A. Toothbrushing technique
    B. Position of the frenal attachment
    C. Oral dosing of medications
    D. Alignment of the teeth in the arch
    E. Gingival inflammation caused by plaque biofilm

8. The mandibular anterior central incisors are at increased risk for each of the following EXCEPT one. Which one is the EXCEPTION?
    A. Accumulation of biofilm
    B. Sensitivity
    C. Wear
    D. Decay
    E. Trauma

OBTAINING AND INTERPRETING RADIOGRAPHS
Basic Level Questions

9. The most likely cause of the overlapped image of the maxillary left premolar region is
    A. Malaligned teeth
    B. Incorrect horizontal angulation
    C. Excessive vertical angulation
    D. Inadequate coverage of the film with x-ray beam
    E. Poor retention of the film holder by the patient

10. What caused the radiolucent artifact present on the left molar bitewing radiograph?
    A. Accidentally tearing the film packet exposing the film to white light
    B. Bending the film packet when positioning into the film holder
    C. Touching the film with a latex-gloved finger when opening the film packet
    D. Sliding the film out of the film packet too quickly creating static electricity
    E. Positioning the film packet in the oral cavity backwards resulting in a herringbone image

Competency Level Questions

11. Each of the following teeth present with caries radiographically EXCEPT one. Which one is the EXCEPTION?
    A. Maxillary right canine
    B. Maxillary left lateral incisor
    C. Maxillary left first molar
    D. Mandibular left first premolar
    E. Mandibular right first premolar

PLANNING AND MANAGING DENTAL HYGIENE CARE
Basic Level Questions

12. Which of the following is the recommended technique for pain control for scaling this patient's mandibular left quadrant?
    A. Local infiltration
    B. Field block
    C. Nerve block
    D. Supraperiosteal injection
    E. Intraligamentary injection

13. Each of the following specific local injections may be required to provide anesthesia for scaling this patient's maxillary left premolar and molar sextant EXCEPT one. Which one is the EXCEPTION?
    A. Middle superior alveolar nerve block
    B. Posterior superior alveolar nerve block
    C. Greater palatine nerve block
    D. Inferior alveolar nerve block

14. After treatment in a supine position, this patient should be allowed to sit upright for 2 minutes before standing up to avoid which of the following medical emergencies?
    A. Syncope
    B. Diabetic coma
    C. Hypoglycemia
    D. Respiratory difficulty
    E. Anesthesia toxicity

Competency Level Questions

15. Which of the following would be the best choice of local anesthetic for this patient?
    A. Lidocaine HCl 2%
    B. Lidocaine HCl 2% with epinephrine 1:50,000
    C. Lidocaine HCl 2% with epinephrine 1:100,000
    D. Mepivacaine HCl 3%
    E. Bupivacaine HCl 0.5% with epinephrine 1:200,000

PERFORMING PERIODONTAL PROCEDURES
Basic Level Questions

16. Which of the following terms best applies to this patient's periodontal disease status?
    A. Early
    B. Moderate
    C. Advanced
    D. Aggressive
    E. Refractory

17. Which of the following handheld instruments would be the best choice for removing the calculus deposit from the distal surface of the maxillary right molar observed in the radiographs?
    A. Straight shank Gracey 7/8
    B. Rigid Gracey 9/10
    C. Mini Gracey 11/12
    D. Standard series Gracey 15/16
    E. Extended shank Gracey 17/18

Competency Level Questions

18. The distance measured from the cementoenamel junction to the free gingival margin on the facial surface of the mandibular right central incisor is 4 mm. What is the clinical attachment loss in this region?
    A. 2 mm
    B. 4 mm
    C. 6 mm
    D. 8 mm

USING PREVENTIVE AGENTS
Competancy Level Questions

19. Which of the following is the recommended treatment for the brown discolored areas observed on the facial surfaces of the maxillary right anterior teeth?
    A. Scaling with hand instruments
    B. Application of tooth whitening
    C. Topical fluoride application
    D. Polishing with a power-driven instrument
    E. Burnishing with a desensitizing agent

PROVIDING SUPPORTIVE TREATMENT SERVICES
Basic Level Questions

20. Each of the following is a reason to employ selective polishing for this patient EXCEPT one. Which one is the EXCEPTION?
    A. Communicable disease
    B. Areas of demineralized enamel
    C. Cemental caries
    D. Spongy, bleeding gingiva
    E. Probable xerostomia

21. To assist this patient in following the dietary recommendations he most likely received to help manage his medical conditions, each of the following should be reinforced EXCEPT one. Which one is the EXCEPTION?
    A. Eat small, frequent meals and snacks
    B. Monitor intake of carbohydrates
    C. Limit alcohol intake
    D. Consume less fats
    E. Eliminate sucrose

Competency Level Questions

22. Which of the following is the best recommendation for this patient's xerostomia?
    A. Xylitol gum
    B. Saliva substitute
    C. Frequent sips of water
    D. Home fluoride rinses
    E. Limit salt in diet

DEMONSTRATING PROFESSIONAL RESPONSIBILITY
Basic Level Questions

23. Each of the following is applicable and appropriate to approach a discussion with this patient EXCEPT one. Which one is the EXCEPTION?
    A. "Diets high in carbohydrates associated with weight gain also put you at risk for caries."
    B. "Poor plaque control has contributed to the crowding and malalignment of your teeth."
    C. "Uncontrolled diabetes has most likely played a role in the progression of your periodontal disease."
    D. "Maintaining your oral health has the potential to reduce your risk of coronary artery disease."
    E. "Some of the medications you are taking have the potential to reduce salivary flow."

Competency Level Questions

24. Which of the following is the most likely reason this patient's physician has recommended periodontal assessment and treatment?
    A. Improving his periodontal condition may assist this patient with his goal of weight reduction.
    B. Reducing periodontal inflammation may help this patient better control his diabetes.
    C. Nonsurgical periodontal therapy may indirectly help to lower this patient's blood pressure.
    D. Restoring his oral health may eliminate this patient's need for medications.
    E. Eliminating this patient's periodontal disease may reduce his low-density lipoprotein levels and increase his high-density lipoprotein levels.

25. The need for local anesthesia was not determined during the assessment and therefore was not in the treatment plan to which the patient consented. Because the need for local anesthesia arose after the scaling procedure began, the dental hygienist should

A. Use topical anesthesia only at this appointment and secure the patient's written consent for use of local anesthesia at the next appointment.
B. Obtain the patient's verbal permission to administer the anesthesia before continuing with treatment.
C. Sit the patient up in the dental chair to allow him to ask questions regarding anesthesia options and obtain additional written consent.
D. Reschedule the patient after he has had the opportunity to weigh anesthesia options.

SETTING PATIENT GOALS

ESTABLISHING A DENTAL HYGIENE CARE PLAN

To assist this patient in meeting his needs, develop a dental hygiene care plan that establishes a framework within which to help him identify goals for obtaining oral health. In addition to the clinical assessment, a well-prepared dental hygiene care plan should take into account the patient's age, gender, lifestyle, culture, attitudes, health beliefs, and knowledge level. To help link this patient's needs for overall well-being with his oral conditions, and to provide motivation for achieving better health, the following is a partial list of possible deficits based on the Human Needs Conceptual Model to Dental Hygiene Practice. (See the appendix for an explanation of the Human Needs Conceptual Model to Dental Hygiene Practice to help you identify additional unmet needs.) Use this partial list of unmet needs or deficits as a guide in preparing a dental hygiene care plan for this patient. One set of goals and dental hygiene actions/implications has been completed as an example.

Deficit identified in Protection from Health Risks

Due to: overweight, diet, lifestyle
Evidenced by: diabetes, secondary hypertension, multiple medications

Goals: _____

Dental hygiene actions/implications: _____

Deficit identified in Freedom from Head and Neck Pain

Due to: gingival inflammation and periodontal disease
Evidenced by: hypersensitivity to periodontal instrumentation

Goals: *provide comprehensive pain-free, nonsurgical periodontal therapy.*

Dental hygiene actions/implications: *discuss pain control options with the patient; provide information that assists the patient with making an informed decision; together with the patient select the appropriate pain control method; secure patient's consent; initiate pain control; periodically evaluate efficacy of pain control; assess verbal and nonverbal reactions to procedures to determine the need for administration of additional or alternate methods of pain control; perform instrumentation procedures carefully with precise adaptation.*

Deficit identified in Skin and Mucous Membrane Integrity of the Head and Neck

Due to: bacterial plaque accumulation and moderate subgingival calculus
Evidenced by: periodontal disease and subsequent attachment loss

Goals: _____

Dental hygiene actions/implications: _____

Deficit identified in Conceptualization and Problem Solving

Due to: lack of knowledge regarding the interrelationships of oral and general health
Evidenced by: inadequate oral health behaviors

Goals: _____

Dental hygiene actions/implications: _____

Deficit identified in Responsibility for Oral Health

Due to: lack of knowledge regarding oral health condition
Evidenced by: no regular dental hygiene care

Goals: _____

Dental hygiene actions/implications: _____

REFLECTIVE ACTIVITIES

1. **Determine this patient's level on the Learning Ladder** (*Unawareness, Awareness, Self-Interest, Involvement, Action, Habit*) **or decision-making continuum as it pertains to his oral self-care. Then develop a plan for assisting him with moving up through each level in sequence.**

2. **Plan an oral self-care session with this patient where you teach him self-assessment methods for determining the health of the gingiva and the efficacy of dental biofilm infection control. Role-play the implementation of your plan with another student playing the role of the patient.**

3. **Prepare a fact sheet that a dental hygienist may use for sharing information with patients regarding the warning signs for diabetes and the recommendations for testing an individual at risk for the disease.**

REFERENCES

American Academy of Periodontology: Periodontal disease, C-reactive protein and overall health. www.perio.org/consumer/happy-heart.htm. Accessed April 20, 2007.

Cooper MD, Wiechmann L: *Essentials of Dental Hygiene. Clinical Skills.* Upper Saddle River, NJ: Prentice Hall, 2006, pp. 30–36, 52–56.

Gurenlian JR: Overweight and obesity: A challenging eating disorder. *Access,* 8(16), 46–49, 2002.

Hupp JR, Williams TP, Firriolo FJ: *Dental Clinical Advisor.* St. Louis: Mosby (Elsevier), 2006, pp. 72–75.

Johnson ON, Thomson EM: *Essentials of Dental Radiography for Dental Assistants and Hygienists,* 8th ed. Upper Saddle River, NJ: Prentice Hall, 2007, pp. 121–122.

Lyle DM: Diabetes mellitus. *RDH,* 23(3), 54–56, 88, 2003.

Malamed SF: *Handbook of Local Anesthesia,* 5th ed. St. Louis: Mosby (Elsevier), 2004, pp. 55–75, 189–190, 275–276.

Mealey BL, Rose LF: Periodontal inflammation and diabetes mellitus. Recognizing the relationship. *Contemporary Oral Hygiene,* 7(1), 23–29, 2007.

Moritz AJ, Mealey BL: Periodontal disease, insulin resistance, and diabetes mellitus. *Grand Rounds in Oral-Systemic Medicine,* 1(2), 13–20, 2006.

Nield-Gehrig JS, Willmann DE: *Foundations of Periodontics for the Dental Hygienist,* 2nd ed. Philadelphia: Lippincott Williams & Wilkins, 2008, p. 168.

Palmer CA: *Diet and Nutrition in Oral Health,* 2nd ed. Upper Saddle River, NJ: Prentice Hall, 2007, pp. 87–95.

Perry DA, Beemsterboer PL: *Periodontology for the Dental Hygienist,* 3rd ed. St. Louis: Saunders (Elsevier), 2007, pp. 105–106, 128–131.

Pickett FA, Terezhalmy GT: *Lippincott Williams & Wilkins' Dental Drug Reference with Clinical Implications.* Baltimore: Lippincott Williams & Wilkins, 2006, pp. 477–478, 539–540, 681–682, 691–692.

Spolarich AE: The top most commonly prescribed medications for 2005. *Access,* 20(10), 39–49, 2006.

Stefanac SJ, Nesbit SP: *Treatment Planning in Dentistry,* 2nd ed. St. Louis: Mosby (Elsevier), 2007, pp. 79–80.

Wilkins EM: *Clinical Practice of the Dental Hygienist,* 9th ed. Philadelphia: Lippincott Williams & Wilkins, 2005, pp. 208, 378, 592–597, 726–730, 1043–1045, 1072–1089.

CASE O

Eileen Olds

SITUATION

Eileen Olds works part time as a paralegal in the community legal services office, which provides assistance to the poor, elderly, minorities, and middle-income families. Her diagnosis of chronic renal failure progressed to end stage renal disease (ESRD) and 9 months ago she began dialysis. She is receiving hemodialysis at a health care facility on Monday, Wednesday, and Friday afternoons each week. She has presented today to restore her oral health, to get on the waiting list for a kidney transplant.

LEARNING GOALS

Following integration of core scientific concepts and application of dental hygiene theory to the care of this patient, you will be able to

1. **Assess patient characteristics.**
   A. Apply correct terminology to oral examination findings.
   B. Distinguish between normal anatomy and pathology found upon oral examination.
   C. Describe the appearance of gingival tissues using appropriate terms.
   D. Determine the nature of oral conditions upon visual inspection.
   E. Utilize appropriate techniques when measuring blood pressure on the medically compromised patient.

2. **Obtain and interpret radiographs.**
   A. Identify normal radiographic anatomy.
   B. Interpret radiographic findings.
   C. Identify the cause of radiographic error.
   D. Examine radiographic images for possible manifestation of systemic disease.

3. **Plan and manage dental hygiene care.**
   A. Investigate possible contraindications to treatment of the medically compromised patient.
   B. Plan appointment schedule for nonsurgical periodontal therapy for the patient receiving dialysis.
   C. Identify adverse oral effects of medications taken by the medically compromised patient.
   D. Recommend oral self-care aids based on patient needs.

   E. Identify oral signs of systemic disease and its treatment modalities.
   F. Identify the interrelationship between ESRD, its treatment, and oral health.

4. **Perform periodontal procedures.**
   A. Select the appropriate instruments for periodontal debridement.
   B. Predict outcomes of nonsurgical periodontal therapy.
   C. Identify etiology of probe reading changes observed at 6-week reevaluation following initial therapy.

5. **Use preventive agents.**
   A. Recognize contraindications of treatment modalities and preventive products for the medically compromised patient.
   B. Recommend the appropriate oral self-care agent for home use for the medically compromised patient.

6. **Provide supportive treatment services.**
   A. Determine what conditions prompt the use of the pulp vitality test.

7. **Demonstrate professional responsibility.**
   A. Provide the patient with correct information regarding the use of oral self-care products.
   B. Differentiate between ethical responsibility and contraindications to treat the medically compromised individual.

MEDICALLY COMPROMISED PATIENT—*Eileen Olds*
PATIENT HISTORY SYNOPSIS

Age	*50 years*	
Gender	*female*	
Height	*5' 7"*	
Weight	*132 lbs.*	

VITAL STATISTICS

Blood Pressure	*154/102 mm Hg*
Pulse Rate	*74 bpm*
Respiration	*14 rpm*

1. Under care of physician
   Yes [X]   No [ ]   Condition: *end stage renal disease (ESRD)*

2. Hospitalized within the last 5 years
   Yes [X]   No [ ]   Reason: *surgical placement of arteriovenous shunt in right forearm for dialysis*

3. Has or had the following conditions
   chronic renal insufficiency
   chronic renal failure
   renal osteodystrophy
   secondary hyperparathyroidism
   hypertension
   anemia

4. Current medications
   enalapril maleate (Vasotec)—antihypertensive, ACE inhibitor
   losartan potassium (Cozaar)—antihypertensive, angiotensin-II antagonist
   furosemide (Lasix)—loop diuretic
   epoetin alfa (Procrit)—erythropoietin
   fluoxetine (Prozac)—antidepressant
   calcitriol (Calcijex)—fat-soluble vitamin D
   calcium carbonate (Calcichew)—calcium-containing phosphate binder
   heparin (Hep-Lock)—anticoagulant (IV administration during dialysis only)

5. Smokes or uses tobacco products
   Yes [ ]   No [X]

6. Is pregnant
   Yes [ ]   No [X]   N/A [ ]

MEDICAL HISTORY
Hemodialysis for the past 9 months. Currently undergoing tests to determine if she is a candidate for a kidney transplant. Has dietary phosphate and salt restrictions and chews ice to manage her restricted oral fluid intake.

DENTAL HISTORY
Oral health status screened by the medical transplant team and deemed in poor condition. Her last dental hygiene appointment was 5 years ago. Has recently started using tartar control toothpaste stating that she wanted to remove the deposits on her teeth.

SOCIAL HISTORY
Kidney disease has significantly altered her lifestyle, and although Medicare pays for 80% of her expenses for dialysis, she is overwhelmed with the enormous cost of her disease. Her physician prescribed an antidepressant to help with depression.

CHIEF COMPLAINT
Wants a kidney transplant and was told that her oral health must be improved to qualify for a place on the wait list for a donated organ.

CURRENT ORAL HYGIENE STATUS
Heavy, generalized calculus
Heavy, generalized plaque biofilm

SUPPLEMENTAL ORAL EXAMINATION FINDINGS
Moderate, generalized bleeding upon probing
Moderate xerostomia

ADULT CLINICAL EXAMINATION

	1	2	3	4	5	6	7	8	9	10	11	12	13	14	15	16
Probe 2	X	1086	X	524	X	323	324	514	614	323	314	414	425	636	738	X
Probe 1		1087		624		324	425	626	726	523	446	323	326	527	748	

(F / P)

	1	2	3	4	5	6	7	8	9	10	11	12	13	14	15	16
Probe 1	X	976	X	444	X	333	333	535	755	755	335	535	556	757	568	X
Probe 2		866		434		323	323	434	535	322	335	423	445	645	547	

R   **L**

	32	31	30	29	28	27	26	25	24	23	22	21	20	19	18	17
Probe 2	X	857	744	545	555	434	434	434	434	334	323	535	645	549	968	758
Probe 1		977	855	757	774	656	311	211	212	223	324	543	657	758	1069	9710

(L / F)

	32	31	30	29	28	27	26	25	24	23	22	21	20	19	18	17
Probe 1	X	729	1024	726	625	545	524	525	625	735	525	636	524	529	739	738
Probe 2		627	823	525	523	343	423	313	323	524	424	524	423	417	727	627

Legend:
- Clinically visible carious lesion
- Clinically missing tooth
- △ Furcation
- ▲ "Through and through" furcation
- Probe 1: Initial probing depth
- Probe 2: Probing depth 6 weeks after periodontal therapy

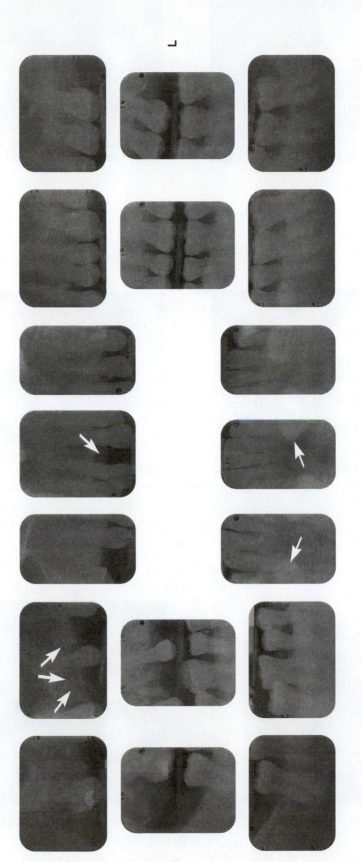

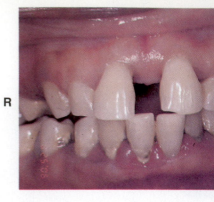

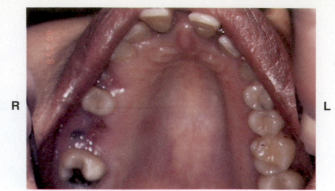

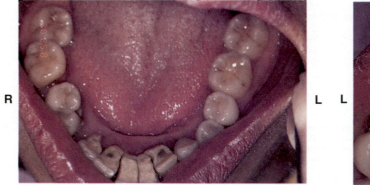

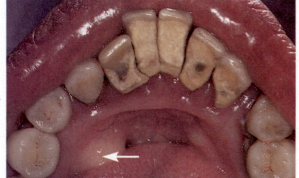

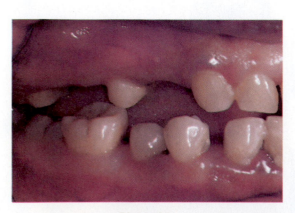

Right side

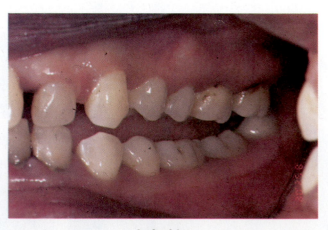

Left side

CASE QUESTIONS

ASSESSING PATIENT CHARACTERISTICS
Basic Level Questions

1. Which of the following terms applies to the space between the maxillary central incisors?
   A. Centric relation
   B. Open bite
   C. Diastema
   D. Parafunctional
   E. Fremitus

2. The clinical observation noted in the mandibular sublingual region near the left canine and first premolar (arrow) that is hard when palpated is most likely a
   A. Torus
   B. Polyp
   C. Mucocele
   D. Cyst
   E. Ranula

3. Which of the following best describes the papillary gingiva between the mandibular right central and lateral incisors?
   A. Knife-like
   B. Cratered
   C. Blunted
   D. Rolled
   E. Bulbous

4. What is the clinical observation contributing to the appearance of the lingual surfaces of the mandibular anterior teeth?
   A. Developmental anomalies
   B. Periodontal splinting
   C. Composite restorations
   D. Dental calculus
   E. Hypercementosis

Competency Level Questions

5. Which of the following blood pressure cuffs and area to which it is applied is correct for taking this patient's blood pressure?
   A. Child-size cuff applied to the left arm
   B. Regular adult-size cuff applied to the left arm
   C. Regular adult-size cuff applied to the right arm
   D. Adult thigh-size cuff applied to the left leg
   E. Adult thigh-size cuff applied to the right leg

OBTAINING AND INTERPRETING RADIOGRAPHS
Basic Level Questions

6. What is the most likely interpretation of the oval-shaped radiolucency observed between the maxillary right and left central incisors (arrow)?
   A. Infraorbital foramen
   B. Incisive foramen
   C. Incisive fossa
   D. Canine fossa
   E. Nasal fossa

7. What is the most likely interpretation of the round radiopacities observed near the teeth roots of the mandibular right and left canine and premolar regions (arrows)?
   A. Osteosclerosis
   B. Hypercementosis
   C. Mandibular tori
   D. Condensing osteitis
   E. Fingerprint artifacts

8. What is the most likely interpretation of the findings observed in the maxillary right posterior region? (arrows)
   A. Retained root tips
   B. Supernumerary teeth
   C. Microdont molars
   D. Implants
   E. Retention pins

Competency Level Questions

9. The lack of image contrast and overall gray appearance of this patient's radiographs may have resulted when the film packets were stored under each of the following conditions EXCEPT one. Which one is the EXCEPTION?
   A. Stray radiation
   B. High humidity
   C. Excessive heat
   D. Physical pressure
   E. Long wavelength light

10. The slight ground glass appearance to the mandibular posterior regions and the disappearance of the lamina dura and narrowing of the pulp chambers observed on this patient's radiographs is most likely the result of
    A. Lack of professional dental hygiene care
    B. Adverse effects of medications
    C. Trauma from her habit of chewing on ice
    D. Renal osteodystrophy
    E. Significant calculus at the base of deep pockets

PLANNING AND MANAGING DENTAL HYGIENE CARE
Basic Level Questions

11. Each of the following must be discussed with this patient's nephrologist before quadrant scaling EXCEPT one. Which one is the EXCEPTION?
    A. Need for prophylactic premedication
    B. Determination of blood clotting time
    C. Adequacy of salivary flow
    D. Assessment of vital signs
    E. Pain management doses and contraindications

12. Quadrant scaling appointments for this patient should be scheduled in the mornings, before her afternoon dialysis session.

    An appointment for extraction of the fractured teeth should be made on Saturday morning.
    A. The first sentence is true, the second sentence is false.
    B. The first sentence is false, the second sentence is true.
    C. Both sentences are true.
    D. Both sentences are false.

13. Which of the medications prescribed for this patient does NOT increase the risk of dry mouth and taste disturbances?
    A. Vasotec
    B. Cozaar
    C. Lasix
    D. Procrit
    E. Prozac

14. Which one of the following would be the least helpful recommendation for assisting this patient with her goal of improved oral health?
    A. Power toothbrush
    B. Interproximal brush
    C. Dental floss
    D. Toothpick-in-holder
    E. Floss threader

Competency Level Questions

15. The pale appearance of the gingiva and lessening demarcation of the mucogingival junction may be attributed to
    A. Anemia
    B. Hypertension
    C. ESRD
    D. Dialysis
    E. Periodontal disease

16. Even with improved self-care, this patient's medical conditions put her at an increased risk for each of the following EXCEPT one. Which one is the EXCEPTION?
    A. Development of halitosis
    B. Increase in dental calculus accumulation
    C. Rampant decay
    D. Demineralization of alveolar bone
    E. Increased gingival bleeding

PERFORMING PERIODONTAL PROCEDURES
Basic Level Questions

17. Which of the following is the best choice to begin initial periodontal debridement in the mandibular right quadrant?
    A. Sonic scaler
    B. Ultrasonic scaler
    C. Sickle scaler
    D. Chisel scaler
    E. Universal curet

18. Which of the following ultrasonic instrument tip designs would be the best choice for initial periodontal debridement of the lingual surfaces of the mandibular anterior teeth?
    A. Beavertail tip
    B. Standard-diameter universal tip
    C. Standard-diameter triple bend tip
    D. Slim-diameter straight tip
    E. Slim-diameter curved tip

Competency Level Questions

19. Which of the following is NOT a likely adverse outcome of scaling this patient's mandibular anterior teeth?
    A. Tooth mobility
    B. Root sensitivity
    C. Gingival recession
    D. Risk of tooth fractures
    E. Longer appearance of the teeth

20. Which of the following is the most likely explanation for the mandibular anterior region probe reading changes seen at the 6-week reevaluation appointment?
    A. Patient failed to stay motivated to follow oral self-care instructions given at initial appointment.
    B. Complex medical conditions that compromise this patient's immune system have limited the healing process.
    C. Rapid reaccumulation of dental calculus after the initial scaling appointment has most likely prevented tissue shrinkage.
    D. Probing was done with greater than 10 to 20 g of pressure causing the probe to penetrate the junctional epithelium.
    E. Heavy calculus limited access to the base of the pocket for accurate probe readings at the initial appointment.

USING PREVENTIVE AGENTS
Basic Level Questions

21. Which of the following would be approved for use in treating this patient?
    A. Air-powder polishing with sodium bicarbonate to remove stain
    B. Controlled-release local delivery of tetracycline-containing fibers or doxycycline hyclate gel to periodontal pockets not responding to treatment
    C. Sodium fluoride varnish application for prevention of caries and management of tooth sensitivity
    D. Subgingival oral irrigation with saline solution for treatment of edematous gingival tissues
    E. Aspirin or ibuprofen for postscaling pain management

Competency Level Questions

22. Which of the following mouth rinses would be the best to add to this patient's long-term daily oral self-care routine?
    A. Listerine® Antiseptic (essential oils)
    B. PerioGard® (chlorhexidine gluconate)
    C. Biotene Mouthwash (lactoperoxidase enzyme)
    D. Scope (cetylpyridinium chloride)
    E. Oral-B Fluorinse (0.2% sodium fluoride)

PROVIDING SUPPORTIVE TREATMENT SERVICES
Competency Level Questions

23. The pulp vitality test may play a role in diagnosing the condition affecting which of the following teeth?
    A. Maxillary right first molar and first premolar
    B. Maxillary left and mandibular right second molars
    C. Maxillary right and left central incisors
    D. Mandibular right and left central and lateral incisors
    E. Mandibular right first molar and first premolar

DEMONSTRATING PROFESSIONAL RESPONSIBILITY
Basic Level Questions

24. Which of the following should be communicated to this patient regarding her use of tartar control toothpaste?
    A. Tartar control toothpaste will help prevent additional buildup of subgingival dental calculus.
    B. Tartar control toothpaste will help prevent additional buildup of supragingival dental calculus.
    C. Tartar control toothpaste will help remove the subgingival dental calculus formed on her teeth.
    D. Tartar control toothpaste will help remove the supragingival dental calculus formed on her teeth.

Competency Level Questions

25. This patient has an increased risk for contracting hepatitis B.

    If the dental hygienist has not received the hepatitis B vaccine, he/she can legally refuse to treat this patient.
    A. The first sentence is true, the second sentence is false.
    B. The first sentence is false, the second sentence is true.
    C. Both sentences are true.
    D. Both sentences are false.

SETTING PATIENT GOALS

ESTABLISHING A DENTAL HYGIENE CARE PLAN

To assist this patient in meeting her needs, develop a dental hygiene care plan that establishes a framework within which to help her identify goals for obtaining oral health. In addition to the clinical assessment, a well-prepared dental hygiene care plan should take into account the patient's age, gender, lifestyle, culture, attitudes, health beliefs, and knowledge level. To help link this patient's needs for overall well-being with her oral conditions, and to provide motivation for achieving better health, the following is a partial list of possible deficits based on the Human Needs Conceptual Model to Dental Hygiene Practice. (See the appendix for an explanation of the Human Needs Conceptual Model to Dental Hygiene Practice to help you identify additional unmet needs.) Use this partial list of unmet needs or deficits as a guide in preparing a dental hygiene care plan for this patient. One set of goals and dental hygiene actions/implications has been completed as an example.

Deficit identified in Protection from Health Risks

Due to: professional oral treatment potential to exacerbate medical condition
Evidenced by: life-threatening diseases and multiple medications

Goals: _____

Dental hygiene actions/implications: _____

Deficit identified in Skin and Mucous Membrane Integrity of Head and Neck

Due to: bacterial biofilm accumulation; lack of regular professional care
Evidenced by: periodontal disease

Goals: *improve periodontal status to obtain access to the organ donor wait list.*

Dental hygiene actions/implications: *educate patient on the disease process; assess patient's ability to perform oral self-care recommendations; plan, implement, and evaluate nonsurgical periodontal therapy.*

Deficit identified in Biologically Sound Dentition

Due to: lack of functioning dentition on the right side
Evidenced by: badly decayed, broken down maxillary teeth; supereruption of the opposing mandibular teeth

Goals: _____

Dental hygiene actions/implications: _____

Deficit identified in Conceptualization and Problem Solving

Due to: lack of knowledge regarding oral disease processes
Evidenced by: misconception of the action of tartar control toothpaste

Goals: _____

Dental hygiene actions/implications: _____

REFLECTIVE ACTIVITIES

1. Currently in the United States there are over 95,000 patients on the wait list for an organ donation. Nearly 4,000 new patients are added to this list each month, and every day 17 people die while waiting for a transplant. Prepare a presentation for your class or other group that provides information to enlighten and inspire your listeners to become organ donors.

2. Together with a partner prepare and present for the class a role-play scenario between the dental hygienist and this patient in which you explain the interrelationship between the patient's medical conditions and her oral health. Each student partner group should choose a different topic to role-play. Examples of topics include the importance of regular professional dental hygiene treatment; oral self-care products to use/avoid and why; what causes halitosis/xerostomia and the steps she can take to manage these; certain medications used in dental hygiene treatment that she must avoid; and the oral manifestations of her medical condition/treatment.

3. Organize a training group with your classmates to participate in the next National Kidney Foundation's Kidney Walk for dialysis patients, organ transplant recipients, donor families, living donors, the medical communities, and the general public to come together to celebrate life and to support the foundation's mission. Go to www.kidney.org to find out when the next event will be held in your area.

REFERENCES

Bots CP, Pooterman JHG, Brand HS, Kalsbeek H, Van Amerongen BM, Veerman ECI, Nieuw Amerongen AV: The oral health status of dentate patients with chronic renal failure undergoing dialysis therapy. *Oral Diseases*, 12(2), 176–180, 2006.

Darby ML, Walsh MM: *Dental Hygiene Theory and Practice*, 2nd ed. St. Louis: Saunders (Elsevier), 2003, p. 107.

Gudapati A, Ahmend P, Rada R: Dental management of patients with renal failure. *General Dentistry*, 50(6), 508–510, 2002.

Haveles EB: *Applied Pharmacology for the Dental Hygiene*, 1st, 5th eds., St. Louis: Mosby (Elsevier), 2007, pp. 287–303.

Ibsen OAC, Phelan JA: *Oral Pathology for the Dental Hygienist*, 4th ed. St. Louis: Saunders (Elsevier), 2004, pp. 59–60.

Johnson ON, Thomson EM: *Essentials of Dental Radiography for Dental Assistants and Hygienists*, 8th ed. Upper Saddle River, NJ: Prentice Hall, 2007, pp. 91, 225, 273–274, 277–279.

Kerr AR: Update on renal disease for the dental practitioner. *Oral Surgery Oral Medicine Oral Pathology Oral Radiology Endodontology*, 92(1), 9–16, 2001.

Kho HS, Lee SW, Chung SC, Kim YK: Oral manifestations and salivary flow rate, pH, and buffer capacity in patients with end-stage renal disease undergoing hemodialysis. *Oral Surgery Oral Medicine Oral Pathology Oral Radiology Endodontology*, 88(3), 316–319, 1999.

Klassen JT: The dental health status of dialysis patients. *Journal of the Canadian Dental Association*, 68(1), 34–38, 2002.

Knevel RJM: Is your knowledge up-to-date? *International Journal of Dental Hygiene*, 1(3), 183, 2003.

National Kidney Foundation: 25 facts about organ donation and transplantation.http://www.kidney.org/news/newsroom/fsitem.cfm?id=30. Accessed April 30, 2007.

Nield-Gehrig JS: *Fundamentals of Periodontal Instrumentation and Advanced Root Instrumentation*, 5th ed. Baltimore: Lippincott Williams & Wilkins, 2004, p. 554.

Nield-Gehrig JS, Willmann DE: *Foundations of Periodontics for the Dental Hygienist*, 2nd ed. Baltimore: Lippincott Williams & Wilkins, 2008, pp. 147–148.

Pickett FA, Terezhamlmy GT: *Lippincott Williams & Wilkins' Dental Drug Reference with Clinical Implications*. Baltimore: Lippincott Williams & Wilkins, 2006, pp. 375–376, 381–382, 418–419, 431–432, 514–515.

Proctor R, Kumar N, Stein A, Moles D, Porter S: Oral and dental aspects of chronic renal failure. *Journal of Dental Research*, 84(4), 199–208, 2005.

Rethman J: Mouthrinse table. A listing of therapeutic and cosmetic mouthrinses. *Dimensions of Dental Hygiene*, 5(4), 34–35, 2007.

Thomas C: Transplanted. *RDH*, 24(2), 76–81, 2004.

White SC, Pharoah MJ: *Oral Radiology. Principles and Interpretation*, 5th ed. St. Louis: Mosby (Elsevier), 2004, pp. 362, 492–495.

Wilkins EM: *Clinical Practice of the Dental Hygienist*, 9th ed. Philadelphia: Lippincott Williams & Wilkins, 2005, pp. 134, 279–280, 618–619, 943–944.

Human Needs Conceptual Model to Dental Hygiene Practice

Dental hygiene care must meet the needs of the whole patient. Oral health needs cannot be separated from the total health of the patient. In fact, a patient's attitude, lifestyle, culture, and health beliefs are often interrelated with oral health. Because a perceived need often motivates the patient to action, the Human Needs Conceptual Model to Dental Hygiene Practice[1] is one way to assist with identifying the patient's needs through the identification of deficits in the following eight areas.

- **Freedom from Health Risks**—The need to avoid medical contraindications related to dental hygiene care.
- **Freedom from Head and Neck Pain**—The need to be exempt from physical discomfort in the head and neck area.
- **Freedom from Stress**—The need to feel safe and to be free from fear and emotional discomfort in the oral healthcare environment, and to receive appreciation, attention, and respect.
- **Skin and Mucous Membrane Integrity of the Head and Neck**—The need to have an intact and functioning covering of the person's head and neck area, including the oral mucous membranes and gingivae, which defend against harmful microbes, provide sensory information, resist injurious substances and trauma, and reflect adequate nutrition.
- **Biologically Sound Dentition**—The need for intact teeth and restorations that defend against harmful microbes, provide for adequate function, and reflect appropriate nutrition and diet.
- **Conceptualization and Problem Solving**—The need to grasp ideas and abstractions to make sound judgments about one's oral health.
- **Responsibility for Oral Health**—The need for accountability for one's oral health as a result of interaction between one's motivation, physical capability, and social environment.
- **Wholesome Facial Image**—The need to feel satisfied with one's oral-facial features and breath.

Some of the patient needs, called deficits, are identified in each of the cases. The cause of the deficit is identified by the presence, or evidence of, a condition or sign or symptom. For example, a patient with gingival attachment loss of 4 to 6 mm (evidence) would have a deficit in Skin and Mucous Membrane Integrity of Head and Neck (one of the eight areas identified by the Human Needs Conceptual Model to Dental Hygiene Practice) caused by (due to) the presence of bacterial plaque accumulation. This model is presented here as the basis of organizing the comprehensive data gathered in the assessment phase of dental hygiene care planning. The purpose of organizing data in this manner is to provide the student with a systematic method for developing a dental hygiene care plan that integrates the patient's needs, and assists with strategies that lead the patient to meeting these needs.

---

[1] Reprinted from M. L. Darby and M. L. Walsh, *Dental Hygiene Theory and Practice*, 2nd ed., p. 23, copyright 2003, with permission from Elsevier.

Answers and Rationales

CASE A PEDIATRIC PATIENT MAYA PATEL

1.
   A Perikymata refers to horizontal developmental lines seen on the facial surface of anterior teeth and is not evident here.

   B Enamel hypoplasia appears as pitting in the enamel surface and is not evident in this patient.

   C Depending on the stage, fluorosis appears as parchment-white spots, lines, or as a white "snow capping" along the incisal edges of anterior teeth and is not evident in this patient.

   (D) The scalloped appearance of the incisal edges of the anterior teeth is characteristic of mamelons, developmental lobes found on the incisal edges of newly erupted teeth.

   E Attrition appears as the wearing away of the incisal edge as a result of contact with the teeth of the opposing arch. In fact, over time, this contact may result in the attrition of the mamelons.

2.
   A,B Normal respiratory rate for children at age 9 years can range from 18 to 20 rpm.

   (C) Normal resting pulse rate for children at age 9 years can range from 70 to 100 bpm.

   D This patient's pulse rate of 110 bpm indicates a higher than normal range for children at age 9 years.

   E Normal blood pressure readings for children at age 9 years can range from 95 to 105/57 to 65 mm Hg.

3.
   A The hard tissue appearance of the erupting tooth indicates that this finding is not an aphthous ulcer. Additional indicators for identifying an aphthous ulcer include a red (erythematous) halo surrounding a yellowish-white area of irritation and pain.

   B A mandibular torus appears in varying sizes as a bony outgrowth on the lingual surface of the mandibular arch. A mandibular torus would not appear to protrude through the soft tissues of the dental arch.

   C,D The radiographs confirm the erupting mandibular left first premolar and not the presence of a developmental cyst or a retained root tip.

   (E) The cusp of the mandibular left first premolar appears to be erupting into its appropriate position in the arch. The radiographic appearance of this area confirms this clinical assessment.

4.
   (A) The dorsal surface of this patient's tongue appears to have a yellow coating indicating a need for oral self-care instruction in tongue cleaning.

   B A fissured tongue occurs infrequently in children, and is often considered a condition of aging.

   C A coated tongue should not be mistaken for a disease state such as lymphangioma, which would manifest in enlarged lymphoid aggregates. Lymphangioma appears as a raised yellow-pink swelling frequently located on the lateral posterior of the tongue.

   D,E This patient's tongue does not appear to be enlarged (macroglossia) or ulcerated.

5. A,B,C,D Xerostomia, taste changes, increased anxiety, and sore throat are all possible adverse effects of Proventil HFA.

E Gingival bleeding is a result of bacterial plaque accumulation and is not a side effect of Singulair or Proventil HFA.

6. A,C,E The incisive foramen, nasal fossae, and median palatine suture would all appear radiolucent.

B This radiopaque horizontal band represents the dense, bony structure of the hard palate.

D Although the dense, bony structure of the nasal septum would appear radiopaque, it is imaged vertically between the paired oval radiolucent nasal cavities.

7. A Although there is a possibility that this patient may experience an asthma attack during treatment, choosing to expose a panoramic radiograph instead of intraoral films will neither increase nor decrease this risk.

B Both the panoramic and intraoral radiographs would most likely be exposed with the patient in an upright position. Additionally, there is nothing in this patient's health history indicating that she cannot be placed in a supine or semi-supine position during dental hygiene treatment.

C This patient has a hypersensitive gag reflex that most likely made it difficult to place a film packet intraorally.

D The pairing of fast film with intensifying screens allows panoramic radiographs to use a significantly lower dose of radiation to image the teeth and supporting structures. However, this fact is not the reason a panoramic radiograph was prescribed. Instead, the panoramic radiograph enabled the clinician to produce diagnostic images while managing the conditions and behaviors with which this patient presented.

E This patient's anxious state indicates that she would most likely be nervous of all treatment, including both intraoral and panoramic radiographs. Either procedure would require a thorough explanation and demonstration to gain patient confidence and cooperation.

8. A When an object is positioned outside of the panoramic focal trough, or the imaginary zone of sharpness, the object will not be imaged on the film. The natural tilt of the anterior teeth in the arches sometimes places the apices of these teeth outside the focal trough, in this case, causing the tooth roots to be distorted and appear short on the film.

B The concept of the focal trough and the resulting phenomenon of panoramic imaging should not be mistaken for shortened teeth roots due to external physiologic resorption or incomplete root formation.

C The root(s) of an erupting tooth continues to develop and calcify after the crown appears in the oral cavity. During this stage of development, the apical foramen of a tooth with incomplete roots will appear widened at the apex. The radiolucency of the dental sac is often visible as well. Whereas several other teeth such as the mandibular premolars exhibit this stage of development, the mandibular incisors do not. Instead, the incisors appear shorter than normal, as if cut off. This appearance is the result of the teeth roots being located outside the panoramic focal trough.

D Microdontia refers to a tooth that develops a smaller size than normal. The crowns of the mandibular anterior teeth appear normal and the roots of these teeth appear to be of normal width. The shorter than normal length of the roots is the result of the panoramic imagining concept where these teeth roots were located outside the panoramic focal trough and therefore did not image onto the film.

E Directing the vertical angulation of the x-ray beam incorrectly may result in a foreshortened or elongated image on an intraoral radiograph. However, the panoramic x-ray machine has a PID in a fixed position, which is correct for producing a diagnostic image. The vertical angulation cannot be changed.

9.   A Based on this patient's health history, an asthma attack is a likely occurrence. Although symptoms vary with the patient, rapid breathing and/or shortness of breath may indicate a possible attack. Additionally, difficulty talking and stiffness that may be due to tightening neck muscles indicate signs that an attack is eminent.

(B) This patient's culture should not be expected to predispose her to display these physical symptoms of anxiety, shortness of breath, and possible impending asthma attack.

C This patient has indicated nervousness regarding dental treatment. The nervous patient typically presents with an increased pulse rate, dry mouth, and shortness of breath.

D Symptoms of nervousness and increased anxiety are possible adverse effects of Proventil HFA.

10.   A A tray that is too large may impinge on the soft tissue in the back of the oral cavity, exciting a gag reflex. Trying the tray in the mouth before loading with impression material will allow for the selection of a comfortable size.

B,C Concentration on controlled breathing can help the patient control a gag reflex. Humming and deep breathing exercises can assist in maintaining an airway to prevent a gag reflex.

(D) Pressing down on the anterior region of the tray first when seating in the mouth will most likely cause excess impression material to accumulate in the posterior region and initiate a gag reflex. The tray should be seated by pressing down on the posterior region first.

E The patient is more likely to cooperate with the procedure when she knows what to expect. Additionally, a confident operator is more likely to instill confidence and trust in the patient.

11.   A Oral rinses do not debride the tongue.

B Tongue scraping, although often recommended, may be more difficult for a child of this age level and manual dexterity.

(C) Brushing the tongue is the recommended daily oral hygiene instruction for this patient.

D Oral irrigation is recommended for cleansing subgingivally.

E Chewing sugar-free gum with xylitol after meals has been shown to reduce levels of *Streptococcus mutans* and promote remineralization of potential carious lesions, but will not remove microorganisms from the tongue.

12.   (A) Show-tell-do is the simplest and most effective way to ease apprehension in all patients who appear nervous of treatment procedures.

B Oral sedation may be an extreme measure for managing this patient. Additionally, adding another drug to this child's current medications may not be prudent.

C Papoose board restriction is used to control physical movements for a patient who may be spastic or unruly.

D,E Hypnosis and biofeedback are management techniques generally used for adult dental phobic patients.

13.   A Premedicating a patient before oral prophylaxis is prudent when there is risk of developing infective endocarditis. Nothing in this patient's health history indicates the need for antibiotic premedication.

B Although her pulse rate is rapid, this patient's other vital signs are within normal ranges. Nothing in her health history would necessitate that vital signs be continuously monitored during treatment.

C When uncontrolled bleeding is a risk factor, a recent prothrombin time can help determine whether it is safe to continue with dental hygiene treatment. Nothing in this patient's health history indicates the need for this test.

D The emergency response anticipated is an acute asthma attack. Having a history of past dental experiences, at age 9, it is highly unlikely that this patient would be put any more at ease by the physical presence of her mother in the treatment room.

(E) Albuterol is often administered in an acute asthmatic attack. This patient has a prescription for albuterol as the drug Proventil HFA, which is administered using a metered-dose inhaler. Patients with asthma should be instructed to bring their inhalers with them to the dental hygiene appointment. The inhaler should be placed on the bracket table ready for emergency use.

14. A,B,C Given this patient's health history, the breathing difficulty is most likely the result of an asthma attack. The clinician should discontinue treatment and provide verbal reassurance to this patient.

(D) The difficulty in breathing is most likely a symptom of an asthma attack. The Trendelenberg position with the feet elevated 10 to 15 degrees to increase blood flow to the brain is better suited to a situation involving vasodepressor syncope and is contraindicated in this situation. The patient should be placed in a comfortable position to ease breathing which almost always involves sitting, with the arms forward.

E Given this patient's health history, an asthma attack may become evident, at which time a bronchodilator should be administered.

15. A *Streptococcus salivaris* is usually found in high proportions on the tongue and in the saliva and is less concentrated on the teeth.

(B) These three species of bacteria have strong association in the etiology of gingivitis observed in this patient.

C *Fusobacterium nucleatum* and *Prevotella intermedia* are strongly associated with chronic periodontitis.

D *Streptococcus mutans* and lactobaccilli are the etiologic bacteria in dental caries.

E *Actinobacillus actinomycetemcomitans* has a strong association in the etiology of aggressive periodontitis.

16. A The use of the ultrasonic scaler is contraindicated for this patient with asthma. Additionally, the large pulp chambers of primary teeth and newly erupted permanent teeth would also contraindicate using the ultrasonic scaler.

B,D The design characteristics of sickle scalers with pointed tips, triangular working ends, and straight lateral surfaces make these instruments a less desirable choice for instrumentation subgingivally.

C Area-specific curets are more often the instruments of choice for accessing the root surfaces in periodontal pockets. Multiple instruments would be required to complete the whole mouth.

(E) The rounded toe, curved back, and complex shank of the universal curet allows for adaptation near the gingival margin and when necessary, subgingival instrumentation in shallow sulci, throughout the entire mouth without having to stop and change instruments when progressing to different regions.

17. A The right maxillary primary first molar presents with caries and the left maxillary primary first molar presents with a restoration. Additionally, according to the radiographic interpretation, each of these teeth will be exfoliated soon. The mandibular primary first molars have exfoliated.

B The primary second molars do not present with developmental pits in the occlusal anatomy and would not need sealant placement. Additionally, according to the radiographic interpretation, these teeth will be exfoliated soon.

C,E The permanent first premolars and permanent second molars have not yet erupted.

(D) The pits and fissures of the occlusal surfaces of the permanent first (and second) molars are considered to be the most susceptible to caries and therefore this patient's erupted first molars present as ideal candidates for sealants.

18. **A** The use of xerostomia-causing medications and mouth breathing puts this patient at an increased risk for caries. A self-applied home-use fluoride should be recommended.

 B Mouth rinses containing phenolic-related essential oils are often recommended for patients with gingivitis because of their demonstrated ability to reduce bacterial biofilms. Daily fluoride would better meet this patient's needs.

 C Mouth rinses containing oxygenating agents are often recommended for the short-term treatment of oral infections such as pericoronitis not evidenced in this patient.

 D Although not proven as effective as chlorhexidine gluconate and essential oils, mouth rinses containing quaternary ammonium compounds are sometimes recommended for patients with gingivitis. Daily fluoride would better meet this patient's needs.

 E Although chlorhexidine gluconate use has been shown to be effective at reducing bacterial plaque and *Mutans streptococcus* infections, a self-applied home-use fluoride is a better recommendation for this patient. Chlorhexidine gluconate's adverse effects of irritation to the soft tissues and a change in taste sensations may be compounded by the taste changes and xerostomia this patient experiences as a side effect of her medication.

19. A The highly acidic acidulated phosphate fluoride is often contraindicated for use in this patient with xerostomia.

 B Because of her reduced salivary flow, a neutral sodium fluoride is the agent of choice.

 C Because of its adverse effects such as gingival sloughing, bitter taste, and teeth staining, stannous fluoride's use as a professional topical fluoride application has decreased.

 D Sodium monofluorophosphate is a fluoride preparation found in over-the-counter dentifrice, and is not used for professional applications.

20. A Weakening the fluoride-rich enamel surface by polishing is particularly detrimental to the patient who presents with xerostomia.

 B,E Power-driven scaling and polishing instruments are contraindicated for the patient who presents with asthma.

 C Scaling is an effective method of removing stain, when power-driven polishing is contraindicated for the patient exhibiting signs of respiratory difficulty.

 D Toothbrushing alone is not likely to remove the brown stain.

21. A The cause of the gingival sensitivity in the area distal to the mandibular left permanent canine is most likely the erupting premolar. Although this temporary sensitivity might be a patient complaint, it is not anticipated to be a complication for impressions.

 B,C,D This patient's tongue thrust may be a contributing factor to the pronounced overjet and occlusal open bite, but none of these findings is anticipated to be a complication for impressions.

 E This patient presents with a hypersensitive gag reflex that can be anticipated to make impressions difficult to take.

22. A,D,E The amounts and frequency of eating fermentable carbohydrates has the greatest potential for decay and may be a factor in cultural food preference and eating habits.

 B Understanding the risk potential for caries and explaining the importance of a well-balanced diet from all food groups would be important nutritional counseling information to share with the preparer of the child's food.

 C This patient's medications do not interfere with nutrient absorption or utilization.

23. **A,D** The actual time specified to maintain a patient's dental records, which include the radiographs, varies from state to state. Most states require radiographs to be retained 7 to 10 years. Often this statement means that records should be retained for 7 to 10 years after the patient ceases to be a client of the practice. However, it is prudent risk management to retain the radiographs indefinitely, especially when the patient is a minor.

   B Although it is equally important that all radiographs be retained indefinitely as a prudent risk management strategy, the statute of limitations for a minor patient begins at 18 years of age. Therefore, the radiographs should be kept past the time when the patient turns 18.

   C In addition to the risk management strategy that radiographs be retained indefinitely, radiographs can provide documentation of the progress of disease and conditions that have existed previously. Previous radiographs provide documentation with which to compare subsequent radiographs.

   (E) Although most states require a practice to keep a patient's dental records, which include the radiographs, for a minimum of 7 to 10 years, the statute of limitations for minors does not usually begin until the patient turns 18 years of age. Additionally, the statute of limitations may not run until the patient discovers a problem, which could occur at some future date. Because of this variability, prudent risk management suggests that the radiographs should be retained indefinitely.

24. **A,C,D** These answers are incorrect.

   (B) The second part of the Health Insurance Portability and Accountability Act (HIPAA) which went into effect in 2003 helps ensure privacy of an individual's health information. However, this patient's mother is responsible for her wellbeing as long as she is a minor and has a legal right to knowledge regarding her daughter's oral health.

25. **A** Because placing the sticker in this manner is in violation of HIPAA, it would be considered a risk for legal repercussions regarding the handling of a patient's private health information.

   B,C These answers are incorrect.

   (D) It is a violation of the Health Insurance Portability and Accountability Act (HIPAA) to identify a medical condition with an individual in this manner. Although the chart will most likely only be handled by individuls within the oral health practice, placing a sticker with this information on the outside of the file clearly alerts all who see it to the condition and the patient's name.

CASE B PEDIATRIC PATIENT ZACK WARE

1. **A,D** Mesognathic and orthognathic profiles are demonstrated by a harmonious facial profile in which the maxilla and mandible appear balanced and the lips sealed lightly at occlusal rest without muscle strain.

   (B) This patient's facial profile is best described as retrognathic, where the chin appears retruded, giving the mandible a small appearance. Contributing further to a retrognathic profile, to keep the lips closed at rest, this patient presents with an unbalanced facial musculature. The decreased maxillary lip thickness is indicative of lip strain to achieve a lip seal at occlusal rest.

   C A prognathic profile appears as a reverse of the retrognathic profile, with the chin protruded, giving the mandible a larger or longer appearance when compared with the maxilla.

2. **(A)** Although the anterior teeth appear crowded and malaligned in the arch, the mesiobuccal cusp of the permanent maxillary first molar occludes in line with the buccal groove of the permanent mandibular first molar, and the permanent maxillary canine occludes with the distal half of the permanent mandibular canine and the mesial half of the first premolar indicating a Class I malocclusion.

B When the buccal groove of the permanent mandibular first molar is distal to the mesiobuccal cusp of the permanent maxillary first molar and the distal surface of the permanent mandibular canine is distal to the mesial surface of the permanent maxillary canine, a Class II malocclusion is indicated. Class II, Division 1 is indicated when all of the maxillary incisors protrude forward.

C When the buccal groove of the permanent mandibular first molar is distal to the mesiobuccal cusp of the permanent maxillary first molar and the distal surface of the permanent mandibular canine is distal to the mesial surface of the permanent maxillary canine, a Class II malocclusion is indicated. Class II, Division 2 is indicated when some but not all of the maxillary incisors protrude forward.

D When the buccal groove of the permanent mandibular first molar is mesial to the mesiobuccal cusp of the permanent maxillary first molar and the distal surface of the permanent mandibular canine is mesial to the mesial surface of the permanent maxillary canine, a Class III malocclusion is indicated.

3. A,B,D These answers are incorrect.

C The physiologic external root resorption evident on the primary mandibular left second molar viewed in the panoramic radiograph indicates that this tooth will be exfoliated next. Although the primary maxillary left second molar also exhibits physiologic external root resorption, it appears less advanced. Additionally, the maxillary teeth usually follow the mandibular teeth in a normal exfoliation and eruption pattern. The exfoliated primary mandibular left second molar will be replaced by the developing permanent mandibular left second premolar viewed in the panoramic radiograph.

4. A Although stress and nervousness may play a role in bruxism in children and adolescents as well as adults, occlusal interference is often thought to be the trigger. In this case, the patient has recently undergone the initial stages of orthodontic intervention making occlusal interference the better answer in this case.

B The uneven, scalloped appearance of the incisal edges of the anterior teeth is characteristic of mamelons, developmental lobes found on the incisal edges of newly erupted teeth that have not yet been worn away by normal mastication.

C Chewing bubble gum is not likely to contribute to this patient's bruxism. Occlusal interference is the better answer in this case.

D The most likely cause of this patient's nocturnal bruxism is occlusal interference. Malocclusion may cause grinding or clenching outside the normal range of chewing. Because this patient is undergoing orthodontic treatment, his occlusion is in transition and discrepancies in centric occlusion and centric relation are thought to be a cause of noctural bruxism.

E Although the retained primary teeth may contribute temporarily to occlusal disharmonies, it is highly unlikely that the primary teeth are the cause of the bruxism.

5. A The radiographs indicate that all of the permanent teeth are present and developing normally. Additionally, there are no congenitally missing teeth or supernumerary teeth evident. However, the lack of arch space is evidenced by significant anterior crowding.

B,C,D These answers are incorrect.

6. A Acids produced by bacteria break down or demineralize enamel, producing a white spot carious lesion that eventually becomes chalky and then detectable as a rough spot by an explorer. The parchment-white color of fluorosis should not be mistaken for caries.

B Demineralized enamel may be remineralized by components in the saliva and/or by exposure to fluoride. The parchment-white color of fluorosis should not be mistaken for demineralized or remineralized enamel.

C These teeth do not exhibit the wearing away of the enamel surface that is characteristic of abrasion.

D Fluorosis refers to the parchment-white color representing hypocalcification of tooth enamel. This patient's history of exposure to a high concentration of fluoride during tooth development further indicates the diagnosis of fluorosis.

E Wear facets, abrasion characterized by flat facets that reflect light, usually result from a mechanical force such as bruxism or other occlusal disharmonies. These teeth do not exhibit wear facets. The unique scalloped edges of the anterior teeth are mamelons, developmental lobes found on the incisal edges of newly erupted teeth that have not yet been worn away by normal mastication.

7.   A Caries appears radiolucent.

B Enamel pearls appear as small round or oval radiopacities within the pulp chambers of affected teeth. Although dense radiopaque structures, enamel pearls would not appear as radiopaque as metallic restorations.

C This characteristic appearance of buccal pit amalgam restorations should not be confused with processor artifacts.

D The photographic observation of amalgam restorations rule out the possibility of orthodontic brackets. The size, shape, and location of these radiopacities indicate amalgam restorations.

E The radiopacities indicate the radiographic appearance of buccal pit amalgam restorations. The dense nature of amalgam causes these restorations to appear radiopaque on the resultant radiographs.

8.   A Periodontal status is best evaluated with intraoral radiographs such as periapicals and vertical bitewings.

B A cephalometric radiograph is most often used to evaluate growth and development and is especially useful in assessment of the dentition and the relationship of the arches for orthodontic intervention and treatment.

C The radiograph most often used to image caries is the horizontal bitewing. Other intraoral radiographs such as the vertical bitewing, periapical, and occlusal would all be better choices then extraoral radiographs for imaging caries

D The cephalometric radiograph images a lateral view of the skull, superimposing the right and left structures making evaluation of the sinus cavities difficult. The better choice for imaging the sinus is the Water's extraoral projection.

E The cephalometric radiograph images a lateral view of the skull, superimposing the right and left structures making evaluation of specific areas for the detection of a specific condition difficult. The panoramic radiograph is often used as a survey film for the detection of occult disease, although this use is questionable. When a condition or disease is suspected, a radiograph specific for the site of interest should be recommended.

9. A,D,E The cephalostat uses two plastic ear rods to stabilize the skull into position. The penetrating x-ray beam will image the ear rods onto the resultant film. Knowledge of the equipment used to image a cephalometric radiograph will help distinguish these parts from foreign objects such as a metal earring stud or film label or by artifacts produced by fixer contamination.

B The location of the image of the ear rods used for imaging a cephalometric radiograph near the auditory meatus should not be confused with an orthodontic bracket that would be located on or near the dentition to which it is applied.

C A cephalometric radiograph utilizes a cephalostat or head holder to stabilize the patient in position. The cephalostat has two plastic ear rods. To stabilize the skull into position and to provide a basis for standardization of subsequent radiographs, one plastic ear rod is inserted into each ear. As the x-ray beam penetrates the cephalostat, a portion of the beam is blocked by the ear rods, leaving less x-rays to strike the film. The result is an image of a radiopaque object resembling the shape of the ear rods.

10.   A   The midsaggital plane is an imaginary vertical line that divides the left and right sides of the body.

(B) Proper positioning for cephalometric radiographs requires the location and alignment of skeletal landmarks. The device imaged on this radiograph is assisting with aligning the Frankfort plane. The Frankfort plane or orbitomeatal line, extends from the superior border of the external auditory meatus to the infraorbital rim and should be positioned parallel to the floor.

C   The occlusal plane is an imaginary line drawn horizontally across the chewing surfaces of the teeth. The occlusal plane is usually placed into a position that is parallel to the floor for intraoral radiographs.

D   Using the terminology *vertical plane* simply implies any dimension that is positioned up and down, or vertical to the floor.

E   Using the terminology *mandibular plane* implies reference to the occlusion plane, an imaginary line drawn horizontally across the chewing surfaces of the teeth.

11.   A   During internal resorption, as the tooth structure demineralizes, the pulp chamber and root canals widen as a result. The normal development of this patient's teeth at this age should not be confused with internal resorption.

B   During external resorption, as the tooth structure demineralizes, the tooth roots appear to get shorter as a result. The normal development of this patient's teeth at this age should not be confused with external resorption.

C   Cervical burnout refers to the radiolucent optical illusion at the cervical region of the tooth that presents when a very radiopaque structure is imaged next to a very radiolucent structure. Cervical burnout mimics decay and can be a hindrance when interpreting caries.

(D) The tooth root continues to develop after the appearance of the crown clinically. At first the pulp chamber appears wide and open at the apex. As the root develops, the pulp chamber narrows and then closes at the apex. Additionally, this patient's mandibular canines are malpositioned, in torsoversion and appear rotated, giving a particularly wide appearance to the root canal.

E   Over time, depending on the severity, bruxing can lead to tooth changes such as attrition and the formation of secondary dentin. However, the radiolucent appearance of these tooth roots is the result of normal development and not a result of nocturnal bruxism.

12.   **(A)** Effective toothbrushing is this patient's greatest immediate need. Because he indicates distress over brushing around his braces, a power toothbrush could be an effective plaque removal alternative to a manual brush.

B   An oral irrigation device is recommended as a useful adjunct to toothbrushing, but this patient's primary problem must first be addressed. Oral irrigation can be added later, once brushing effectiveness is achieved.

C,D   Floss threaders and the use of a sulcus brush are time consuming. Motivation to use additional oral hygiene aids will be possible in the future if the dental hygienist can first reinforce this patient's plaque removal success with the power toothbrush.

E   Wooden wedges for cleaning proximal tooth surfaces in regions where the interdental gingival is missing would not be recommended for this patient.

13.   A   Incomplete development of a sense of logic and parental dependence would be more characteristic of preschool children. Characteristics of this patient's age group include a fully developed sense of logic evidenced as the patient begins to view the world around him with a more critical eye.

B   An increasing independence from parental influence probably began in this patient as he entered elementary school. At this stage, the patient assumed more control over his self-care.

C   By age 12 this patient has developed a sense of reality and conceptualization of the scientific principles of cause and effect.

D   Adults who have passed through the teenage years, where a sense of invincibility rules, will more readily accept preventive regimens for preventing later health problems. However, a patient in middle school and entering the teenage years will be less likely to listen to self-care instructions that focus on benefits at a future date.

E   Convincing adolescents to accept and comply with preventive regimens is difficult because of their orientation to present-time activities and lack of concern for preventive health care in general. Discussion of developing important health habits for the future, such as the need for orthodontic intervention, protection from risks of athletic activities, and tobacco cessation programs, may not seem pertinent to youth in this age group.

14.   A   Because adolescents are striving for independence from parental control, parents play a minimal role in motivating oral self-care of these patients.

B   Finding out what interests the adolescent patient and linking oral health to that interest would be more likely to motivate this patient than showing him the chart. Additionally, adolescents are less motivated by what has happened and what might happen at a future date to their teeth if they do not improve self-care.

C   Although adolescents generally possess the dexterity to perform a self-care regime that will maintain their oral health, they typically lack the motivation to perform these skills on a regular basis. First, appealing to their perceived needs motivates them to act on new, healthy behaviors. Secondly, providing a new or unique oral hygiene aid that appeals to the adolescent, such as a power toothbrush, can provide an additional motivator to perform the desired healthy behaviors.

D   Adolescents are likely to react adversely to being told what to do by an authority figure.

15.   A   Knife-like describes marginal gingiva that contours flatly to the tooth.

B   Rolled marginal gingiva appears as an enlarged doughnut-shaped ring of gingiva around the teeth.

C   Cratered papillae describes a cupping out of the normal papillary shape.

D   The term *clefting* is used to describe a V-shaped or slitlike indentation in the marginal gingiva.

E   Normal pointed or slightly rounded papillae that become increasing rounded and no longer fill the interproximal space are described as blunted.

16.   A   During the eruption of the teeth, the appearance of the gingiva is often described as thickened, rounded, or rolled. As the eruption process continues, the gingiva appearance flattens out and the marginal gingiva takes on a more knife-like appearance. This can be observed when comparing this patient's photographs 1 month later.

B   It is unlikely that subgingival calculus is present on the facial surfaces of these erupting teeth. Although it is possible, the better explanation for the appearance of the facial gingiva in this region is the eruption process.

C   The effects of spit tobacco are likely to be leukopakia in the region the tobacco is held and not a thickened, rolled appearance to the facial gingiva in this region. The rolled appearance of the facial gingiva is due to the eruption process.

D   Mouth breathing may cause irritating drying conditions in the anterior region leading to increased redness and gingivitis. However, the rolled appearance of the facial gingiva is due to the eruption process.

E   Frequently ingesting sports drinks that are high in fermentable carbohydrates puts this patient at risk for caries. However, the thickened, rolled appearance of the facial gingiva in this region is due to the eruption process.

17.   A As a prudent measure for this patient entering orthodontic treatment, all teeth exhibiting pits and fissures should be recommended for sealants.

B,D Fluoride application in the form of varnish and oral irrigation will benefit the orthodontic patient.

(C) Enamel microabrasion is used to esthetically treat discrete white spots on the teeth. Microabrasion removes a shallow surface of enamel that is replaced with composite resin. This patient's white spots are the result of fluorosis and would not be treated in this manner.

E To avoid caries and periodontal problems during the course of orthodontic treatment, strict attention to dietary habits such as snacking and types of foods consumed is required. Additionally, there should be an investigation into whether the sports drinks he consumes throughout the day contain sugar.

18. A,C,D,E Sodium fluoride, acidulated phosphate fluoride, and stannous fluoride treatments are applied under dry conditions and require that the patient not drink for 30 minutes following application.

(B) Fluoride varnish sets rapidly in the presence of saliva and although the patient should be advised not to eat, brush, or floss for a period of 4 hours following application, fluoride varnish does not require abstinence from drinking for a period of time following application.

19.   A Rubber cup polishing would be difficult around the orthodontic brackets and may not be completely effective at stain removal.

B Powered polishing would be the better choice over manual toothbrushing for removing the stains.

(C) This patient's teeth are indicated for air-powder abrasive polishing to effectively remove plaque and stain around his orthodontic appliances. Because he has his permanent dentition and no respiratory illnesses this procedure is not contraindicated.

D Although time consuming, the porte polisher can be an effective device when professional powered stain removal techniques are contraindicated, which is not the case for this patient.

20.   A The casts have not been trimmed appropriately so that an imaginary line drawn at the occlusal planes of the arches would be parallel to the bases.

B The posterior borders of the casts do not appear to be at right angles to the bases.

C The casts would not remain balanced to rest together naturally if stood on the posterior bases.

(D) Although the maxillary cast is not appropriately trimmed out from the canines to a point in the midline, the anterior border of the mandibular cast is appropriately trimmed to an arc shape.

E The bases appear to be larger than the appropriate one-third art portion of the casts.

21. A,C,D These answers are incorrect.

(B) Nicotine, found in all tobacco products, is a highly addictive drug that acts in the brain and throughout the body. Dip and chew contain more nicotine than cigarettes. Initiation of tobacco use is highly correlated in the adolescent age group as a result of the insecurity and rebellious characteristics of this age group. Media stereotypes and star athletes are powerful influences in teenagers' behaviors and self-image.

22.   A Nicotine, found in all tobacco products, is a highly addictive drug.

B Spit tobacco contains more nicotine than cigarettes.

(C) Patients this age and their friends are often misinformed regarding the relationship of spit tobacco and athletic performance. Although this patient most likely receives an abundance of health information, media and athletic role models often impress children and adolescents with misinformation. However, in a major league baseball poll, not one player who used dip or spit tobacco said that the tobacco improved his game or sharpened his reflexes.

D   In addition to the health problems associated with cigarette smoking, spit to-bacco contributes to periodontal disease, caries, and oral cancer.

E   Spit tobacco increases risk of oral cancer and leukopakia, considered to be pre-cancerous.

23. A,B,C,E A hard plastic thermoset resin mouthguard is used to treat adult nocturnal brux-ism and would not be the material used to fabricate a mouthguard for this patient.

(D) Because the Academy of Sports Dentistry recommends mouth protection for patients who skateboard, this patient should be using a mouth protector specif-ically designed for adolescents who engage in sports and/or recreational activi-ties that increase the risk for trauma to the oral cavity. A thermoplastic boil-and-bite mouth protector is the appropriate appliance choice for a patient in orthodontic brackets.

24.   (A) This patient is a minor, under 18 years of age, and cannot legally give informed consent to undergo nonurgent care such as dental hygiene treatment.

B   Allowing the patient to participate in completing his health history may elicit more information than if his parent completed the form alone.

C   To assist in gaining the patient's cooperation with the care plan, it is important for the dental hygienist to gain his understanding of what is required and his trust in the treatment. However, because this patient is a minor, the dental hy-gienist is obligated to explain oral health findings and the care plan to both the patient and his parent.

D   Providing an opportunity for the patient to contribute to the health history alone, away from his parent, is likely to elicit additional important information regarding his oral health and other behaviors, in this case, his spit tobacco use.

E   The health history of all patients should be kept current.

25. A,B,D These answers are incorrect.

(C) Because of the seriousness of this finding, the dental hygienist is obligated to re-port this patient's use of spit tobacco to his mother and to assist with resources and recommendations for intervention for cessation. The term *paternalism* refers to actions taken by the health care provider in the best interest of the pa-tient, without giving the patient a choice in the matter.

CASE C PEDIATRIC PATIENT ANDREW CHRISTIANSON

1.   A   When present, linea alba refers to a raised, horizontal line on the buccal mucosa corresponding to the region where the teeth meet in occlusion.

(B) The mucogingival line marks the junction between the pale pink attached gin-giva and the darker red alveolar mucosa.

C   The free gingival margin refers to the crest of the free gingiva nearest the incisal/occlusal surface of the tooth.

D   Bone exotosis refers to a raised excess of bone, called tori when present on the lingual aspect. Although pronounced, the mucogingival line is a soft tissue junction and should not be confused with hard tissue exotosis.

E   The normal mucogingival line should not be confused with scaring that results from wound healing.

2.   (A) Excessive wear, most likely the result of chronic bruxing, has worn away the sur-face enamel to reveal the dentin.

B   The yellow color represents the exposed dentin that has resulted from excessive wear and not from caries.

C The excessive wear noted in these regions indicates worn enamel that has exposed the underlying dentin.

D The teeth surfaces have been worn away, exposing the underlying dentin. Food debris would appear on top of the tooth.

E Cementum covers the root surface.

3. A Abfraction refers to cervical destruction of the tooth structure, purported to occur when occlusal forces cause stress on the tooth.

B Abrasion refers to a mechanical wearing away of the tooth surface by a foreign object such as toothbrushing.

C Attrition refers to a mechanical wearing away of the tooth surface by the forces of occlusion, such as bruxing.

D Erosion refers to a chemical wearing away of the tooth surface, such as when stomach acids are regurgitated into the oral cavity.

(E) The incisal edge of the permanent maxillary left central incisor appears chipped.

4. A Hidden or backward caries refers to caries that seems small, detected only as a pinpoint lesion clinically. However, the spread of caries along the dentino-enamel junction creates a much larger lesion that often undermines the tooth surface.

B Early childhood caries refers to caries that develops in the first 3 years of the child's life.

(C) This patient's chronic caries have been progressing over time. The dentin in the large lesions appears stained brown-black and the soft dentin appears as if it could be scooped out.

D Arrested caries refers to lesions that become remineralized.

E Recurrent caries describes caries that reoccurs around the margins of previously placed restorations. The brown-black stained dentin on the affected teeth should not be mistaken for metallic restorations.

5. A Intrinsic stains occur within the tooth and endogenous stains are caused by factors within the tooth.

B Intrinsic stains occur within the tooth and exogenous stains are caused by factors external to the tooth.

C Extrinsic stains, resulting from factors outside the tooth, can only be caused by factors external to the tooth or exogenous.

(D) Poor self-care has resulted in the extrinsic staining present on the facials of the mandibular anterior teeth. The staining is caused by factors outside the tooth (biofilm and materia alba accumulation) and is therefore referred to as exogenous.

6. (A) A side effect of Adderall is dry mouth, or xerostomia.

B,C,D,E The only oral adverse effect of Adderall is dry mouth and possible unpleasant taste. Early tooth loss, risk of congenitally missing teeth, tooth staining, and mouth breathing are not side effects of this medication. Possible systemic side effects of this medication include a modest increase in blood pressure and heart rate.

7. (A) These stains are the result of overlapped films which prevented chemicals and rinse water from reaching this area. Upon careful examination an outline can be observed which represents the outline of the edge of the overlapping film.

B Opening the film packet would result in a black, overexposed region.

C If excess saliva is not removed from paper film packets, over time the moisture can penetrate and cause the black paper inside the film packet to stick to the film.

D Static electricity creates a white light spark that can expose the film. The result is a radiolucent spark or lightening-pattern artifact imaged on the film.

8.   A,B The completely developed roots of the primary canines are resorbing in response to the erupting permanent canines and not in the process of forming and not congenitally missing.

     C The erupting permanent canines are causing the primary canines to undergo normal physiologic external resorption.

     D Internal resorption is characterized by a widening of the pulp and/or root canal chambers as the hard tooth structure demineralizes. The shortened, or disappearing root structure observed here is external resorption.

9.   A The normal appearance of the dental sac should not be confused with a dentigerous cyst that surrounds the crown portion only of an unerupted, often impacted tooth.

     B This tooth is unerupted. The radiolucency represents the dental sac that surrounds a developing tooth.

     C The normal appearance of the dental sac should not be confused with an abscess that would appear as a radiolucency at the apex of the affected erupted tooth.

     D The dental sac surrounds the dental papilla where the dentin and the pulp structures of the erupting tooth develop.

     E Sharpey's fibers refer to the part of the periodontal fibers that attaches to the tooth by embedding into the cementum. Sharpey's fibers are not imaged on radiographs.

10.   A A condition of overgrowth of cementum, called hypercementosis, manifests as a wider than normal, often bulbous tooth root.

     B Newly erupted teeth are formed of primary dentin. As the tooth comes in contact with teeth in the opposing arch, secondary dentin begins to form and continues throughout life. As secondary dentin continues to form, the pulp chambers and root canals of these teeth will gradually appear smaller and narrower.

     C The pathologic condition known as internal resorption will create a widened appearance to the pulp. However, the age of this patient indicates that these newly erupted teeth have not yet formed the secondary dentin that will cause the appearance of these wide root canals to narrow over time.

     D Sclerotic dentin, where the dentinal tubules fill with a dentin material, is formed in response to trauma or decay. This condition is determined from a histological examination and does not appear on radiographic images.

     E A pulpal infection such as an abscess would be observed as a radiolucency at the apex of the tooth.

11.   A, B The primary maxillary left first molar and the primary mandibular right canine appear to be undergoing physiologic external resorption at the apices.

     C The permanent maxillary right canine is unerupted.

     D The permanent mandibular left second molar is unerupted. The radiolucency observed in the apex region is the dental sac of this developing tooth.

     E Radiolucencies can be observed at the apices of the permanent mandibular right first molar, the cause of which is most likely the large caries observed on this tooth.

12. A,B,C The physiologic external root resorption evident on the primary mandibular right first molar is more advanced than the resorption observed on the primary maxillary right first molar, the primary maxillary right canine, and the primary mandibular left second molar.

     D Although the mandibular left canine also exhibits physiologic external root resorption, it appears less extensive than the primary mandibular right first molar. Additionally, the molars usually follow the canines in a normal exfoliation and eruption pattern.

E The physiologic external root resorption evident on the primary mandibular right first molar indicates that this tooth will be exfoliated next. Although the primary mandibular left canine also exhibits physiologic external root resorption, it appears less extensive. Additionally, the molars usually follow the canines in a normal exfoliation and eruption pattern.

13.   A   The gingivitis evident is due to this patient's lack of effective self-care that has allowed the accumulation of biofilms. The presence or absence of gingivitis will not have an effect on the gag reflex.

        B   Color and consistency of this patient's hard palate rugae appears within normal limits. Although palpation of the posterior region of the soft palate may stimulate a gag reflex, in most patients the hard palate, particularly the anterior region, is less likely to do so.

        C   Although physical stimulation of the posterior region of the tongue may elicit a gag reflex, a white coating on the dorsal surface indicates this patient's lack of effective self-care.

       D The enlarged tonsils and uvula have the potential to affect the sensitivity of this patient's gag reflex.

        E   Depending on the stage of eruption, certain teeth may interfere with the clinician's fulcrum, or the placement of a radiographic film packet, but the pattern of eruption will not have an effect on the gag reflex.

14.   A   Short appointments are recommended for the pediatric patient with ADHD.

        B   Rampant caries, poor oral self-care, and xerostomia are indications for administering a professional fluoride treatment.

       C Scheduling back-to-back long scaling appointments within 24 hours, called full-mouth disinfection, would not be indicated for this pediatric patient.

        D   Multiple severe caries and this patient's medical and social history indicate a need for nutritional counseling.

        E   Due to a possible increase in blood pressure and heart rate, patients taking Adderall should have their vital signs monitored at each appointment.

15. A,C,D,E   Only the nitrous oxide sedation would be contraindicated.

       B Patients whose tonsils narrow the airway are at increased risk for airway obstruction when administering nitrous oxide sedation.

16.   **A** Children are less likely to be motivated by being told of consequences of today's action on a future event. Additionally, verbal instructions without a demonstration of the technique or without the use of media that enhances the instruction is less likely to be understood and remembered.

        B   Using the patient's mouth to demonstrate the technique helps make the skill more realistic for the patient. The use of disclosing solution can help gain the patient's attention and make learning fun. Additionally, having the patient try the technique in his own mouth provides an opportunity for the dental hygienist to observe his grasp of the skill and helps to provide feedback that specifically targets his needs.

        C   All patients respond favorably to positive feedback. Complimenting the patient on not only his performance but also on his desire to want to learn better self-care for healthier teeth may help to motivate him to better oral health.

        D   Children respond well to a reward system and often find competition for a prize fun and challenging. Placing a star sticker in the patient record or using a visual reward system that this patient can relate to his love of video games can help make learning and performing the desired behaviors fun and challenging.

        E   Repeating instructions multiple times and in multiple ways will help to make the message more likely to be interpreted correctly and will provide reinforcement for the patient with a short attention span.

17.   A The translucent, thin acquired pellicle that covers the teeth has aided the attachment of the microbial biofilm to these teeth surfaces.

B The thickness of this biofilm at the cervical third of these teeth indicates that bacteria have attached to the pellicle and have multiplied. The significant staining and the gingival inflammation in this region indicate that this microbial biofilm has remained in this region undisturbed for several days.

C Materia alba refers to a collection of living and dead bacteria, desquamated epithelial cells, salivary proteins, and leukocytes that adhere loosely to the teeth in a white or grayish bulky soft deposit. Materia alba would appear to be readily removed by rinsing or water irrigation.

D Similar to materia alba in its ease of removal by rinsing and irrigation, food debris consists of loose food particles that wedge between the teeth, in embrasures and in areas lacking occlusal contact, and in large caries.

E Calculus consists of mineralized bacterial biofilm.

18.   **A** The maxillary right first molar is the only permanent molar that does not exhibit caries that would contraindicate sealant placement.

B,C,D Each of these teeth exhibits caries that contraindicate sealant placement.

19.   A An adjunct to brushing with dentifrice, brushing with 0.4% SnF_2 gel is an effective supplement to professional fluoride treatments and often prescribed to avoid white spot lesions in orthodontic patients. However, given this patient's caries history, the custom tray application of 0.05% APF is the better recommendation. Additionally, patient compliance is likely to be low, because this technique requires the patient to brush twice, once with a dentifrice and then again to apply the fluoride gel. Involving the patient and his mother in learning the tray application method may challenge the patient to take an active role in performing a special procedure to benefit his oral health.

B Daily rinsing with 0.05% NaF is recommended for the general prevention of caries. Given this patient's caries history, the custom tray application of 0.05% APF is the better recommendation. To gain maximum benefit with a fluoride rinse, significant patient compliance is required. The patient must be instructed to swish properly and for the recommended time. Additionally, many over-the-counter rinses contain alcohol that should be limited to use by adult patients and patients without xerostomia.

C Custom or disposable tray application of prescription strength 0.5% APF once daily is recommended for this patient with rampant caries and reduced salivary flow.

D Weekly, high potency oral rinses containing 0.2% NaF are most often used for professionally administered community, group, or school-based fluoride treatment, and would not be recommended for this patient's daily home use.

E Brushing with dentifrice containing Na_2PO_3F is recommended for all patients. This patient is most likely already using a commercial product that contains Na_2PO_3F. He should be encouraged and supervised to increase brushing frequency. However, another home fluoride application should be introduced in addition to his toothpaste.

20.   A This patient's restricted airway has a potential to limit his breathing, contraindicating the use of air-power polishing.

B The porte polisher can be an effective alternative if the power-driven rotary instrument was contraindicated for this patient.

C Oral irrigation will not remove the thick biofilm and stain.

D Scaling will most likely be needed to remove the thick biofilm present on the facial surfaces of the mandibular anterior teeth. Any remaining stain can be removed by selective polishing.

E Toothbrushing is not likely to remove this patient's stain.

21.   A Increased frequency of eating cariogenic foods decreases the opportunity for remineralization between consumption, aiding the caries process.

        B Snacking on fermentable carbohydrates, including soda and sugary drinks, increases the risk for caries.

        C Soft, highly retentive foods are more likely to be retained in the oral cavity, contributing to conditions conducive to producing caries.

        D The sequence of when fermentable carbohydrates are consumed plays a role in the risk for caries.

        (E) Although the number of calories consumed per day is important for weight management and developing lifelong good eating habits, daily caloric intake does not play a direct role in managing the diet for the purpose of caries control.

22.   A,B Sticky snacks such as cookies and pretzels are retained longer in the oral cavity, thus increasing the risk for caries.

        C The fermentable carbohydrates in ice cream lower plaque pH and put teeth at risk for caries.

        D In addition to the fermentable carbohydrates found in sugary soft drinks that lower plaque pH and put teeth at risk for caries, sodas are often consumed over a longer period of time, thus increasing the length of time that the teeth are at risk.

        (E) Sticky foods are more likely to be retained in the oral cavity longer and increase the time of an acid attack on the teeth. However, chewy carbohydrates, such as gummy bears, increase mastication and stimulate salivary flow, making this snack less damaging to the teeth than the others listed.

23.   A The smaller size and less dense tissue of children require less radiation exposure compared to the adult patient.

        B A reduction by one-fourth of the exposure setting used for dentate adult radiographs is recommended for exposure of edentulous adults or edentulous regions of the oral cavity of adult patients.

        C A reduction by one-third of the exposure setting used for adult radiographs is recommended for children between the ages of 10 and 15.

        (D) ALARA stands for "as low as reasonably achievable" and is the ethical principle endorsed by health professionals to reduce radiation exposure to patients. According to ALARA, a reduction by one-half of the exposure setting used for adult radiographs is recommended for children under 10 years of age.

24.   **(A)** Willfully and deliberately not attending to a child's needs to maintain oral health is neglect and considered to be a form of abuse. However, care should be taken not to confuse neglect with this patient's parent's inability to afford the costs involved with restoring oral health. Additionally, this patient's mother lacks the knowledge of the importance of his primary teeth and most likely did not know that his permanent teeth were in need of professional care. Her actions seem rooted in ignorance and not a deliberate desire to harm her child.

    B,C,D These answers are incorrect.

25.   A Threatening or bullying this patient's mother is less likely to produce acceptance of the needed treatment. Threats that make her feel as if she has no choice but to accept the treatment plan may produce a situation where she refuses all treatment.

        (B) Patients generally respond more favorably to positive statements than to negative threats. Additionally, this patient's mother is more likely to accept a recommended treatment plan when she feels in control of the decision. Pointing out that she is now more knowledgeable of the role primary teeth play in future oral health, she is likely to see the value in the recommended treatment.

C Demonstrating moral superiority over this patient's mother is likely to produce a negative response and is less likely to help her feel empowered to make decisions that she will need to help carry out.

D Pressuring this patient's mother or pushing her into accepting treatment before she has processed all the needed information to make her own decision is less likely to produce the desired result.

E Blaming the child's mother for his poor oral health is not likely to create acceptance of a treatment plan that will surely include a commitment from her, not only to keep future appointments but also to help foster a change in oral health care habits, diet, and to supervise better self-care.

CASE D ADULT-PERIODONTAL PATIENT KATHERINE FLYNN

1. **(A)** G. V. Black established the standard for classifying caries in the early 1900s. This system has since been customarily used for describing cavity preparations and restorations as well. The amalgam restoration observed on the lingual surface of the maxillary left lateral incisor is classified as a Class I restoration. A restoration that involves only one surface of the tooth, such as the occlusal surface only of posterior teeth; facial and lingual surface only of molars; and/or the lingual surface only of incisors is classified as Class I.

   B A Class III restoration involves the proximal surface, but not the incisal angle of incisors and canines.

   C A Class IV restoration involves the proximal surface and the incisal angle of incisors and canines.

   D A restoration placed along the cervical one-third of a tooth's facial and/or lingual surfaces (but not the pits or fissures) is classified as a Class V restoration.

   E A restoration placed at the incisal edge only of anterior teeth and/or on the cusp tips only of posterior teeth is classified as a Class VI restoration.

2. A The maxillary first molars are missing and therefore are not available to support the removable partial denture. The denture serves to provide functional replacement of these missing teeth.

   B The maxillary anterior teeth support the major connector of the partial denture. The denture clasps do not rest on these teeth.

   C The mandibular left first premolar and first molar teeth are restored with a fixed three-unit bridge that is not removable. The first premolar and first molar have been restored with crowns that make up the abutment teeth. The second premolar is missing and has been restored with a pontic as part of the fixed bridge.

   (D) As seen in the photographs, preparations have been made on the distal portions of the occlusal surfaces of the maxillary second premolars, allowing the removable partial denture clasps to rest in position on the abutment teeth and lend support for the partial denture.

3. A Prosthetic devices and restorations often provide plaque retentive areas that may be difficult for the patient to keep clean, increasing the risk for caries development.

   B Xerostomia, a risk factor for caries development, is a side effect of the medications taken by this patient.

   C Gingival recession exposes the cemental surface to *Streptococcus mutans* and *lactobacilli,* the primary organisms associated with root caries. This patient's extensive gingival recession is a significant risk factor for caries.

   D Plaque is a significant risk factor for root caries. Although this patient is meticulous with oral self-care aids, the oral photographs reveal plaque accumulation in the cervical regions of several teeth. This finding is further supported by the appearance of gingival redness. She may be avoiding brushing cervical areas where root sensitivity presents, thus allowing the accumulation of microbial biofilm.

(E) As a lifelong residence in a community with near-optimal levels of water fluoridation, this patient can expect to experience a significant reduction in the incidence of root caries when compared to individuals who reside in communities with nonfluoridated water supplies. This patient also reports using fluoride rinses along with her dentifrice, further reducing her risk for root caries.

4.   A Frictional hyperkeratosis is a trauma lesion, usually a white patch that results from chronic rubbing of an ill-fitting denture.

   B An ill-fitting denture may produce a proliferation of flabby hyperplastic tissue. Denture-induced fibrous hyperplasia often results in asymptomatic, single or multiple folds of soft tissue that overgrow the denture flange.

   (C) Denture stomatitis is a local inflammation in response to the partial denture not being removed periodically. Continuous wearing of the partial denture has stressed the tissue. This is especially likely to occur if salivary flow has been decreased; a common occurrence in menopausal women on hormone replacement therapy.

   D Typical papillary hyperplasia results from denture irritation and occurs under a full denture, in the middle of the palate within the bony ridges leading to the palatal side of the teeth.

   E The red appearance of the tissue and the rolled outline of the denture embedded in the tissue of the hard palate are indicators that this condition is denture stomatitis. Although it is highly unlikely that trauma from a partial denture will result in squamous cell carcinoma, the patient should be instructed to remove the denture periodically and the area should be monitored after 2 weeks.

5.   A A post-and-core restoration would appear significantly larger (a bulkier, wider object) than retention pins. Additionally, the post section of this type of restoration would appear to penetrate the pulp chamber, giving support to the tooth upon which a crown may be affixed. To be placed within the pulp chamber, the tooth would show evidence of endodontic therapy; endodontic filling materials would be imaged on the radiographs.

   (B) The radiographs reveal the presence of retention pins that appear as radiopaque thin lines on the radiograph. Retention pins are distinguished from the other materials by their size, shape, and position within the dentin of the teeth. They do not penetrate the pulp chamber or root canal.

   C Silver points are used as an endodontic filling material. This material would appear to fill the pulp chamber and root canals of the tooth. Silver points appear distinctly radiopaque.

   D Gutta percha is used as an endodontic filling material. As with silver points, gutta percha would appear to fill the pulp chamber and root canals of the tooth. Gutta percha appears less radiopaque than silver points.

6.   A Cone cut or clear, blank areas on the film result when a portion of the film was not exposed to x-rays due to not centering the film within the x-ray beam. A cone cut error would appear more uniform, representing the edge of the PID (position indicating device).

   B A radiopaque artifact would result if a metal clasp of the partial denture blocks a portion of the x-ray beam, leaving the area directly behind the metal portion of the denture unexposed. However, the partial denture, if mistakenly left in the patient's mouth during the exposure, would not appear in this region on the film.

   C Although metal scraps from amalgam also will block the x-ray beam and leave a radiopaque artifact on the image, an amalgam fragment, which embeds in the gingiva, would not appear on the edge of the film in this manner or size.

D A radiopaque appearance indicates no exposure to radiographs. In this case the metal arm of a film holding device appears to have blocked a portion of the x-ray beam, leaving the area directly behind the device unexposed. When subjected to processing chemistry, the unexposed area will result in a radiopaque artifact imaged onto the film.

7.   A Radiographically, the increased radiopacity of the material present on the mesial, occlusal, and distal surfaces of the maxillary right first premolar indicates an amalgam restoration. Metal restorations will appear more radiopaque than composite restorative materials. The slightly less radiopaque cusps are visible superior to the restoration. The use of amalgam in this restoration can be confirmed in the photographs which image a MOD restoration.

B Radiographically, the increased radiopacity of the material present on the distal and occlusal surfaces of the maxillary left first premolar indicates an amalgam restoration. Metal restorations will appear more radiopaque than composite restorative materials. The slightly less radiopaque cusps are visible superior to the restoration. The use of amalgam in this restoration can be confirmed in the photographs which image a DO restoration.

C Radiographically, the size, shape, and appearance of metal and porcelain indicate a porcelain-fused-to-metal crown present on the maxillary left second premolar. Metal restorations will appear more radiopaque than composite restorative materials and the smooth margins of this radiopacity indicate a crown and not an amalgam restoration (which would have irregular margins). The radiopaque smooth metal outline of the restoration does not contour to the anatomical shape of the tooth. A close examination of the radiographs indicates the presence of slightly less radiopaque porcelain used to shape cusps to restore the tooth to the correct anatomic shape for mastication. The presence of a porcelain-fused-to-metal crown can be confirmed in the photographs.

D Radiographically, the size, shape, and appearance of metal and porcelain indicate a porcelain-fused-to-metal crown present on the mandibular left first premolar. Metal restorations will appear more radiopaque than composite restorative materials and the smooth margins of this radiopacity indicate a crown and not an amalgam restoration (which would have irregular margins). The radiopaque smooth metal outline of the restoration does not contour to the anatomical shape of the tooth. A close examination of the radiographs indicates the presence of slightly less radiopaque porcelain used to shape cusps to restore the tooth to the correct anatomic shape for mastication. The presence of a porcelain-fused-to-metal crown can be confirmed in the photographs. The photographs indicate a spot on the occlusal surface where the porcelain has been eroded to reveal the metal portion of the crown.

E Radiographically, the slightly increased radiopacity visible on the distal and occlusal surfaces of the mandibular right second premolar indicates the presence of a composite restoration. This finding can be confirmed in the photographs, which image a tooth-colored MODL restoration.

8.   **A** The classic appearance of the mental foramen is a round or oval radiolucency located near the apex of the mandibular first or second premolar. A close examination of the radiographs indicates that the lamina dura of the first premolar is intact, separating the round radiolucency from the apex of the tooth. This separate radiolucency is not associated with the tooth and should not be confused with apical pathology.

B It is possible for a residual cyst to be located in this area of the missing mandibular second premolar. A cyst often appears radiographically as a round radiolucency. However, the classic appearance of the mental foramen in this area of the mandibular first or second premolar must be considered first. A cyst, if present in this area, would most likely appear in addition to the mental foramen and not in place of it. Additionally, careful examination of the radiograph of the mandibular right first and second premolar region reveals a similar looking round radiolucency. Comparing both the left and right radiolucencies can be helpful in determining the presence of a normal anatomical landmark such as the mental foramen.

C,D It is usually not possible to distinguish a periapical abscess and granuloma based on radiographic findings alone. A histological examination would be required. However, both these pathological conditions would be distinguished from the mental foramen by an examination of the lamina dura of the bony tooth socket. The cortical plate of bone that makes up the lamina dura would appear to engulf the radiolucency when a pathological condition presents. A close examination of the radiographs indicates that the lamina dura of the first premolar is intact, separating the round radiolucency from the apex of the tooth. This separate radiolucency is not associated with the tooth indicating the mental foramen, which should not be confused with apical pathology.

9.   A   A periodontal abscess may be imaged radiographically as a large diffuse radiolucency in a lateral position to the tooth. A periodontal abscess is not evident on these radiographs.

B When assessing bone loss evident on radiographs, it is important to determine whether the bone loss is horizontal or vertical. Use the CEJ (cementoenamel junction) of adjacent teeth to form an imaginary line. When bone loss is parallel to this imaginary line connecting adjacent teeth at the CEJ, horizontal bone loss is indicated. When the bone loss is not parallel, but angular to the imaginary line connecting adjacent teeth at the CEJ, vertical bone loss is indicated. In the area distal to the mandibular right first molar, the crestal bone is angular and therefore considered to be vertical bone loss.

C   Furcation involvement would appear as a radiolucency between the roots of multirooted teeth. The mandibular right first molar does not appear to have bone loss involving the furcation region.

D   Horizontal bone loss is associated with several other teeth. However, in the area distal to the mandibular right first molar the crestal bone loss appears angular and therefore is considered to be vertical bone loss. The bone loss in this region is not parallel to an imaginary line connecting the mandibular right first and second molars at the CEJ (cementoenamel junction) indicating vertical bone loss.

10.   A   Allowing time for adjustment to a change in chair position may help to avoid orthostatic hypotension of which the occurrence is an adverse effect of the drug Cardizem.

B   Considering this patient's history of syncope, having ammonia capsules available would allow the dental hygienist to arouse an unconscious patient, thus avoiding a more serious situation.

C This patient does not present with a condition indicating a need for antibiotic prophylaxis.

D   The dental professional can help avoid an emergency situation by requiring that this patient bring the nitroglycerine to the appointment in case an angina attack was to occur.

E   Given this patient's history of syncope and ischemic heart disease, care should be taken to provide a stress-free environment to avoid a fainting episode or the onset of an angina attack.

11.   A,C Periodontal maintenance appointments should include removal of biofilm. The purpose of deplaquing and removing calculus is to disrupt the biofilm and create an environment that contributes to a reduction in inflammation.

B Periodontal maintenance instrumentation for this patient should be limited to deplaquing and instrumental debridment that results in a favorable tissue response. Scaling should be limited to removing detected calculus deposits. Scaling the exposed root surfaces would unnecessarily remove cementum.

D All areas of the mouth must be reprobed at the periodontal maintenance appointment to determine the progression or stabilization of the disease.

E Periodontal maintenance depends on patient compliance with self-care and her ability to be effective. This patient's level of effectiveness with daily oral self-care must be determined at each periodontal maintenance appointment.

12.   A One of the adverse effects of the estrogen is an increase in nervousness.

B This patient presents with a history of past dental experiences that involved pain where her response was fainting. It can be expected that these past experiences will affect her response and apprehension levels regarding today's visit.

C This patient's need to be self-reliant may be adding to her overly enthusiastic apprehension regarding her ability to control her reactions to treatment.

D This patient reports that pain experienced at past dental appointments caused her to faint. Lack of pain control can contribute to her dental anxiety.

E Vital signs such as blood pressure may be an indicator of a patient's anxiety levels but not the cause.

13.   A Oral benzodiazepines such as diazepam have a wide margin of safety when prescribed appropriately. In fact, orally ingesting 2 to 5 mg diazepam will highly reduce the patient's perception of pain and level of anxiety; both are considered mandatory for successful management of the patient with ischemic heart disease and significantly sensitive root surfaces.

B The use of nitrous oxide would not compromise any of the medications this patient is taking nor would it be contraindicated when nitroglycerin is administered. When combined with drugs producing oral sedation, nitrous oxide has the potential to induce unconscious sedation. The dental hygienist must be prepared for this potential.

C The topical application of benzocaine would be contraindicated for patients with a history of allergy or a sensitivity to ester-type anesthetics. This patient's medical history does not indicate a past allergic response to benzocaine.

D Oraqix contains 2.5% lidocaine and 2.5% prilocaine. The effect of prilocaine in combination with nitroglycerin may increase the risk of developing methemoglobinemia, a condition that reduces the ability of the blood to circulate oxygen. Although this patient is not currently taking nitroglycerin, it should be available for use during the appointment should a medical emergency arise. The possible need for nitroglycerin should be considered a caution for use of Oraqix.

E The patient's medical history does not note a sensitivity to amide anesthetics. In fact, Mepivacaine 3% does not contain vasoconstrictors, the use of which should be limited in patients with angina pectoris.

14.   **A** Although gingival diseases have been linked to medications, drug allergies are not associated with increased risk for periodontal breakdown. This patient's tetracycline allergy is not a risk factor for her periodontal condition.

B Periodontal diseases have been linked to endocrine changes. Hormonal therapies based on estrogens and progestin have an influence on the inflammatory response of periodontal tissues.

C Restorations with poorly contoured or rough margins that make oral self-care difficult and lead to plaque retention are considered a local contributing factor for periodontal disease. This patient has several large restorations that appear bulky and may be difficult to clean around.

D This 53-year-old female adult belongs to a demographic cohort with an increased risk of periodontal disease.

E Because prolonged physical and/or psychological stress is a risk factor for periodontal diseases, this patient's life-changing situation (coping with the death of her husband) is likely to increase her susceptibility.

15. A,C,E These answers are incorrect.

B The amount of recession in this area is 4 mm. The measurement of the recession alone (without the pocket depth) is not an accurate measurement of the total loss of attachment in this area.

(D) The clinical attachment level is determined by the probe depth and assessment of the position of the gingival margin in relation to a fixed point, the CEJ. When recession is present, the attachment loss is equal to the amount of recession plus the periodontal probe depth reading. With 4 mm of recession and a 2 mm facial probing depth, the loss of attachment would be 6 mm in this area.

16. A Although the probe reading at the facial of the maxillary right first premolar increased from 1 mm at the initial appointment to 2 mm at the reevaluation appointment, there appears to be a significant amount (more than 2 mm) of attached gingiva in this region.

B The maxillary right lateral incisor appears to have several millimeters of attached gingiva between the mucogingival line and the free gingival margin. Additionally, the probe reading on the facial of this tooth is only 1 mm.

C Based on the location of the mucogingival line and the 1 mm probe reading at the facial point of the maxillary left second premolar, there appears to be 1 or 2 mm of gingival attachment in this area. Although this would be classified as inadequate attached gingiva, the mandibular right lateral incisor would be considered more at risk.

D Even though the appearance of the facial gingiva of the mandibular left first molar is significantly bulbous, the 1 mm facial probe reading and the location of the mucogingival line indicate a significant amount of attached gingiva, putting this tooth at less risk for mucogingival involvement.

(E) Mucogingival involvement is determined by measuring the width of attached gingiva and subtracting the periodontal probe reading. When the resulting measurement is less than 1 mm there is mucogingival involvement. The mandibular right lateral incisor exhibits apparent recession that has progressed almost to the mucogingival line. With a 2 mm pocket depth at both the initial and reevaluation appointments, this area is most at risk for mucogingival involvement.

17. A,B,C,D The other teeth listed do not have sufficient pocket depths for placement of locally applied drug therapies.

(E) With an 8 mm pocket that did not decrease at the 6-week reevaluation appointment, the mandibular right first molar is an ideal candidate for locally applied drug therapy. The evidence that this area did not positively respond to mechanical therapy makes local drug delivery an ideal optional treatment for this region.

18. A Minocycline hydrochloride (syringe-delivered Arestin) contains derivatives of tetracycline as the active ingredient and therefore is contraindicated for this patient.

B Doxycycline hyclate (syringe-delivered Atridox) contains derivatives of tetracycline as the active ingredient and therefore is contraindicated for this patient.

(C) Because the patient is allergic to tetracycline, 2.5 mg chlorhexidine gluconate (PerioChip delivered in a resorbable gelatin wafer) is the only medicament listed that is not contraindicated for this patient.

D Actisite contains fibers that deliver tetracycline directly to the pocket. The patient's tetracycline allergy contraindicates its use.

19.   (A) This patient's lifelong residence in a community with optimal levels of fluoride in the water would not add to the reasons for recommending fluoride therapies.

B The areas of demineralization represent the initial stage of caries development. Fluoride therapy may assist with remineralization that leads to prevention of the development of frank carious lesions.

C The large number of exposed root surfaces are at risk for caries, indicating that fluoride therapy should be recommended for this patient.

D Dry mouth or xerostomia plays a role in the increased incidence of dental caries. Stress and menopause have demonstrated a risk for changes in salivary composition and decreased salivary flow or drying oral conditions indicating that fluoride therapies are a good recommendation for this patient.

E Multiple and complex restorations make plaque control difficult, adding to the risk for dental caries. Additionally, a primary risk factor for future caries is the presence of caries. This patient's history of decay indicates that she is at risk for future decay and would benefit from fluoride therapies.

20.   A Use of 1 ppm fluoridated water is recommended for all patients regardless of caries risk.

B A daily low-potency 520 ppm fluoride rinse is recommended for patients with moderate caries risk.

C Weekly high-potency 900 ppm fluoride rinses are primarily used in school-based programs for children with moderate to high risk for caries.

(D) Brush-on 1,000–1,500 ppm fluoride gel is recommended for this patient with a high caries risk.

21. A,C,D,E Each of the other chemical agents listed is found in professional treatments and not in self-applied agents available for home use.

(B) Potassium nitrate is the active ingredient found in at-home-use toothpaste with the American Dental Association (ADA) seal for treatment of hypersensitive teeth.

22.   (A) Night guard therapy is recommended to reduce the parafunctional habit of nocturnal bruxism and can help prevent further tooth mobility resulting from a decreased functional demand. An additional potential outcome of this therapy would be arrested periodontal destruction in the area.

B,C Biofeedback and therapeutic massage may help the patient reduce bruxism but will not provide treatment for tooth mobility.

D Splinting the teeth will provide stabilization of tooth mobility; however, it does not eliminate the bruxism and attrition that will continue to occur.

23.   A Autonomy is defined as self-determination. After informing the patient about the effects and consequences of treatment, the patient has the right to accept or refuse the procedure.

B Beneficence means doing what will benefit the patient. An ethical dental hygienist will be compelled to design treatment plans (in this case, thorough instrumentation of all areas necessary for comprehensive periodontal maintenance) that benefit the patient.

(C) The definition of nonmaleficence is to do no harm to the patient. By not doing something (instrumenting all areas necessary), the dental hygienist may in fact cause harm (progression of periodontal disease).

D Justice or fairness refers to providing all people, regardless of ethnicity, socioeconomic standing, and education level access to quality preventive oral hygiene care.

E Fidelity is the belief that the dental hygienist is morally obligated to keep promises and commitments communicated or implied.

24. A This patient's blood pressure is considered within normal limits.

(B) The patient's chief complaint, especially when the need is freedom from pain, should be addressed first.

C Immediately after addressing the patient's chief complaint, the treatment plan should address eliminating or reducing predisposing factors for periodontal disease such as nocturnal bruxing.

D Providing the patient with a new soft toothbrush and self-care instructions would occur after conditions that predispose the patient for periodontal disease are eliminated or reduced.

E The periapical radiographs supplement the horizontal bitewings by providing adequate information regarding the periodontium. It is not necessary to expose the patient to additional radiation at this appointment. At a future appointment, when radiographic need is assessed, vertical, instead of horizontal, bitewings would provide an increased image of the supporting bone.

25. A Allowing the patient to stop treatment at any time will help give her a sense of control. However, this action may not be enough to eliminate her anxiety based on her past dental experience that predisposes her to anticipate pain at this appointment.

B,D Relaxation and distraction techniques are effective for some patients. However, based on her past dental experience that predisposes her to anticipate pain at this appointment, recommending the dentist prescribe an antianxiety premedication oral sedative may be the better action for managing this patient's anxiety.

(C) Reduction of anxiety is important for successful management of the patient with angina pectoris to avoid a medical emergency during treatment. This patient presents with a dental experience history that predisposes her to anticipate pain at this appointment. Therefore, consultation with the dentist regarding a prescription for an antianxiety premedication oral sedative would most likely manage this patient's anxiety.

E Careful instrumentation is paramount in helping to reduce pain during instrumentation. However, based on her past reaction (syncope) to dental treatment recommending the dentist prescribe an antianxiety premedication oral sedative may be the better action for managing this patient's anxiety.

CASE E ADULT-PERIODONTAL PATIENT LOUIS RIDDICK

1. A,E When underjet or anterior crossbite present, the maxillary anterior teeth are in a position lingual to the mandibular anterior teeth.

B In an edge-to-edge relationship, the anterior teeth occlude on the incisal edge.

C An open bite indicates a lack of contact (vertical opening) between the maxillary and mandibular anterior teeth.

(D) Overjet, underjet, and anterior crossbite refer to the horizontal distance between the labioincisal surfaces of the maxillary anterior teeth and the linguoincisal surfaces of the mandibular anterior teeth. When overjet presents, the maxillary anterior teeth are in a position labial to the mandibular anterior teeth as evidenced on the study model taken on this patient.

2. (A) Normal melanin pigmentation occurs in persons of color and should not be mistakenly identified as a disease or condition requiring attention. This patient does not present with additional symptoms or a history of pain associated with these regions of the mouth.

B Normal melanin pigmentation should not be mistaken for smoker's melanosis, a brownish discoloration of the oral mucosa that usually occurs in the mandibular anterior region.

C The chronic inflammatory disease, lichen planus, causes bilateral white striations, papules, or plaques on the buccal mucosa, tongue, and gingivae. Erythema, erosions, and blisters may or may not be present.

D Possible clinical presentations of contact stomatitis include erythematous lesions, erosions/ulcerations, leukoplakia-like lesions, oral lichenoid reactions, contact urticaria, and burning mouth syndrome contact stomatitis. This patient does not present with clinic symptoms associated with the dark appearance of the facial gingiva.

E Oral lesions associated with discoid lupus erythematosus usually appear on the buccal mucosa as small (less than 1 cm), painful aphthous ulcerations. The lesions tend to last up to 2 to 3 weeks.

3.   A Although the patient presents with a tongue thrust, this condition may be contributing to his pronounced overjet through forces inflicted anteriorly, but not the diastema which is the result of forces inflicted laterally.

B The enlarged papilla, unlike the frenal attachment, is not involved in mechanical movement and therefore would not be exerting force on the tooth structure to cause displacement.

C Destruction of bone and the development of infrabony defects as the result of periodontal disease will cause tooth mobility and displacement. However, probe depths and radiographic assessment of the maxillary central incisors do not reveal conditions conducive to distal drift of these teeth.

D Although a growing cyst or tumor may indeed displace structures in its path, the radiolucency between the maxillary central incisors is the incisive foramen and should not be mistaken for a pathologic condition.

(E) The maxillary frenum functions to hold the lip in place. The size and location of the labial frenal attachment may affect the position of the maxillary central incisors laterally. This band of connective tissue is so firm that erupting central incisors may not penetrate through it, but will be pushed aside so that a diastema results.

4.   A Leukoedema, Fordyce's granules, nicotinic stomatitis, and candidiasis can usually be distinguished by their characteristic appearances and the location in which they are noted. Leukoedema, found in approximately 80% of the black population, appears as a milky, white-blue striated lesion of the buccal mucosa. Leukoedema is considered normal and no treatment is necessary.

(B) Leukoplakia is the term given to white patches found intraorally that usually cannot be clinically identified as a specific disease entity. Although smoking may have initiated the epithelium in this area to increase in thickness, trauma created by movement of the upper lip over this tissue could also produce the hyperkeratinization. The etiology may not be readily discernable and a histological exam may be ordered for differential diagnosis.

C Candidiasis, representing the overgrowth of *Candida albicans*, may result when the normal flora of the oral cavity is altered as when the patient is taking antibiotics, is immune suppressed, presents with endocrine diseases, or has a hereditary predisposition to fungal infections. The white lesion associated with pseudomembranous candidiasis may be easily wiped off with gauze.

D Nicotinic stomatitis can result in hyperkeratosis of the mucosa of the hard palate in response to the heat introduced into the oral cavity from smoking. The palate usually appears white with small red points.

E   Fordyce's granules, sebaceous glands choristomas, appear yellow in color and are usually found near the maxillary vermilion border and labial mucosa. Fordyce's granules are also considered normal and no treatment is necessary.

5.   A   The mental foramen may be imaged on a mandibular periapical radiograph near the apex of the mandibular first or second premolar.

B   Because of its posterior–superior location in the ramus of the mandible, the mandibular foramen may appear on a panoramic radiograph, but not on an intraoral radiograph.

(C) The incisive foramen is anatomically located between the maxillary central incisors.

D   The lingual foramen may be imaged on a periapical radiograph of the mandibular anterior region. The lingual foramen often appears as a small radiolucent dot within the radiopaque circle of genial tubercles.

E   Because of its superior location, the infraorbital foramen may be imaged on a panoramic radiograph, but not on an intraoral radiograph.

6.   (A) If significantly dense, calculus deposits will appear on radiographs about the same radiopacity as dentin. This deposit located in the furca appears as a "bump" or spur between the roots of the tooth.

B   Pulp stones present within the pulp chamber.

C   Although an enamel pearl may present in this area between the roots, it would appear the same radiopacity as enamel and would be attached to, or appear as an extension of, the enamel.

D   Hypercementosis would appear as a radiopaque overgrowth of excess cementum creating an enlarged or bulbous root structure.

E   Composite restorations would not be placed in this area and would appear in a prepared cavity within the tooth structure rather than an attachment to the root.

7.   A   A nonvital tooth may take on a darkening appearance. However, the hue produced by this tooth is the result of the large metallic restoration showing through the thin enamel.

B   Staining from systemic ingestion of tetracycline would affect all teeth that were forming at the time of ingestion, and not this single tooth.

C   Dentinogenesis imperfecta is a developmental disturbance affecting the dentin that usually produces thinner than normal enamel. Although dentinogenesis imperfecta can result in a translucent blue-gray hue to the teeth, all teeth that were forming at the time of the disturbance would be affected.

(D) The radiographs reveal that this tooth as been restored with endodontic filling material and a metallic restoration. The dark metal materials appear to be showing through the thin enamel, giving the tooth the gray hue.

E   Hypocalcified enamel results from a defect of the ameloblast of the enamel and the affected tooth fails to develop to its normal thickness resulting in a yellow-brown hue, and enamel pitting or roughness. The tooth may also appear smaller in size than a normal tooth. However, this condition should not be mistaken for the appearance of metallic restorations through the enamel as demonstrated by this tooth.

8.   A   This patient does not present with a need for application of desensitizing agents.

(B) To help the patient meet his goals of improving oral health and to encourage success of nonsurgical periodontal intervention, the first step must be patient education in the disease process and explicit instruction in oral self-care. Before any therapeutic intervention, instruction in oral self-assessment and discussion of the relationship between preventive measures and periodontal disease must occur.

C   The difficult prognosis of the furcation involvement of the maxillary first molars makes extraction a likely treatment. However, the patient has not presented with pain at this initial appointment; therefore, before any treatment occurs, a comprehensive treatment plan should be discussed with the patient.

D   The success of periodontal scaling and root debridement depends on the role the patient plays in oral self-care on a daily basis. Prior to treatment, this patient must understand this role, be interested in the treatment plan, and be motivated to comply with recommendations.

E   The most likely diagnosis of the white patches is leukoplakia and not a fungal infection. Because smoking is most likely the cause, the area should be monitored to see if the tissue improves now that this patient has stopped smoking. If available, a brush-biopsy can remove a few cells for testing to determine if cancer cells are present, or the patient may be referred to an oral pathologist for a biopsy.

9.   A   Because the power toothbrush is a new self-care aid for him, his skill at using this device should be reinforced. He may be less motivated to listen to manual brushing instructions, knowing that he will be using the power toothbrush at home.

B,C   At this time, reinforcing the use of his new power brush would be more likely to produce better results. The spaces between his teeth suggest that an interdental brush, which could be introduced after he masters power brush instructions, may be more effective than floss or an end-tuft brush.

D   An interdental brush would be ideal to introduce after this patient masters the use of his new power brush. However, simply providing a brochure is not likely to inspire this minimally motivated patient to begin to use this new device effectively.

(E)   This patient reports that he recently began using a power toothbrush. Because effective use of a power toothbrush requires practice, his technique with this device should be evaluated versus teaching him another new method or aid at this time.

10.   A   Although furcation involvement is present, it is the result and not the cause of the hypereruption of the maxillary molars.

B   The length of the junctional epithelium (1 to 2 mm in coronoapical dimension) is not responsible for the supereruption of the teeth. As this patient's molar teeth continue to erupt, the junctional epithelium migrates down the root surfaces, exposing more of the root surfaces of the teeth.

(C)   Premature loss of mandibular teeth may result in the hypereruption of the opposing maxillary teeth.

D   This patient has no history of surgical intervention for periodontal disease.

E   Attached gingival widths vary among patients naturally and as a result of periodontal diseases. The amount of attached gingiva on these molars is not related to the supereruption of these teeth.

11.   (A)   The calibrated markings on this instrument indicate that it is a probe. The curved working end and insertion into the furcation area shown in the photograph indicates that this instrument is a furcation probe. A furcation probe is used to gage the depth of penetration through the furcation area of periodontally involved teeth.

B   A treatment instrument such as a scaler or curet does not have the calibrated markings of a probe. Additionally, the instrument in the photograph would demonstrate a shank that terminated into a working end that would appear balanced or centered in line with the long axis of the instrument handle.

C   Explorers do not have the calibrated markings of a probe. Additionally, the tactile sensitivity required for the detection of calculus requires that an explorer be thin, slender, and wirelike.

D Periodontal probes used to measure pocket depths contain calibrated markings. However, these instruments have a straight, tapered, round shank and working end. A periodontal probe used to measure pocket depths would be adapted so that the side of the probe tip is inserted into the pocket with the terminal shank parallel to the long axis of the tooth.

E Subgingival irrigation agents are introduced into periodontal pockets via a cannula attached to a syringe or an air-driven handpiece.

12. A The mini Gracey 1/2 curet is designed specifically for instrumentation and removal of light calculus in deep, difficult to access pockets of anterior teeth.

B Rigid Gracey curets are site-specific periodontal instruments used to remove moderate calculus. The 11/12 Gracey curet is designed specifically for instrumentation of the mesial surfaces of posterior teeth.

C The standard flexible shank Gracey 13/14 curet is designed specifically for instrumentation of the distal surfaces of posterior teeth with light calculus.

D The design of a universal sickle scaler prohibits its use subgingivally to access the calculus at the base of this periodontal pocket. Additionally, the pointed tip of a scaler will not allow for adequate adaptation to the curved root surface of this second molar for thorough removal of the calculus.

E A chisel scaler is effective at removing heavy supragingival calculus from exposed proximal surfaces of anterior teeth and possibly premolars when access is not limited by the patient's cheeks.

13. A,B When the alveolar bone crest does not appear parallel to an imaginary line imaged on radiographs connecting adjacent teeth at the CEJ, the bone loss is considered vertical or angular.

C Dehiscence refers to bone loss that manifests as a resorbed cleft, a condition not associated with these teeth.

D Fenestration refers to bone loss that creates an opening or "window" through the bone covering the facial root surface; a condition not associated with these teeth.

E Horizontal bone loss is differentiated from a vertical or angular defect by comparing the bone crest imaged on radiographs to an imaginary line connecting adjacent teeth at the cementoenamel junction (CEJ). When the alveolar bone crest appears parallel to this imaginary line, horizontal bone loss is noted.

14. A Grade I furcation involvement is characterized by a detectable depression in the furcation opening only. Radiographic changes are not evident at this early stage.

B Grade II furcation involvement is characterized by bone loss that allows the probe to detect a cul-de-sac under the dome of the furcation. Radiographs may or may not depict the involvement at this stage.

C Significant bone loss in the furcation area in which the bone is not attached to the roof of the furcation and the probe may pass through the roots is classified as a Grade III. However, soft tissue would prevent clinically visualizing the furcation.

D In the 1950s, Glickman developed a classification of furcation involvement identified by grades. Significant bone loss in the furcation area in which the bone is not attached to the roof of the furcation and the probe may pass through the roots is classified as a Grade III. If the soft tissues have receded apically so that a Grade III furcation involvement is clinically visible, then Grade IV is the appropriate classification. Although plaque appears to block this area, the photograph of the maxillary right first molar appears to reveal a Grade IV furcation involvement.

15. A Because the pocket depth was 5 mm at the initial appointment, it would be tempting to say that the initial clinical attachment level was 10 mm; however, we do not know what the position of the free gingival margin was at that appointment.

B The clinical attachment level is calculated by measuring (in millimeters) the distance from the CEJ to the free gingival margin and by measuring the pocket depth. The recession and the pocket depth measurements are added together. The sum is the total loss of attachment. The facial surface of the maxillary right first molar demonstrates 4 mm of recession plus a 5 mm pocket depth at the reevaluation appointment. Therefore, the measurement of the clinical attachment level at the reevaluation appointment is 9 mm.

C   This answer is not correct.

D   The pocket depth at the initial appointment was 6 mm. Pocket depth alone is not a measurement of clinical attachment level.

E   The pocket depth at the reevaluation appointment is 5 mm. Pocket depth alone is not a measurement of clinical attachment level.

16.   A   This tooth has undergone endodontic therapy; however, this procedure is limited to the pulp chamber and does not have an implication in periodontal disease.

B,D,E   Overhanging restorations, caries, and occlusal trauma are all local contributing factors for periodontal disease; however, these conditions are not evident in this area.

C The concave root morphology on the mesial surface of the maxillary first premolar provides a protected environment for bacteria to accumulate. The severity of the concavity is demonstrated on the radiographs.

17.   **A** Although tooth mobility may result from various conditions, such as trauma or periapical pathology, only one of the conditions listed here is directly responsible for this patient's tooth mobility. The significant bone loss associated with periodontal disease is responsible for the mobile teeth.

B   Although some systemic diseases, such as diabetes mellitus and HIV/AIDS, are systemic contributing risk factors for periodontal diseases, which in turn is responsible for tooth mobility, hypertension is not related to the condition of the periodontium.

C   Tooth mobility is not an adverse effect of Zyban or Nicorette.

D   Premature loss of permanent teeth may cause adjacent teeth to shift position. The patient reports that several teeth were extracted many years ago. Mobility during the shift of adjacent remaining teeth may have occurred at that time. Any mobility detected at this appointment is the result of bone loss caused by periodontal disease.

E   Smoking has been documented as a risk factor for periodontal disease; however, it is this patient's periodontal disease that has caused the teeth mobility.

18.   A   Although this patient's brushing habits have not been effective at plaque control, studies have indicated that even when self-care is ideal, smokers exhibit deeper periodontal pockets and significantly more bone loss than nonsmokers with similar self-care abilities.

B   This patient is not taking any medication associated with an adverse effect of increasing risk for periodontal diseases.

C   Stress can elevate susceptibility to periodontal diseases, but it is highly unlikely that stress plays a role in this patient's life. The greater risk from this list is smoking.

D   Prehypertension is not associated with an increased risk for periodontal diseases.

E It has been established that tobacco smoking may be the most important environmental factor in the United States associated with periodontal disease.

19.   A   The photographs reveal gingival tissue that appears edematous and bulbous. An expected outcome of removal of calculus and disruption of biofilms at the reevaluation appointment is tissue shrinkage, possibly accompanied by recession resulting in a 1 to 2 mm reduction in pretreatment probing depths.

B Debridement results in a renewal of epithelial cells in contact with the tooth surfaces to improve integrity of the clinical attachment demonstrated at the reevaluation appointment.

C Following scaling and root planing, healing takes place by the formation of a long junctional epithelial attachment resulting in a closure to the pocket.

D Regeneration of new bone, cementum, and periodontal ligament is a more likely outcome of periodontal surgery.

E Following calculus removal and disruption of biofilms, reformation of gingival collagen may stop the probe tip at a more coronal point in the pocket, resulting in a reduction in probe readings.

20. **A** Maintenance appointment intervals as short as 1 month should be recommended for this level of disease. Aggressive attachment loss and the patient's ability to perform effective plaque control will need to be monitored. Additionally, success with smoking cessation has not yet been established.

B,C Research indicates that patients with a history of periodontal disease should be on a maintenance schedule that is no longer than 4 months. However, based on the severity of the periodontal condition this patient presents with, he should be monitored in 1 month.

D,E Patients with a history of periodontal disease should be on a maintenance schedule that is no longer than 4 months.

21. A Essential oils are also effective at reducing bacterial plaque and gingivitis but with less substantivity than chlorhexidine gluconate. Less substantivity requires more frequent use for optimal results, in turn requiring a bigger commitment from the patient to comply with recommendations.

B Zinc chloride has been used in many products to reduce the formation of calculus and reduce mouth malodor. Limited studies are available that substantiate the link between using these products and an effective reduction in bacterial plaque.

C Evaluation of cetylpyridinium chloride products currently on the market has produced mixed results on their efficacy. Given this patient's advanced periodontal condition, recommending an agent with proven efficacy would be the better choice.

D Currently chlorhexidine gluconate is the most effective antiplaque and antigingivitis agent approved for short-term clinical use.

E Although demonstrated to be a temporary debriding agent in the oral cavity, especially for conditions such as acute necrotizing ulcerative gingivitis and periocoronitis, the use of hydrogen peroxide as an antiplaque/antigingivitis agent has not be confirmed.

22. A To get the maximum benefit from nicotine gum, the patient may need to be reminded of the instructions on its use. Nicotine gum should be used whenever the urge to smoke occurs. Nicotine gum should be chewed slowly for 30 minutes and then "parked" inside the cheek against the oral mucosa. Every few minutes, he may repeat slow, gentle chewing.

B Because nicotine addiction is so difficult to overcome, positive reinforcement and complimenting the patient on his success so far can often be an impetus to continued success.

C Slipping, or smoking again, can be very discouraging to the patient trying to quit. Making the patient aware that he can try to stop again, and has not failed, if he smokes one or a few cigarettes, may provide needed motivation.

D Overcoming nicotine addiction can be especially difficult in the beginning, because it may take 1 or 2 weeks for withdrawal symptoms to subside. Providing the patient with this information along with encouragement and support from the dental hygienist will aid in his success.

E This negative approach will most likely stimulate patient denial and may result in tuning out advice.

23.   A As tissue shrinkage takes place, recession and papillary shape changes can result in the appearance of a longer clinical crown. The patient should be educated regarding this possible outcome.

B It is important that the patient understand the healing process that follows scaling and root planing. Increased dentinal sensitivity as a result of tissue shrinkage that exposes root surfaces can play a role in patient compliance with self-care and satisfaction with treatment. Additionally, the patient needs to be aware that treatment is available should this condition arise.

C Because this patient reports that tooth mobility prompted him to make this initial appointment, he needs to be prepared for a possible increase in tooth mobility following treatment. The dental hygienist must be sure that effective communication occurs regarding this possibility.

(D) It is important that the patient understand the possible outcomes of his treatment, especially when changes to the oral cavity are likely. This patient may not be expecting to experience a possible change in the appearance of gingival tissues or possible discomfort from roots exposed by gingival recession. He should be prepared for these outcomes. Although statistics on success rates of treatment should be considered when treatment planning for the patient, this is not an outcome of his treatment.

E As tissue shrinkage occurs, additional blunting of papillae is likely. The patient must be made aware not only of the possible change in appearance of the gingiva, but also of methods to clean these areas. The dental hygienist must stress the importance of patient compliance with self-care that will be required following treatment.

24.   A There is a possibility that tooth mobility will increase following scaling. The dental hygienist should be cautious about offering false assurance, especially given the periodontal involvement exhibited by this patient.

B Given the periodontal involvement of both maxillary first molars, the prognosis is less than ideal, indicating a possible need for extractions. However, the dental hygienist should refrain from making this dental diagnosis. Instead, the patient should be referred for evaluation.

(C) The dental hygienist is educated to make decisions to recommend referrals to other professionals. The type and severity of the periodontal condition this patient presents with and the presence of periodontal pockets greater than 5 mm at the reevaluation appointment indicate a necessity to be evaluated by a periodontist.

D The wording of this statement is outside the realm of the dental hygienist's scope of practice. Additionally, having recently undergone a complete physical by his physician, and taking into consideration the diagnosis of prehypertension, his physician's recommendations are sound. If the dental hygienist discovers something incongruent with the physician's recommendations and dental hygiene treatment, the physician can be contacted for clarification, or the patient may be referred back to the physician for evaluation.

E Implants may indeed be an option for this patient, but the dental hygienist should be cautious about offering false assurance, especially given this patient's circumstances, such as the severity of active periodontal disease, lack of established smoking cessation at this point in time, and need for an assessment by a periodontist.

25.   (A) This patient may be reluctant to accept preventative treatment because he does not see himself as someone who invests time and money in dental treatment. The dental hygienist can help him make a connection between what steps he takes now toward good oral health and how this will contribute to maintaining his oral health in the future. Voicing confidence in the patient's abilities can help

him take responsibility for what happens to his teeth and will encourage him to accept the recommended treatment plan.

B Blaming the patient for his periodontal condition and for failing to deal with the worsening condition is not likely to contribute to a change in his behavior to comply with treatment.

C The patient should not be pushed into treatment decisions before he has an understanding of the situation, has agreed that he has a need, and can value the treatment enough to be able to comply.

D Threatening the patient with negative consequences may cause him to tune out the message. This is especially true when the patient is not in pain, or does not perceive his poor oral health as causing him any immediate discomfort.

E Humor, when used correctly, can contribute to developing a rapport with this easy-going patient. However, at this point the dental hygienist would not want to validate the patient's point of view, possibility casting a negative shadow over the need for extensive, and possibly expensive, treatment.

CASE F ADULT-PERIODONTAL PATIENT BANU RADPUR-ANSARI

1.   A An overgrowth of bone, or bony exostosis, beginning in the midline of the palatal vault would be indicative of a torus palantinus.

(B) The term *ruga* means a ridge or fold. Although seemingly pronounced in this view of her palate, this is the normal appearance of palatal rugae.

C There are no major salivary glands located in this region.

D The normal appearance of the rugae should not be confused with pathology. Blisterform lesions would appear as fluid-filled pustules or vesicles.

E Although trauma that may occur when eating very hot or crunchy foods can sometimes irritate this region of the palate, there is no evidence of irritation.

2.   A Erosion refers to the wearing away of the tooth structure via chemical means.

B Abrasion refers to a wearing away of the tooth structure by forces other than mastication. This term is most often applied to wear that results from incorrect tooth brushing.

(C) Attrition refers to the wearing away of the tooth surface via tooth-to-tooth contact or chewing habits that include nail biting and chewing course foods. In this case uneven, moderate wear is exhibited on the incisal edges of both the maxillary and mandibular teeth.

D The incisal edges of these teeth present with wear that should not be mistaken for caries activity.

E Abfraction presents as a wedge-shaped notch in the cervical region of the tooth, often resulting from parafunctional occlusion.

3.   **(A)** Because the opposing maxillary teeth have been extracted, the possibility exists that the mandibular teeth will supererupt into an extruded position.

B Ankylosed teeth remain embedded, or fused to the supporting bone. Teeth that are ankylosed usually do not fully erupt into their natural position in the arch.

C Both the mandibular right second and third molars appear to be fully erupted into their natural position. Neither one of these teeth is impacted, or embedded in the bone.

D Hypercementosis is a condition of an overgrowth of cementum that makes the roots of the teeth appear enlarged and bulbous. Hypercementosis is not evident radiographically, nor are these teeth at risk for this condition.

E Fusion occurs when unerupted adjacent teeth become joined with cementum. Fusion is not evident, nor are these teeth at risk for this condition.

4.   A The size of the distal occlusal defect on the mandibular right first molar would indicate caries as the reason for food impaction. Mobility is not noted in this region.

B Blunted papilla can contribute to food accumulation in the embrasures. However, the size of the distal occlusal defect on the mandibular right first molar is the overriding reason for food impaction between these teeth.

C The facial recession noted does not contribute to food impaction between the teeth.

(D) Recurrent decay most likely caused the loss of the distal portion of the amalgam restoration, creating the potential for food impaction.

E A diastema refers to a natural space created when two adjacent teeth are situated in the arch without contacting. The space created between the mandibular right first and second molar is not naturally occurring, but due to the distal occlusal defect of the first molar.

5.   A Calculus deposits appear radiographically on the mesial and distal of the maxillary right first molar. This observation should not be confused with composite restorations.

(B) The radiographs indicate that the maxillary right central incisor has been restored with composite material.

C The mandibular left first molar has been restored with amalgam.

D Overlapping error on the radiograph of the mandible left lateral incisor should not be confused with composite restorative material.

E The mandibular right first molar has been restored with amalgam. The distal occlusal portion of the amalgam appears less radiopaque on the radiograph. A clinical examination of the photographs reveals that this restoration is missing because of recurrent decay.

6.   A The radiolucency observed on the maxillary right central incisor has the prepared look of a composite restoration.

B The radiolucency observed in the region of the maxillary left second molar roots is furcation involvement.

(C) The radiographs reveal a radiolucency on the distal of the mandibular left first molar that should be suspected as caries.

D The radiolucency observed around the cervical region of the mandibular right canine is the radiographic optical illusion cervical burnout. This optical illusion should not be confused with caries.

E The mandibular right second molar has deep pits and fissures that are evident on the occlusal surface. However, when examining radiographs for occlusal caries, the dentin apical to the occlusal enamel should be observed. The dentin under the enamel of this tooth appears normal.

7.   A The Water's technique is an extraoral radiograph used for imaging the sinus.

B Posterior-Anterior radiographs are an extraoral technique often used by oral surgeons and orthodontists to aid in examination of growth and development, disease, trauma, and developmental anomalies.

C The occlusal radiograph utilizes a variation of the bisecting technique to image a large area of pathology. On an adult, a film size #4 would most likely be used.

D Localization techniques usually utilize two radiographs, taken with two different angles to determine the buccolingual position of an object.

(E) When posterior film packet placement is difficult, or placement will not adequately image the posteriorly located structure, the disto-oblique periapical radiographic technique can be used. Using the disto-oblique technique allows the x-ray beam to be directed toward the film obliquely from the distal for the purpose of imaging the posterior structure. The result is more of the posterior structure being imaged, but a side effect is the production of increased overlapping, evident in this film.

8.   A   The lingual foramen when observed radiographically appears as a small radiolucent dot usually surrounded by the radiopaque genial tubercles, inferior to the mandibular anterior teeth apices.

       (B) This is the normal appearance of the mental fossa and should not be confused with pathology.

       C   Although early periapical cemental dyplasia appears radiolucent, the normal appearing mental fossa should not be confused with this condition.

       D   The reduced amount of cancellous bone of osteoporosis is difficult to assess from dental radiographs. With special techniques, the loss of density of the cortical plate of bone of the inferior border of the mandible may indicate osteoporosis. However, the normal appearing mental fossa should not be confused with oral manifestations of this disease.

       E   A periapical abscess would manifest within the lamina dura of the affected tooth. In each of the radiographs of the mandibular anterior region, all teeth present with intact lamina dura.

9.   **(A)** The American Heart Association recommends that patients with a history of infective endocarditis be premedicated before procedures likely to induce gingival bleeding.

       B   Hypothyroidism controlled with medication does not require alterations in dental hygiene treatment.

       C   A sinus infection does not require premedication with antibiotics before nonsurgical periodontal therapy. However, the amoxicillin she is taking for her sinus infection is not considered significant premedication to prevent infective endocarditis. Another antibiotic such as clindamycin or cephalexin should be prescribed.

       D   There are some indications that being born in certain countries puts an individual at risk for certain diseases, such as tuberculosis. However, place of birth does not play a role in determining the need for antibiotic premedication.

       E   Antibiotic premedication is not required for any condition relating to blood pressure. Additionally, this patient's blood pressure reading is normal.

10.   A   The American Heart Association recommends 2 g amoxicillin orally 1 hour before treatment for patients at risk for infective endocarditis. However, this patient is currently taking amoxicillin for a sinus infection. Therefore, another antibiotic, such as clindamycin, should be prescribed.

     B,D   The American Heart Association recommends administering ampicillin or cefazolin intramuscularly or intravenously when patients cannot tolerate oral medications.

       (C) Because this patient is already taking amoxicillin for her sinus infection, another antibiotic should be prescribed as a premedication for prevention of infective endocarditis. The American Heart Association recommends 600 mg clindamycin orally 1 hour before treatment.

11.   A   Prescribing antibiotics over the course of time required for one-quadrant treatment each week increases the risk of creating antibiotic-resistant microorganisms and should be avoided.

       B   Because this patient presents with no conditions that contraindicate long appointments, one-half of the mouth can be treated at each appointment avoiding prolonged treatment over the course of one quadrant every 2 weeks.

       C   Because antibiotic resistance is unlikely to continue 9 to 14 days after stopping the antibiotic, it is advised that appointments requiring premedication be spaced 2 weeks apart.

D Prolonged antibiotic use is discouraged, as this can create the proliferation of antibiotic-resistant microorganisms. Because resistance is unlikely to continue 9 to 14 days after stopping the antibiotic, it is advised that appointments requiring premedication be spaced 2 weeks apart. Additionally, completing as much treatment as possible at one appointment will reduce the number of times that the patient must take the antibiotic. Because this patient presents with no conditions that contraindicate long appointments, one-half of the mouth can be treated at each appointment.

E Although completing as much treatment as possible at one appointment will reduce the number of times that the patient must take antibiotics, this patient presents with heavy subgingival calculus and an advanced periodontal disease condition that requires comprehensive nonsurgical periodontal treatment. Treatment of one-half the mouth will involve a long appointment that is best scheduled twice.

12.   A Nitrous oxide–oxygen analgesia would be acceptable when only slight discomfort was anticipated. Comprehensive treatment of the periodontal abscess would be better achieved through the use of a block anesthesia.

B Topical anesthetic such as benzocaine would not provide the profound anesthesia required to treat the periodontal abscess especially when discomfort will most likely be felt in the teeth and soft tissue.

C Infiltration anesthesia alone is not likely to produce the desired amount of comfort required to treat the periodontal abscess. Infiltration with short-acting prilocaine may not provide the level of anesthesia for the duration of the procedure as the lack of epinephrine allows the anesthetic to be diffused rapidly away from the region. Additionally, without epinephrine there is likely to be increased bleeding.

D Noninjectable anesthetic lidocaine 2.5% and prilocaine 2.5% gel provides very good anesthesia for a short (10 to 20 minutes) duration. It is most likely that profound anesthesia for a medium to long duration would better allow treatment in the region of the periodontal abscess.

E A block anesthesia is required to debride the area affected by the periodontal abscess to provide drainage. Long-lasting bupivacaine allows ample time to complete the scaling, debridement, and irrigation of the quadrant. The added benefit of a long-lasting anesthetic is pain control following the procedure. The addition of epinephrine will control bleeding throughout the procedure.

13.   A,C Endocrine system problems such as diabetes and hormone fluctuation have been shown to play a role in increasing risk for periodontal disease. However, this patient does not present with evidence of these conditions. Her thyroid condition is controlled with medication and does not play a role in increasing her risk for periodontal disease.

B Susceptibility to periodontal disease seems to increase with long-term stress. It is most likely that this patient's pursuit of a doctoral degree and work on her research project has created a stressful situation for her over time.

D Although risk for developing periodontal disease appears to increase with age, this patient's age would seem to place her into a category of being less likely to have the disease.

E Although genetics may play a role in developing periodontal disease, there is no evidence that this patient's race predisposes her for the disease.

14.   A Pocket formation, bone loss, and inflammation categorize this patient's periodontal disease as chronic periodontitis.

B Aggressive periodontitis usually results in localized rapid destruction of the periodontium and is more commonly found in patients under age 30. Although this patient presents with severe bone loss in the molar regions, the radiographs reveal generalized varying levels of bone loss.

C   This patient is not taking any medications that would result in drug-induced gingival disease.

D   This patient does not present with a systemic disease that would predispose her to a compromised host response for periodontal disease.

E   Necrotizing periodontitis is often seen in patients with compromised immune systems, not evident in this patient's health history.

15.   (A) The probe reading on the facial aspect of the maxillary left canine is 2 mm. Although there is recession in this area, an estimate of the distance from the mucogingival line to the free gingival margin indicates that there is still adequate attached gingiva in this region.

B   The facial aspect of the maxillary left second molar appears to be where a periodontal abscess is draining. Taking into consideration the deep probe readings in this region, there is likely to be inadequate attached gingiva here.

C   The probe reading on the facial aspect of the mandibular left central incisor is 2 mm. Taking into consideration the recession observed in this area, an estimate of the distance from the mucogingival line to the free gingival margin indicates the likelihood of inadequate attached gingiva in this region.

D   The probe reading on the facial aspect of the mandibular right canine is 1 mm. Taking into consideration the recession observed in this area, an estimate of the distance from the mucogingival line to the free gingival margin indicates the likelihood of inadequate attached gingiva in this region.

E   The probe reading on the facial aspect of the mandibular right second molar is 1 mm. Taking into consideration the recession observed in this area, an estimate of the distance from the mucogingival line to the free gingival margin indicates the likelihood of inadequate attached gingiva in this region.

16.   A   Although the increased probe readings obtained at the reevaluation appointment in three of the posterior quandrants indicate a need for retreatment, the decreased probe readings obtained at the reevaluation appointment in the mandibular right quandrant indicate a favorable response to treatment.

B   Although the increased probe readings obtained at the reevaluation appointment in the area of the mandibular central and lateral incisors indicate a need for retreatment, the decreased probe readings obtained in the other regions of the mandibular indicate a favorable response to treatment.

C   Although the increased probe readings obtained at the reevaluation appointment in the maxillary right and left posterior regions indicate a need for retreatment, this answer does not include other nonresponsive regions.

D   Although the increased probe readings obtained at the reevaluation appointment in the area of the mandibular central and lateral incisors indicate a need for retreatment, the decreased probe readings obtained in the maxillary anterior sextant indicate a favorable response to treatment.

(E) The increased probing depths assessed at the reevaluation appointment for the maxillary right posterior, the maxillary left posterior, and the mandibular left central and lateral incisor regions all indicate no response to treatment. These unstable sites should be assessed and if calculus is remaining in the pockets, it should be removed.

17.   A   Although flossing would be a better choice for complete interproximal self-care, including removal of the plaque, this patient has most likely discovered that the size and nature of food particles may well be more easily removed by use of the interproximal plastic pick.

B   Food accumulation in the embrasures is more likely to be noticed by the patient than plaque accumulation in the furcation areas.

C   The root surfaces exposed by gingival recession will be increasingly difficult to keep clean. However, these areas would be unlikely to benefit from the use of an interproximal oral hygiene aid.

(D)   The blunted papillae have left the embrasures between the teeth open to food debris accumulation.

E   Although cultural and or familiar use of certain oral self-care devices may influence the patient's choice, it is more likely that annoying food particles accumulating in the embrasures is the reason she has chosen to use this interproximal oral hygiene aid.

18.   (A)   A periodontal abscess is suspected given the symptom of throbbing pain and the enlarged, red appearance with exudate upon probing. The presence of deep pockets, furcation involvement, and mobility of the teeth in this area indicate a periodontal emergency. The radiographs reveal a slight widening of the periodontal ligament space. The reason the radiographs do not play a major role in identifying this condition could be that it is difficult to adequately image intrabony defects involving these multirooted teeth.

B   This patient's symptoms are characteristic of a periodontal emergency. Incorrect use of interdental cleaners may produce trauma, but not of this nature.

C   Bone exostosis, like tori, are considered normal in some patients. These hard, bony extensions of the arches do not cause pain or exude suppuration.

D   Occlusal disharmonies contribute to periodontal disease, and are likely to produce mobility, bone loss, and pain, but not in this acute, throbbing painful manner. Occlusal disharmonies will not produce the extended gingival swelling nor exude purulence.

E   An impacted tooth is not evident on the radiographs.

19.   A   Recurrent periodontal disease refers to disease that has returned after a period of stabilization. This patient's initial periodontal status has not responded to nonsurgical treatment and therefore surgical intervention should be considered.

B   Periodontal diseases that do not respond to treatment are often said to be refractory. Because this patient's initial periodontal status has not responded to nonsurgical treatment, she should now be referred for assessment of surgical intervention options.

(C)   The increased probe depths in three of four posterior quadrants and in the mandibular central and lateral incisor region assessed at the reevaluation appointment indicate no response to treatment. Additional considerations for referral for evaluation for periodontal surgery include periodontal abscess, tooth mobility, and the possibility of refractory periodontal disease.

D   Necrotizing ulcerative periodontitis is characterized by extensive necrosis and pain and usually occurs in patients who are immunosuppressed.

E   This patient does not present with use of a drug linked to gingival enlargement.

20.   A,C,E   This patient does not present with any condition that would contraindicate the use of these self-care products.

(B)   This patient's needs for premedication and degree of inflammation associated with her periodontal condition may contraindicate oral irrigation. The incidence of bacteremia increases with the degree of inflammation and infection present. However, because this patient is likely to benefit from irrigation with chlorhexidine gluconate, her physician should be consulted to determine if this treatment can be prescribed.

D Although use of a whitening product may be contraindicated in this patient with active periodontal disease, it is not necessary to contact her physician to make the decision regarding recommendations for its use.

21. A The systemic use of the antibiotic she is currently taking for her sinus infection may not be providing the level of concentration needed at the site of the periodontal abscess.

B Although the most likely reason for antibiotic failure is inadequate/incorrect dosing required for the periodontal condition, she also presents with local risk factors of deep pockets and furcation involvement that accumulate and trap bacterial plaque. The radiographs also reveal the presence of calculus, a local contributing risk factor that prevents healing.

C It is possible that the microorganisms are not susceptible to the antibiotic chosen. Also, antibiotic-resistant microorganisms may have emerged as a result of long-term use of the amoxicillin.

D It is most likely that the dose of antibiotic she is taking is appropriate for her sinus infection, but not for her periodontal condition.

(E) Because this patient reported taking amoxicillin for her sinus infection on the health history, there is no reason to assume that she is noncompliant. Each of the other factors listed are potential reasons for failure of the antibiotic she is currently taking for her sinus infection to also reduce the periodontal abscess.

22. A Treatment of this acute periodontal abscess should begin with establishing drainage to the area as well as scaling and root planing to remove any calculus. The tissues should be given time to respond to this treatment and can be evaluated after 24 hours to decide on the next phase of treatment.

B The time period within which even the longest-acting anesthesia will wear off is not long enough to allow the tissues to respond to treatment.

(C) If successfully treated with debridement and providing drainage to the area, the patient should report a decrease in the discomfort after 24 hours.

D,E Successful treatment will eliminate the pain within 24 hours. If the patient's symptoms have not subsided within this time frame, periodontal surgery will most likely be needed to access the affected area.

23. A,B This patient should be instructed to avoid whitening products until the periodontal abscess has been treated and her periodontal condition responds to treatment.

C The anterior composite restoration will not whiten.

(D) Adult patients over the age of 16 (who are not pregnant or lactating) may use whitening products.

E This patient's teeth are already very white and her teeth would be at risk for developing a bluish hue that sometimes develops with excessive whitening treatments.

24. A The patient must sign the medical history form verifying that she (as a legal adult) has provided the information. Although the clinician has taken the vital signs as part of the assessment data, the patient's signature is not required to verify this data.

(B) Legally the patient must provide consent to treatment. A signed written informed consent form satisfies this legal requirement.

C A patient need not be a legal resident of the United States to receive dental hygiene treatment.

D Obtaining a patient's signature to validate a commitment to self-care can be a helpful motivator for maintaining good oral health self-care. However, this would not be legally required for treatment.

E Although this question is often included on a dental history as part of the health history, it is not a legal requirement that the patient must sign prior to treatment.

25.   A This patient has been using over-the-counter tooth whitening products that seem to have produced the very white shade observed in the photographs. Because she is still seeking whitening products, it is highly likely that she has unrealistic expectations of the outcome.

B,D,E All whitening products contain either hydrogen peroxide or carbamide peroxide in varying concentrations. Because this patient has been using over-the-counter whitening products without tooth or soft tissue sensitivity or an allergic reaction, it is highly unlikely that these conditions will develop with professionally applied or prescribed products.

C The anterior composite restoration appears to be lingually located, and less visible from the facial aspect and/or appears to match the very white shade of her natural teeth. Additionally, this patient's natural teeth appear to be as white as they can be, making it highly unlikely that additional whitening treatments will produce a significant increase to a whiter shade and increase the visibility of the composite restoration.

CASE G GERIATRIC PATIENT JUAN HERNANDEZ

1.   A Necrosis indicates cell death, which is not present in this area.

B Although cyanosis will appear as a bluish discoloration on the tissue, the cause is an excessive concentration of reduced hemoglobin in the blood not present in this area.

C Leukoplakia appears as a white thickened tissue not present in this area.

D Exostosis appears as a hard outgrowth of bone not present in this area.

E An amalgam tattoo presents lingual to the maxillary right first molar when viewing the intraoral photographs. An amalgam tattoo often appears as a localized gray-blue discoloration due to the inadvertent depositing of amalgam fragments into the gingiva during the cavity preparation.

2.   A Torus palantinus would not resemble a chronic inflammatory lesion such as a granular tumor. Granular tissue is characterized by soft, pink fleshy tissue that forms during wound healing.

B Pseudocyst, a cyst without a lining membrane, is a condition related to the digestive tract, often occurring following pancreatitis.

C The palatal region is not covered with gingival tissue.

D The bony projection in the midline of the palate is characteristic of a torus palantinus and should not be confused with pathosis or conditions requiring further diagnosis.

E There are no salivary duct openings in the midline of the palate.

3.   A An open bite refers to the relationship between maxillary and mandibular anterior teeth that do not contact or overlap in occlusion.

B Edge-to-edge refers to occluding incisal surfaces of anterior teeth.

C As demonstrated on the study model, the maxillary first molar on the left side occludes with the mandibular molar in a cusp-to-cusp, or end-to-end relationship.

D Posterior teeth that are located facial or lingual to their normal position are in cross bite.

E When the maxilla or mandible is protruded, the teeth are located anterior of normal.

4.   A Cervical burnout is the term given to the radiographic optical illusion that results in an increased radiolucency imaged in the cervical region of the tooth. Cervical burnout does not refer to the condition of the tooth itself.

B This region exhibits recession that most likely exposed cementum. This patient's horizontal scrubbing action of toothbrushing may have contributed to abrasion that began on the exposed cementum and extended into a wedge-shaped lesion into the dentin.

C Aggressive scaling over time can lead to a significant loss of cementum, creating the need for these restorations.

D Recession that exposed these root surfaces increased the risk for caries.

E Abfraction lesions occur when mechanical stress of teeth is exceeded during mastication. The maxillary first and second premolars have porcelain fused-to-metal crowns that may have exerted loading pressure on the mandibular teeth, creating flexure at the cervix. This is further evidenced by the fremitis exhibited by these teeth. Repeated flexing results in loss of tooth structure on the buccal surfaces of the cervical one-third of the affected teeth.

5. A,C,D These answers are incorrect.

(B) Although the incidence of gingival recession increases with age and occlusal trauma, this patient's gingival recession is the result of periodontal disease. Gingival recession exposes the cemental root surface, putting the tooth at risk for root caries.

6.   A Stroke often leaves victims debilitated to some degree in motor function, speech, and mental function. However, the temporomandibular joint would not be singled out as a target for dysfunction.

B High blood pressure does not cause TMD.

(C) TMD may be found in 45% to 75% of arthritic patients. Symptoms include pain, stiffness, swelling, and decreased mobility.

D Although the incidence of diseases such as arthritis and conditions such as TMD increase with aging, age itself does not cause TMD.

E Attrition and other changes that may influence occlusion may play a role TMD, but this patient's examination does not indicate occlusal deviations significant enough to create TMD.

7.   (A) The radiopaque appearance of the pulp chambers of this tooth indicate the presence of endodontic filling material. Gutta percha and a post-and-core restoration can be observed on the radiograph of this tooth.

B The spiral pin core restoration is similar in appearance, although much smaller, to an endosseous implant. However, the tooth root is visible indicating that an implant has not replaced a missing tooth.

C Internal resorption appears as a radiolucent widening of the pulp chamber as tooth structure is destroyed.

D The presence of endodontic filling material rules out observing pulp stones.

E The root length and morphology is normal and no apicoectomy is evident.

8.   A,B The required teeth have been imaged on this film. Moving the film posteriorly or anteriorly will omit the required teeth from the image.

C The vertical angulation is correct for this image. Decreasing the vertical angulation will result in not imaging the root apices.

D The vertical angulation is correct for this image. Increasing the vertical angulation will result in not imaging the incisal edges of the teeth.

(E) The technique error evidenced in the maxillary right canine periapical radiograph is cone cutting. Cone cutting is corrected by completely covering the film with the x-ray beam so that the entire radiograph is exposed. In this case, it is the inferior portion of the radiograph that did not get exposed. The PID should be moved inferiorly to completely expose the film.

9.   A The age of this patient would not play a role in the orientation of the film packet.

(B) Vertical bitewing radiographs provide increased imaging in the vertical dimension over horizontal bitewings. Imaging an increased area of alveolar bone is especially valuable for use when periodontal involvement presents.

C The presence of a large torus may be more likely to interfere with a vertical film packet placement than a horizontal film packet placement.

D When opening is painful or difficult, vertical film packet placement may be more difficult than horizontal film packet placement.

E Vertical placement of the bitewing radiograph does not provide information about the apices of teeth and therefore would not replace periapical radiographs.

10.   A Genial tubercles often appear apical to the mandibular central incisors as a radiopaque circle surrounding the lingual foramen.

B Although the mental foramen would also appear as a round radiolucency, the mental foramen is more likely to be imaged near the apices of the mandibular first and second premolars.

(C) The mandibular right lateral incisor appears to have been extensively restored. Given the history of restorative trauma to this tooth, the rounded radiolucency observed at the apex of this tooth should be suspected to be indicative of a periapical abscess.

D The film identification dot should not be confused as an interpretive finding.

E Tori appear radiopaque.

11.   A The diuretic Diuril would not contraindicate treatment.

B The antihyperlipidemic Lipitor would not contraindicate treatment.

C Naprosyn, a nonsteroidal anti-inflammatory, may sometimes increase risk for bleeding. In the absence of symptoms of blood dyscrasias, this patient's use of Naprosyn would not contraindicate treatment.

(D) Coumadin interferes with blood clotting, which may lead to excessive bleeding following scaling. Therefore, a medical consult should determine this patient's prothrombin time or international normalized ratio (INR) status prior to proceeding with subgingival instrumentation. The Coumadin dose may need to be reduced or stopped before scaling to prevent excessive bleeding.

12.   (A) This patient's osteoarthritis is causing morning stiffness in his hips and knees, which makes it difficult for him to walk. A later appointment would allow the stiffness to dissipate and increase his ambulatory capabilities.

B,C,D Assisting with patient comfort will help avoid stress and physical problems that may result from the paresis.

E Short treatment segments are recommended to avoid stress.

13.   A,C If an acceptable prothrombin time indicates that excessive bleeding will not occur, debridement with hand and ultrasonic instrumentation would be acceptable treatment for this patient.

(B) Patients taking a diuretic to manage hypertension are often advised to limit the use of sodium-containing products. Therefore, air-powder polishing with sodium bicarbonate would be contraindicated.

D If necessary, there is no contraindication for use of nitrous oxide sedation with this patient.

E There are no contraindications to using sodium fluoride with this patient.

14.   A The purpose of oral prophylaxis is to prevent gingivitis, or if gingivitis is diagnosed, to prevent periodontitis. Because this patient presents with periodontitis, appointment planning should be based on nonsurgical periodontal therapy. Additionally, a reevaluation appointment 4 to 6 weeks later should be scheduled to assess the need for additional therapy and to determine the length of recall interval that would best manage his disease.

(B) The purpose of nonsurgical periodontal therapy is to treat and manage established periodontal disease. Based on this patient's periodontal condition (4 to 6 mm pockets in the posterior regions) and the slight generalized calculus accumulation at this 6-month recall appointment, complete mouth debridement could be accomplished in one appointment of typical length. A reevaluation appointment scheduled 4 to 6 weeks later is considered appropriate for assessing tissue response.

C The amount of calculus and the depths of the pockets this patient presents with indicate that a complete mouth disinfection is not necessary. A long appointment, or appointments scheduled within 24 to 48 hours, may be planned to complete all aspects of nonsurgical periodontal therapy. This full-mouth disinfection involves scaling, root planing, and removal of local contributing factors that harbor plaque. The purpose of full-mouth disinfection is to reduce the cross-contamination from untreated regions during the time between appointments.

D,E The amount of calculus and the depths of the pockets this patient presents with indicate that a complete mouth debridement could be accomplished in one appointment of typical length.

15. A Aggressive periodontitis is characterized by rapid attachment loss and bone destruction not evident in this patient.

B Slight chronic periodontitis is characterized by probing depths of 4 to 5 mm and clinical attachment loss of 1 to 2 mm; bone loss is less than 20%; and no mobility or furcation involvement.

(C) This patient's probing depths in the posterior regions, probe-depth readings of the anterior teeth combined with the amount of recession in these regions, and furcation involvement indicate a generalized moderate periodontal disease state.

D Severe chronic periodontitis is characterized by probing depths of more than 8 mm and clinical attachment loss greater than 5 mm; bone loss is more than 50%; and mobility and/or furcation involvement is evident.

E Refractory periodontitis is considered resistant to treatment. This term may be given to all types of periodontal disease that do not respond to treatment, for example, refractory chronic periodontitis.

16. A Furcation involvement of the multirooted first molars may make comprehensive instrumentation in these areas difficult.

B Poorly contoured crown margins and amalgam overhanging restorations noted in the radiographs will most likely hinder access to these areas.

C This patient presents with multiple cervical restorations that require increased tactile sensitivity and skill for effective instrumentation.

D Coumadin and Naprosyn taken by this patient are likely to increase bleeding during subgingival instrumentation in inflamed regions that can hinder the ability of the dental hygienist to thoroughly remove all deposits.

(E) An examination of this patient's oral cavity reveals extensive past dental treatment indicating that he does not appear to object to oral health care by professionals.

17. (A) Systemic antibiotic therapy, often prescribed in aggressive periodontitis and acute infections, would not be prescribed for this patient, whose pocket depths may respond better to physical disruption of localized plaque biofilm.

B Patients with generalized moderate chronic periodontal disease should maintain regular appointments with the periodontist. Additionally, this patient requires evaluation of occlusal risk factors for periodontal disease; furcation involvement; and assessment of pocket depths not responding to treatment.

C Unresponsive regions should be assessed for the need for additional scaling to remove calculus deposits still remaining. All areas of inflammation should be instrumented to deplaque and disrupt biofilm to promote healing.

D The effectiveness of a chemotherapeutic agent may be enhanced when delivered to the unresponsive pockets by oral irrigation.

E Pocket depths over 5 mm that did not respond to treatment are good candidates for locally delivered drug therapy.

18. A This patient does not present with the aggressive attachment loss that would require periodontal maintenance appointment intervals as short as 1 month.

   B The probe readings at the reevaluation appointment appear stabilized and in some areas, decreased. Based on his moderate periodontal condition, occlusal problems (fremitus and history of abfraction lesions), and health status that make him an unlikely candidate for periodontal surgery, he should be placed on a 3-month recall interval.

   C A patient with no previous history of periodontal diseases who presents with no risk factors for the disease can be scheduled for up to 6-month recall intervals.

   D Research indicates that this patient, with a history of periodontal disease, should be on a maintenance schedule that is no longer than 3 or 4 months.

19. A,E This patient's arthritis and self-reported difficulty using floss would be indicators for the use of an automatic toothbrush and floss-holding device.

   B To target the accumulation of cervical plaque and marginal bacteria, an oral irrigation device may be useful. A power-driven device may aid this patient with limited manual dexterity.

   C Use of fluoride mouth rinse is a simple, safe, and cost-effective method of increasing caries protection for an aging population. In addition to this patient's generalized recession which increases his risk of root caries, xerostomia associated with antihypertensive medications further indicates the need for home fluoride use.

   D The photographs of this patient reveal intact papilla. The use of interdental brushes for cleaning interproximally would not be indicated.

20. A Diamond finishing strips are difficult to use in the posterior regions of the mouth and are best suited for composite and glass ionomer restorative margination.

   B The flame-shaped silicon carbide bur will not adapt to the tooth surface adequately.

   C A gold knife is better suited for the removal of a composite restorative flange.

   D The margination of an interproximal overhang can best be accomplished with the use of a fine-fluted carbide bur because it fits into the proximal space, adapts to the tooth, and removes the amalgam without much damage to the tooth structure.

21. A,B A soft diet and application of moist heat can help alleviate pain and stiffness.

   C Based on the anti-inflammatory and anticoagulant medications this patient is currently taking, recommending acetaminophen is contraindicated. The patient can be referred to his physician to evaluate the success of his medications at managing his TMD.

   D Fabrication of an occlusal appliance can help manage TMD.

   E This patient's TMD is most likely interrelated with his arthritis. His physician may be able to evaluate the medications he is taking to manage the arthritis and make recommendations that can also help control TMD pain.

22. A,B,C Effective communication for this patient with a history of a stroke requires good communicative techniques that include speaking clearly and slowly, and directly to the patient; providing frequent feedback to ensure that the patient comprehends what is being communicated; and using basic, uncomplicated media to demonstrate instructions and explain treatment.

   D Maintenance of stability is normally a concern of the patient living with effects of a stroke. Moving slowly and deliberately around the patient can help to avoid disorientation.

   E Stroke victims are often unaware of the extent of their paresis. Therefore, it is important to not overestimate this patient's abilities. The dental hygienist should take a proactive stance with this patient and provide assistance when seating or dismissing or changing chair positions.

23. **A,D** Disclosing to determine the presence of biofilms and probing are considered data gathering, necessary to prepare a dental hygiene treatment plan, and as such are considered to be covered by implied consent.

(B) Implied consent is given by the patient's presence in the treatment chair and includes assessment gathering procedures only. This patient would need to grant written and documented informed consent to nonsurgical periodontal therapy after being informed of all options, risks, and potential complications of treatment.

C,E An intraoral examination to determine occlusal relationships and an extraoral examination of the TMJ, necessary to prepare treatment plans and referrals, are considered covered by the patient's implied consent.

24. **(A)** Ethnicity and culture are not likely to play a role in deciding treatment recommendations for this patient. Although knowledge of certain cultural beliefs that aid or hinder outcomes of treatment is helpful, treatment should not be based on ethnic stereotypes.

B To help improve prognosis, this patient's ability to make decisions regarding commitment to treatment and self-care recommendations should be identified.

C,D Determining the geriatric patient's anticipated life span remaining and weighing treatment options at varying financial levels will assist in realistic treatment planning that is prioritized based on the needs of the patient.

E Functional ability of the patient can be used to determine the treatment options with the best prognosis for success.

25. **A** Informed consent requires an explanation of expected outcomes and prognosis of treatment.

B,E Informed consent requires an explanation of possible outcomes of treatment and of possible consequences of no treatment.

C A list of alternative treatments and their costs is required for the patient to make informed decisions about which treatment to consent to undergo.

(D) This patient is considered competent and unless he requests it, his granddaughter need not be involved with his decision to give consent to treatment.

CASE H GERIATRIC PATIENT VIRGINIA CARSON

1. **A** Hypotension refers to a drop in blood pressure below normal rates.

B For adults, a systolic blood pressure reading under 120 mm Hg and a diastolic reading under 80 mm Hg is classified as normal.

C For adults, a systolic blood pressure reading between 120 and 139 mm Hg and diastolic readings between 80 and 89 mm Hg is considered prehypertension.

(D) Systolic blood pressure readings between 140 and 159 mm Hg and diastolic readings between 90 and 99 mm Hg are classified as hypertension stage 1.

E Systolic blood pressure readings over 160 mm Hg and diastolic readings over 100 mm Hg are classified as hypertension stage 2.

2. **A** Grade I furcation is characterized by a detectable depression in the furcation opening only. Radiographic changes are not evident at this early stage.

B Grade II furcation is characterized by bone loss that allows the probe to detect a cul-de-sac under the dome of the furcation. Radiographs may or may not depict the involvement at this stage.

(C) In the 1950s, Glickman developed the classification of furcation involvement identified by Grades I through IV. Grade III is characterized by the absence of interradicular bone visible radiographically where the bone is not attached to the dome of the furcation. The entrance to the furcation remains occluded by the gingiva.

D If the soft tissues have receded apically so that a Grade III furcation involvement is clinically visible, Grade IV is the appropriate classification.

3.   A Primary herpetic gingivostomatitis presents as painful vesicles on the gingiva, mucosa, tongue, or lips. This patient does not exhibit the fever, malaise, and pain that would interfere with eating that accompany this infection.

(B) The round red area in the middle of the palate is the classic appearance of chronic atrophic candidiasis, also known as denture stomatitis. This condition is limited to the mucosa covered by a full or partial denture.

C Herpetiform aphthous ulcers cause pain that is not a complaint of this patient.

D Melanin pigmentation most commonly presents in dark-skinned individuals and appears blue, black, or brown in color.

E Torus palatinus is an overgrowth of bone that presents as a raised surface and a paler diffuse color than the surrounding area.

4.   **(A)** The genial tubercles are seen as a radiopacity on this mandibular incisor periapical radiograph.

B The symphysis is a bony landmark located along the border of the mandible, but is not evident in this projection.

C The mental foramen is a radiolucent circle often observed on mandibular premolar radiographs.

D A retrocuspid papilla is a gingival landmark seen clinically on the lingual gingiva of mandibular canines and is not detectable radiographically.

E Trabeculae are radiopaque areas of bone that give cortical bone the sponge-like appearance. The defined circle seen on this film is characteristic of genial tubercles.

5.   A The cementoenamel junction occurs significantly superior to this dense band of calculus. Additionally, the scalloping continues across the interdental space, ruling out dental anatomy variations of the teeth.

B Enamel would not be present in this root region of the teeth.

(C) Heavy calculus buildup gives the radiopaque appearance seen in these radiographs.

D The clinical appearance of calculus noted in the photographs rules out this being composite resin.

E Cementicles are microscopic calcifications of the periodontal ligament.

6.   A The soft tissue of the nose will sometimes be imaged as an enlarged outline traversing the film in a somewhat horizontal direction. The missing maxillary teeth prevents the film from being positioned where it would image the soft tissue outline of the nose.

B Film fog would appear as an overall graying of the film.

C The region being assessed is the nasal fossa, not the sinus cavity.

D The regions being assessed are the bilateral walls of the nasal fossa, not the nasal septum in the midline of the cavity.

(E) The nasal conchae or turbinates are normal radiographic landmarks that are often observed projecting into the nasal fossa from the more radiopaque lateral walls of the nasal cavity. The conchae are not densely calcified and therefore appear less radiopaque than the surrounding bony structures.

7. A,D Clinically, this tooth does not exhibit wear at the cervical area that would indicate abrasion or abfraction.

B This radiolucency represents an optical illusion of darkness sandwiched between the more radiopaque bone below and the more radiopaque ledge of heavy calculus above. The radiolucency is further enhanced by the morphology of the tooth root, which presents with an increased concavity further contributing to the optical illusion of radiolucency in this area of the tooth. The optical illusion cervical burnout should not be confused with the radiographic appearance of interproximal caries.

C A fracture is not evident clinically or radiographically.

E Caries, when present, will usually appear at the contact point between adjacent teeth or just apical to this area and not under the gingival margin at the alveolar crest.

8.   A Like other respiratory complications, patients with COPD should be treated in an upright chair position. However, antibiotic premedication is not indicated.

B Standard precautions taken to avoid disease transmission will contain exposure to hepatitis C. Antibiotic premedication is not indicated.

C This patient's congestive heart failure should be determined to be medically managed prior to comprehensive nonsurgical periodontal therapy; however, antibiotic premedication is not indicated.

D Antibiotic premedication is not indicated for the spontaneous gingival bleeding resulting from this patient's periodontal disease.

E None of the conditions noted in this question place this patient at a greater risk for infective bacterial endocarditis than the general population.

9.   A,B Medical complications are more likely early in the morning, so appointments during this time should be avoided.

C Midmorning to early afternoon, 11:00 A.M. to 2:00 P.M., is the best time to schedule the older adult patient, especially when medically compromised. Medical complications are more likely early in the morning and the older adult is more likely to be stressed by the happenings of the day in the later afternoon.

D,E Stress can be linked to an increased risk for a medical emergency in the medically compromised, geriatric patient. Because stress tends to increase as the day progresses, these appointment times should be avoided.

10.   A The use of epinephrine in oral health care treatment for the patient on chronic drug therapy for congestive heart failure should be limited or avoided. Epinephrine could cause adverse reactions with her prescribed medications.

B Postural hypotension is a condition associated with the antihypertensive drugs taken by this patient.

C Most patients with chronic obstructive pulmonary disease can breathe more comfortably in a semisupine or upright position. This patient should be asked her preferred position prior to moving the treatment chair.

D Stress reduction protocol can help to avoid triggering a breathing emergency.

E Vital signs should be monitored before and after treatment.

11.   A,C Because this patient exhibits bone loss and gingival recession, an interdental aid that can adapt to wide embrasures and concave proximal tooth surfaces is indicated.

B The blunted papillary shape exposing the wide embrasures are well suited for the use of tufted floss.

D Most patients with a history of congestive heart failure will be on a salt restrictive diet, especially when the underlying cause is hypertension. This patient is taking antihypertensive medication that would most likely prohibit the use of a sodium-based agent.

E A toothpick-in-holder can be an effective tool for removing biofilm in areas of furcation involvement as well as in interproximal regions.

12. A,C,D,E Patients with COPD who are chronic smokers are at increased risk for halitosis, periodontal disease, extrinsic tooth stains, and oral cancer.

B This patient's maxillary full denture will most likely protect her hard palate from the concentrated heat stream created from smoking cigarettes. The lesion noted on the palate is most likely denture stomatitis, the result of an ill-fitting denture.

13. A The gingival sulcus refers to the crevice between the free gingival margin and the tooth. The term *sulcus* is used when no pocketing presents.

B,C A pocket detected when the gingiva has enlarged is called a gingival or pseudopocket. When the free gingival margin is located coronal to the cementoenamel junction (CEJ), a deep probe depth reading would not indicate true loss of attachment. Part of the probe depth reading in a gingival or pseudopocket is actually above the CEJ and does not represent loss of attachment. Although a pseudopocket may be associated with gingivitis, it is not associated with bone loss.

D The bone loss associated with a periodontal intrabony pocket is usually vertical, where the base of the pocket extends apical into the alveolar crest.

E The bone loss associated with a suprabony pocket is usually horizontal and coronal to the alveolar crest.

14. A,B When less than 30% of the sites are periodontally involved, the term *localized* is used. This patient presents with a generalized periodontal involvement.

C Because this patient presents with more than 30% of her remaining teeth periodontally involved, her disease is classified as generalized. However, this patient's loss of attachment is significantly more than the 1 to 2 mm loss that would be categorized as early.

D This patient presents with more than 30% of her remaining teeth periodontally involved, classifying her disease as generalized. However, this patient's loss of attachment is more than the 3 to 4 mm loss that would be categorized as moderate.

E This patient presents with more than 30% of her remaining teeth periodontally involved, classifying her disease as generalized. Advanced periodontitis is characterized by a significant amount of bone loss representing 5 mm or more of attachment loss, areas of significant furcation involvement, and tooth mobility.

15. A,B Curettes will most likely be used to access subgingival deposits once the heavy calculus has been removed by the anterior sickle scaler.

C Although a power-driven scaler would be the first choice for removing heavy calculus, this patient's history of cardiovascular disease coupled with chronic obstructive pulmonary disease contraindicate the use of an ultrasonic scaler. To remove the heavy calculus deposits located in this region, the anterior sickle scaler would be the best hand instrument choice from this list.

D,E Use of a power-driven ultrasonic scaler is contraindicated for this patient who presents with a respiratory risk.

16. A,B Based on the probing depths and radiographic assessment, the mandibular right second molar and mandibular right first premolar would appear to have the better prognosis.

C Clinically and radiographically, the mandibular right central incisor presents with the greatest loss of attachment and bone resorption.

D Clinically the mandibular left lateral incisor does not have the amount of recession observed on the facial of the mandibular right central incisor, indicating less attachment loss.

E The loss of attachment associated with the mandibular left second premolar is not as severe as with the mandibular right central incisor.

17.   A The incidence of periodontal disease seems more prevalent in older populations. The association of periodontal disease with aging may be due to the cumulative nature of the disease. Age also increases this patient's susceptibility to infection and can be expected to lengthen healing time following treatment.

(B) Although gender is a risk indicator for periodontal disease, males tend to present with an increased risk.

C Smoking is a risk factor for periodontal disease and will inhibit tissue response to treatment.

D Poor home care habits that allow bacterial plaque to accumulate increase the risk for periodontal disease.

E A lowered socioeconomic status and reduced access to regular professional dental care are risk indicators for periodontal disease.

18.   (A) Based on this patient's advanced periodontal disease status, and the lack of significant pocket reduction observed at the 6-week reevaluation appointment, this patient should be referred to a periodontist.

B This patient does not present with a condition that would prompt the need for pulp vitality testing.

C Pit and fissure sealants are unlikely to benefit this patient who does not present with a high risk of caries on the occlusal surfaces of the three teeth remaining without restorations.

D This patient does not present with caries requiring dental restorations.

E Currently this patient does not present with a need for desensitization. Tissue shrinkage that exposes sensitive root surfaces may result after scaling. However, based on the information presented and the lack of significant pocket reduction observed at the 6-week reevaluation appointment, the best answer from this list is that the patient be referred to a periodontist.

19.   A Dietary counseling is more commonly performed for caries control that this patient does not exhibit.

B Although this patient should receive instruction in self-examination for oral cancer, the lesion observed on the palate is most likely chronic atrophic candidiasis and would require a denture adjustment and not a referral to a physician. This lesion should be observed again following denture adjustments.

C This patient's mastitory function has recently been restored through the fabrication of the maxillary denture that does not appear to need implants for stabilization. Additionally, implants would not be recommended until her periodontal status is improved and smoking cessation is realized.

(D) Tobacco cessation intervention is the most immediate need, both for the improvement of periodontal status and to eliminate this risk factor for COPD and heart disease.

E There are no advanced or special infection control procedures to be used for patients presenting with communicable infectious diseases. All patients should be treated using standard precautions.

20.   A Bis-GMA acrylics are the main component in composite resins.

B UEDMA acrylics are polyurethane acrylics used to make athletic mouth protectors and soft, flexible dentures.

(C) The denture in the photograph appears to be made of poly methyl methacrylate (MMA) resin acrylic. MMA is the most widely used acrylic in dentistry and is the main component of this denture's base.

D,E HEMA and PENTA-P acrylics are placed in dentin bonding–agent products.

21.   A   Mouth rinses freshen breath, but do not remove plaque and debris from denture surfaces.

   (B)   Daily brushing with a toothbrush and paste made specifically for denture care is recommended to prevent stain accumulation.

   C,E   Immersion in sodium hypochlorite (household bleach) or placing the denture in a dishwasher is not recommended for acrylic dentures.

   D   Brushing with a household scouring powder will damage the acrylic denture base and teeth.

22.   A,D   Repeating self-care instructions, providing written instructions, and using good communication techniques will improve communication with all patients.

   B   Serious, but nonjudgmental recommendations will more likely produce patient compliance.

   C   Eliminating distracting background noise and music will help improve communication with the older adult.

   (E)   These terms may be viewed as condescending to the older adult. Additionally, the patient should not be addressed by her first name unless she has specifically asked to be addressed in an informal manner.

23.   (A)   Assessing the oral health care facility for potentially hazardous barriers is important, especially when serving older patients who may present with diminished senses or limited motor control.

   B,C,D,E   These answers are incorrect. An assessment of safe access to the facility will help avoid potential accidents for all patients.

24. A,C,D   These answers are incorrect.

   (B)   Dental hygiene care planning for the older adult must consist of comprehensive care that helps maintain good oral health for the life of the patient. All treatment options should be presented to the patient so that she can better make informed decisions about what treatment options will best serve her needs.

25.   A   Smoking and stress are two of the risk factors shared by both periodontal disease and cardiovascular disease.

   B   Patients with periodontal disease have demonstrated higher levels of cardiovascular disease, or approximately twice the risk.

   C   Incidence of myocardial infarction has been shown to increase in patients with poor oral health, periodontitis, and oral infections.

   (D)   Periodontal disease has been linked with other chronic inflammatory diseases such as heart disease and diabetes, each affecting the other. However, the cause and effect have not yet been established.

   E   Studies have indicated a link between periodontitis and chronic obstructive pulmonary disease, both chronic inflammatory diseases.

CASE I GERIATRIC PATIENT ELEANOR GRAY

1.   A   Denture stomatitis or chronic atrophic candidiasis manifests as a round, red irritation caused by a full maxillary denture. This patient's partial denture replaces mandibular teeth and therefore would not be likely to affect the tissue of the hard palate.

   (B)   This bony exotosis observed at the midline of the palate is a torus palatinus. Tori vary in size and not all patients present with tori.

   C   The viral infection herpangina would appear as erythematous vesicles or ulcers which would be painful and soft when palpated. The patient presents with no painful symptoms. Additionally, although the manifestation of herpangina is usually observed in the posterior region of the hard palate or on the soft palate, the nodule noted here is hard when palpated.

    D The median palatine suture, an anatomical landmark located in the midline of the palate, would not be clinically detectable. This landmark may be observed on radiographs as a thin radiolucent vertical line extending posteriorly from between the maxillary centrals.

    E Most ulcers present as painful depressed lesions, whereas this patient presents with an asymptomatic raised bony exostosis.

2.   A Green stain results from oral uncleanness not exhibited by this patient.

    B Rarer orange and red stains resulting from chromogenic bacteria often appear on the cervical regions of the teeth.

    C Black line stain often presents as a raised line that follows along the cervical one-third of the teeth. Although black line stain can occur in clean oral conditions such as those exhibited by this patient, the staining in the pits and fissures of these teeth is indicative of brown stains from foodstuffs.

    (D) The teeth surfaces pits and fissures in this region are difficult to clean. As a result, the acquired pellicle has become stained from foodstuffs such as coffee or tea.

    E Although this patient presents with intrinsic yellow staining of all her teeth, the brown staining of the pits and fissures of these teeth is not necessarily associated with the presence of biofilm. Yellow stain associated with the presence of biofilm is more likely to be observed when self-care is not effective.

3.   A Although an acquired pellicle and biofilm may be present, gingival recession has exposed the root surface cementum as indicated by the darker yellow color.

    B Intrinsic stains that occur inside the tooth and endogenous stains that develop from within the tooth often present as changes in the dentin that appear through the enamel. The normal appearance of root surface cementum observed as a result of gingival recession should not be mistaken for abnormal tooth staining.

    (C) Gingival recession has exposed the darker yellow cementum covering the root surfaces of these teeth.

    D None of the medications taken by this patient would result in tooth staining.

    E Enamel hypoplasia results from an ameloblastic disturbance in which the teeth erupt with white spots that over time may become stained from foodstuffs and biofilm. The normal appearance of the exposed cementum of these teeth should not be confused with an abnormal disturbance during the formation of the teeth.

4.   **(A)** The radiographs indicate a metal crown, and the remaining porcelain bonding is evident in the photographs. The oxidized metal is exposed indicating porcelain failure.

    B The appearance of porcelain bonding indicates that this is a porcelain-fused-to-metal crown and not a full metal crown.

    C The defective porcelain on the facial surface of this porcelain-fused-to-metal crown should not be confused with enamel that would be evident in a large, multisurface amalgam restoration. Additionally, the smooth, regular margins and complete crown coverage of the metal observed in the radiographs indicate a crown.

    D Porcelain veneer restorations are often placed on the facial surfaces of anterior teeth to restore esthetics. The tooth-colored material observed in the photographs is porcelain. However, the radiographs reveal the presence of a metal crown, indicating that the porcelain was bonded to the crown and not to the tooth itself.

E The defective porcelain on the facial surface of this porcelain-fused-to-metal crown should not be confused with enamel. Although an onlay can be used to restore a significant amount of the occlusal surface of the tooth, including one or more cusps, this indirect fixed restoration is a crown, completely surrounding the tooth.

5. A The clasp of the removable partial denture attaches to the right second premolar. This tooth serves as a support for the partial denture, but is not termed an abutment.

B The removable partial denture that replaces the mandibular right first and second molars is constructed as a bilateral appliance and is supported by both the teeth and the alveolar ridge. The framework of the appliance also serves to support the periodontally involved mandibular anterior teeth. However, neither the teeth to which to denture is clasped, nor the teeth upon which the framework rest are considered abutments. The term *abutment* refers to a tooth that supports a retainer of a fixed bridge.

C,D The mandibular incisors have been splinted together to assist with stabilizing these periodontally involved teeth. The lingual metal wire is connected to these teeth with a bonding material. The term *abutment* does not apply to this appliance.

(E) The fixed bridge on the mandibular left side consists of two pontics replacing the missing first and second molars and two retainers at each end of the bridge that are attached to the second premolar and the third molar. The teeth that support the retainers are called abutments. In this case, the mandibular left second premolar and the third molar serve as abutments for this four-unit bridge.

6. A A cantilever bridge is supported by an abutment tooth or teeth on only one end.

B,E A Maryland bridge is a resin-bonded cast metal bridge that does not use full crowns over natural teeth as retainers. A Maryland or resin-bonded cast metal bridge uses bonding material to attach the framework of the bridge to the abutment teeth with little or no removal of the natural tooth structure.

(C) The photographs and radiographs indicate that the missing teeth on the mandibular left side have been replaced with a fixed partial denture. The two denture retainers are attached to the abutment teeth at each end of the bridge; and two pontics restore the space left by the missing molars.

D This patient's removable partial denture has been constructed to restore function to the mandibular right side. The radiographs indicate that the left side has been restored with a fixed bridge.

7. A A post is placed into an endodontically treated root canal for the purpose of retaining a core buildup to support a crown restoration. A post-and-core restoration can only be placed into a root canal that has undergone endodontic therapy. The radiographs do not indicate root canal therapy on the mandibular right premolar. Additionally, the core serves to build up the tooth to accept a crown, but once the crown is placed into permanent position, the core would no longer be visible and would not extend out of the top of the metal crown.

B,C,D The metal depression in the crown surface has been specifically constructed to accept the rest of the partial denture clasp to aid in retention of the appliance. This normal appearing construction should not be confused with stain accumulation, an amalgam restoration, or a defect in the crown.

(E) This portion of the crown has been specifically constructed to assist with retention of the partial denture. This precision attachment serves to accept the rest portion of the clasp on the partial denture and should not be confused with a defect of the crown.

8.
A Depending on the size and location, tori may make placing the long dimension of the film packet vertically difficult. When tori are expected to interfere with film packet placement, a horizontal bitewing may be recommended.

B Placing the long dimension of the film packet vertically increases the amount of alveolar bone imaged on a bitewing radiograph. Vertical bitewing radiographs are recommended for the periodontally involved patient when imaging more alveolar bone is desired.

C A hypersensitive gag reflex may be stimulated by placement of the film packet. It is often when the film packet contacts the posterior region of the hard palate or soft palate that a gag reflex is stimulated. The film packet placement most likely to elicit a gag reflex is the posterior periapical radiograph. However, placing a film packet for a vertical bitewing radiograph with the long dimension positioned vertically could increase the likelihood of contacting the sensitive posterior region of the oral cavity, and may actually increase the likelihood of stimulating a gag reflex over a horizontal bitewing.

D The vertical placement of a bitewing radiograph is not likely to increase patient comfort during film packet placement. In fact, placing the longer dimension of the film packet vertical is more likely to decrease comfort.

E Vertical bitewings are recommended for any patient when an increased image of alveolar bone is desired.

9.
A The normal radiographic appearance of the coronoid process of the mandible is a faint radiopaque, sometimes triangular-shaped process observed in the far posterior on maxillary molar periapical radiographs.

B The maxillary tuberosity can be observed in this region posterior to the maxillary second molar. However, the landmark pointed out is the coronoid process of the mandible, superimposed over the maxillary tuberosity.

C The lateral pterygoid plate may be imaged when the maxillary molar periapical radiograph is positioned quite far posteriorly. Often the suture that separates the maxilla and the lateral pterygoid plate can be used to help distinguish between these two structures. However, the lateral pterygoid plate is not imaged on this radiograph.

D The structure pointed out in this radiograph is the normal radiographic appearance of the coronoid process of the mandible. This landmark should not be confused with other structures. This answer tries to wrongly insinuate that the patient's finger was used to hold the film packet in the patient's mouth and therefore was imaged onto the resulting image.

E The mandibular condyle is positioned too far posteriorly to be imaged onto any intraoral radiograph. The mandibular condyle should not be confused with the coronoid process of the mandible.

10.
A Intratoral radiographic film size no. 0 is approximately 7/8" x 1 3/8" (22 mm x 35 mm). This smallest sized intraoral film packet, often called a pedodontic film packet, is usually used to expose periapical or bitewing radiographs on children.

B Intraoral radiographic film size no. 1 is approximately 15/16" x 1 9/16" (24 mm x 40 mm). This smaller sized intraoral film packet, can be used to expose periapical or bitewing radiographs on children and for exposure of periapical radiographs on adult patients, in the narrow anterior regions of the arches. The size no. 1 film packet was used to expose the maxillary and mandibular right and left lateral-canine periapical radiographs and the mandibular central incisor periapical radiograph on this patient.

C Intraoral radiographic film size no. 2 is approximately 1 1/4" x 1 5/8" (32 mm x 41 mm). The size no. 2 intraoral film packet can be used in a variety of situations including exposure of periapical and bitewing radiographs for children who can tolerate the larger film packet and adolescents and adults. The size #2 film packet was used to expose the maxillary central incisor periapical radiograph and all the maxillary and mandibular posterior periapical radiographs and the left and right bitewing radiographs on this patient.

D   Intraoral radiographic film size no. 3 is approximately 1 1/16" x 2 1/8" (27 mm x 54 mm). This size is characteristic of longer dimension film packets used to expose horizontal bitewing radiographs on adult patients. The size no. 3 film packet often comes prepackaged with the bitewing tab attached.

E   Intraoral radiographic film size no. 4 is approximately 2 1/4" x 3" (57 mm x 76 mm). This largest sized intraoral film packet is most often used to expose occlusal radiographs on adult patients.

11.   A   Not aligning the PID perpendicular to the film packet in the vertical dimension would result in cutting the crown or the apices off the teeth in the image (paralleling technique) or elongation or foreshortening (bisecting technique). Not aligning the PID perpendicular to the film packet in the horizontal dimension would result in horizontal overlapping.

B   Although there is often slight elongation or foreshortening inherent in the bisecting technique, correct use of the technique would not be likely to result in this overall gray appearance indicative of a lack of image contrast.

C   Positioning the open end of the PID at an increased distance from the patient decreases the amount of radiation reaching the film resulting in a light, less dense, image.

D   The error created when leaving the partial denture in the mouth during the exposure would be an image of the metal framework on the radiograph and not this overall gray appearance indicative of a lack of image contrast.

(E)   The lack of image contrast that produces an overall gray appearance to this patient's radiographs resulted when the film was fogged. Film fog results when film packets are improperly exposed to stray radiation, white light, heat, humidity, chemical fumes and/or as film ages.

12.   A,B   Aricept and Risperdal put the patient at risk for orthostatic hypotension after laying supine in the treatment chair. Additionally, vital signs should be monitored at each appointment because of the possible effects of these drugs on the cadiovascular system.

(C)   It has been reported that patients taking bisphosphonates such as Fosamax have a low, but significant risk of developing osteonecrosis of the jaws, either after oral surgical procedures or spontaneously.

D   Calcium supplements do not have adverse effects on the oral cavity or dental and dental hygiene procedures.

13.   A,B,D   These answers are incorrect.

(C)   Allowing biofilm and debris to accumulate on the partial denture, especially in the area of attachment to the natural teeth, will most likely contribute to a decline in health for the natural tooth. Because the partial denture depends on the stability of the mandibular right second premolar, maintaining the health of this natural tooth is important.

14.   (A)   A clasp brush is ideal for cleaning the inside surfaces of the metal clasp of the removable partial denture.

B   Using the same toothbrush for cleaning both the appliance and the natural teeth is not recommended. The toothbrush filaments are easily damaged by the metal framework and clasps of the appliance, diminishing the effectiveness of the toothbrush for removing biofilm from the natural teeth.

C A power toothbrush has the potential to catch on the metal framework and clasps and possibly damage the appliance. Therefore, a power toothbrush is not recommended for cleaning a partial denture.

D,E An interproximal brush and an end-tuft brush are designed for specific purposes in removing biofilm from natural teeth. Although these may be considered for use in cleaning removable dentures, the clasp brush, designed specifically for this purpose, is the best choice.

15.   A The patient with AD will require assistance to maintain oral self-care throughout the progression of the disease. Asking permission to include her caregiver in the education process shows respect for, and maintains the dignity of, the patient.

B Because this patient wears glasses, it is important that she use them to better understand the oral self-care instructions given in the treatment chair. The patient should be instructed also to wear her glasses at home during self-care so that she can evaluate her effectiveness.

C Eliminating distracting background noise and facing the patient when speaking assists with communicating with the elderly and with the patient who may be easily confused in the dental hygiene treatment room environment.

(D) Oral self-care instruction should build on what the geriatric patient has spent a lifetime learning. An attempt should be made only to change or stop detrimental habits. Additionally, during the early stages of AD the patient will likely begin to exhibit difficulty in learning and retaining new information. Because this patient is already comfortable using an oral irrigator, she will most likely respond best to encouragement to continue doing what is familiar.

E Implementation of oral self-care at the same times each day helps to maintain a routine that may contribute to a comfortable familiarity with the procedures, and may assist with helping this patient remember to perform the skills.

16.   A This patient's multiple composite and porcelain restorations and the generalized exposed root surfaces contraindicate using the air polisher.

B Because her joint replacement surgery was completed over 2 years ago and she has had no complications or subsequent infections, prophylactic antibiotic premedication is not indicated.

C Because she is taking the bisphosphonate, Fosamax, this patient should be cautioned against elective periodontal surgery such as a dental implant.

D Because of the possible adverse effects of both Fosamax and Risperdal on the GI system, a semisupine position in the treatment chair is recommended. Additionally, Aricept and Risperdal increase the occurrence of orthostatic hypotension, when moving from a completely supine position to sitting upright. Maintaining a more upright position during treatment may help to reduce this occurrence.

(E) If needed, medications such as short-acting benzodiazepines are recommended for the patient with AD prior to the appointment. For the patient with AD, the dental hygiene treatment room can become unfamiliar and the patient can feel threatened or frightened by this disorientation. Reducing the fear experienced through the use of antianxiety medications can help manage treatment.

17.   A Total loss of attachment is calculated by adding to, and not by subtracting from, the loss from recession to the measurement of the pocket depth.

B To determine the total loss of attachment, the 1 mm probing depth must be added to the 6 mm recession measurement.

(C) Total loss of attachment is calculated as the sum of the measurement (in millimeters) of the loss observed from the CEJ (clinically observable due to recession) to the free gingival margin and the measurement (in millimeters) of the depth of the pocket. In this case, 6 mm is given as the measurement of recession (from the CEJ to the free gingival margin.) To this 6 mm, the probing depth (pocket measurement) of 1 mm is added for a total loss of attachment (sum) of 7 mm.

D Adding the 1 mm probing depth measurement to the 6 mm of recession equals a 7 mm total loss of attachment.

18. (A) A periodontal splint has been placed to stabilize the mandibular incisors. The lingual metal wire connected to these teeth with a bonding material is holding the teeth in a fixed position.

B Fosamax, the medication this patient is taking for management of her osteoporosis, inhibits osteoclast cells from breaking down bone. This interruption is directed at preventing further bone loss caused by osteoporosis. Fosamax will not regenerate bone and is not responsible for reducing the mobility of the mandibular incisors.

C Effective oral self-care is certainly important in maintaining the health of the periodontal splint, but is not responsible for reducing the mobility of the mandibular incisors.

D The patient may have had periodontal resective and/or regenerative surgical intervention in this region to reduce pocket depths and provide access for cleaning. However, it is the placement of the periodontal splint that is maintaining the teeth in a fixed and stable position.

E Regular maintenance appointments have helped this patient to maintain her natural dentition in good function. However, it is the placement of the periodontal splint that is maintaining the teeth is a fixed and stable position.

19. A Scrub-method brushing technique often leads to recession and abrasion of the tooth structure, especially on the facial surfaces at the cervical region of the teeth. Although toothbrushing may have contributed to facial abrasion of these teeth, the diminished width contributing to the hourglass shape exhibited by these teeth is the result of aggressive scaling.

(B) Repeated, aggressive scaling over time has diminished the width of these teeth. The goal of scaling and root planing is to remove calculus and cementum from the root surfaces. Although it was thought that bacterial products were held by the cementum, it is no longer considered necessary for aggressive removal of cementum.

C The outer surface of tooth enamel is removed during polishing. The amount removed depends on the coarseness of the polishing agent and the pressure used during polishing. However, the diminished width contributing to the hourglass shape exhibited by these teeth is the result of aggressive scaling and root planing.

D Congenital defects such as enamel hypoplasia that change the shape and appearance of the crowns of the teeth should not be confused with the reduced cementum and dentin that have diminished the width of these teeth as a result of aggressive scaling and root planing.

E Chemical erosion caused by contact of the tooth surfaces with acids such as those found in carbonated beverages, lemons and lemon juice, or via chronic vomiting should not be confused with the characteristic hourglass shape of teeth that have undergone aggressive scaling and root planing.

20. (A) Older adults often do not have the same tooth sensitivity found in younger patients because of the formation of secondary or reparative dentin over many years. Pulpal recession and decreased cellularity contribute to a decrease in the number of nerve fibers in the pulp. Therefore, debridement with hand instruments is not likely to elicit hypersensitivity of tooth root surfaces. This secondary dentin does not protect a patient from decay of the tooth root surfaces. Because root caries account for a large proportion of caries found in older adults, meticulous home care should be maintained and fluoride therapies should be implemented to help minimize this risk.

B,C,D These answers are incorrect.

21.   A,E A 0.05% sodium fluoride over-the-counter mouth rinse and a 0.76% sodium monofluorophosphate dentifrice should be recommended for all patients at risk for caries. This patient's risk factors include root surface exposure due to recession; extensive restorations that have the potential for recurrent decay; difficult to clean and maintain removable and permanent appliances; and potential of AD to diminish her ability to maintain daily oral self-care.

      B,C Because of the risk factors this patient presents with—including root surface exposure due to recession, extensive restorations that have the potential for recurrent decay, difficult to clean and maintain removable and permanent appliances, and potential of AD to diminish her ability to maintain daily oral self-care—she should receive professionally applied fluoride treatments, especially following debridement and polishing procedures that reduce the fluoride-rich outer tooth structure. Two application choices that are appropriate for this patient are 2% sodium fluoride gel tray application and 5% sodium fluoride varnish treatments.

      (D) Acidulated phosphate fluoride should be avoided in the patient with porcelain and composite restorations.

22.   A,B Sodium hypochloride and acetic acid will corrode the metal framework of the appliance and therefore are contraindicated for cleaning this patient's removable partial denture.

      C Hot water may cause warping or distortion of the plastic resin base of the denture and therefore should be avoided.

      (D) An alkaline detergent such as hydrogen peroxide helps to loosen debris and light stains. Many commercially available denture cleaners use sodium perborate or percarbonate and are recommended for regular use to help prevent the buildup of heavy stains.

      E There are a number of safe commercially available products made especially for cleaning removable partial dentures with metal framework and clasps. The use of household scouring abrasive has the potential to scratch the plastic resin base and/or acrylic teeth of the denture and therefore should be avoided.

23.   A Geriatric patients are especially at risk for developing root caries. In addition to instruction on mechanical removal of biofilm and the application of fluorides, the patient and her caregiver should receive information on carbohydrate type and frequency of ingestion and other links between nutrition and root caries.

      B The link between osteoporosis and periodontal disease is still unclear at the present time. Although some studies reveal a connection between alveolar bone lost in proportion to the severity of periodontal disease and the imbalance observed in osteoporosis of resorbing bone and the laying down of new bone, other studies have produced inconclusive results. Until conclusive evidence is presented, the understanding that both periodontal disease and osteoporosis share common risk factors should be communicated to the patient and her caregivers.

      (C) Because this patient's joint replacement surgery was completed over 2 years ago and she has had no complications or subsequent infections, prophylactic antibiotic premedication is not indicated.

      D Although this patient appears to have had her periodontal condition treated and stabilized before beginning bisphosphonate therapy, the importance of maintaining oral health to avoid the need for future invasive treatment should be explained in relation to her risk of developing osteonecrosis of the jaws.

      E Because of the progressive nature of AD and the declining ability to adequately perform oral self-care, both the patient and her caregiver should actively participate in learning how best to manage oral self-care to maintain oral health.

24. A,C,D These answers are incorrect.

B Many terms and categories have been applied to various age groups of older adults. Although traditionally, those aged 65 and older have been referred to as elderly or seniors, with the average age of those 85 years of age and older continuing to rise, several other classifications have developed. Researchers have referred to those aged 65 to 74 as elderly or young old; those aged 75 to 84 have been categorized as old or aged; and those aged 85 and older as old, old or very old. These categories are used to help define demographics and lay the foundations for research, and are not a form of ageism. Ageism refers to negative discrimination toward the aged community. Functionally dependent refers to a person who, like this patient, is able to perform life functions, but must still depend on the supervision of her caregiver to maintain this functionality.

25. A,B Although bonding agent treatments are available to restore an esthetic appearance to this restoration, these treatments do not hold up as well as the original bonded porcelain. If a patient is concerned with the appearance or insists on restoring the appearance of failed porcelain, the best course of action would be to replace the entire bridge, which is not an easy course of action for this patient.

C The stress and risks involved with removing the cosmetically defective crown and replacing with a new fixed bridge outweigh the benefits of this complex and expensive treatment.

D The cantilever bridge was removed from the mandibular right side because it was loose and endangering the periodontal stability of the mandibular right second premolar. The lack of a molar tooth to support the posterior portion of a fixed denture in this region is the most likely reason that a removable partial denture was made to restore function to the patient's right side. In later stages of AD the patient is most likely to find it difficult to care for and keep track of a removable appliance.

E The chipped and fractured porcelain on the facial surface of this porcelain-fused-to-metal crown has exposed the oxidized metal of the crown. The damage to this restoration is cosmetic and not functional. The expenditure for the family in time and travel to accompany the patient to the practice for multiple appointments, the chair time demands on the patient, the possible stress on the patient to adjust to wearing a temporary appliance and to accepting the fit and feel of the new appliance, the stress on the stability of the periodontium, and the financial commitment all must be weighed in relation to the risks and benefits of the treatment plan.

CASE J SPECIAL NEEDS PATIENT THOROUGHGOOD EPPS

1. A The combination of crowns and pontics are fixed into a permanent bridge and are not removable.

B The radiographs reveal the presence of dental implants with a superstructure of a fixed permanent bridge. A metal framework usually refers to the mesh substructure of a removable partial denture, upon which acrylic resin would be used to shape the denture base and teeth. When a complete or full denture is stabilized by natural teeth roots that remain in the arch or by implants that substitute for teeth roots, it is called an overdenture.

C The radiographs reveal the presence of implants as the restorative replacement of the missing teeth. The implants provide the support for the prosthetic, in this case a combination of crowns and pontics fixed into a permanent bridge.

D A periodontal splint uses a prosthetic to hold the natural teeth in a fixed position.

E A lingual retainer is normally used for the stabilization of teeth that have undergone orthodontic intervention.

2. **A** The teeth that support a fixed bridge are called abutments. In this case, both the maxillary second molar and the maxillary second premolar serve as abutments for this three-unit bridge.

B A pontic refers to that part of the bridge that replaces a missing tooth. In this case, the missing maxillary first molar has been restored with the pontic of this three-unit bridge.

C A retainer refers to the crown portion of the bridge that retains or attaches the bridge to the natural tooth, or abutment.

D A cantilever bridge is attached to a fixed crown on only one side.

E A rest refers to that portion of a removable partial denture clasp that contacts the natural tooth for stability.

3. **(A)** G. V. Black established the standard for classifying caries in the early 1900s. This system has since been customarily used for cavity preparations and restorations as well. The mandibular left first molar presents with a Class I restoration, involving the pits and fissures only of this tooth.

B A Class II restoration involves a proximal surface of a posterior tooth.

C A Class III restoration involves the proximal surface, but not the incisal surface of anterior teeth.

D A Class IV restoration involves both the proximal and the incisal surfaces of anterior teeth.

E A Class V restoration involves the facial or lingual smooth surface of a tooth near the cementoenamel junction (CEJ).

4. A,E This permanent restoration is sound and should not be suspected of failure or confused with a temporary restorative treatment. The attachment of the bridge to the adjacent implant/natural tooth on one side only is characteristic of a cantilever bridge.

(B) The left side of the implant consists of a cantilever pontic that is attached to the fixed bridge on only one side.

C The mandibular left first premolar is clinically not present. It is most likely that this tooth was extracted and/or avulsed during trauma and then restored with the placement of the cantilever pontic.

D A cantilever bridge consists of a permanent attachment to the implant or natural tooth on one side only. There is no need for a clasp attachment on this side of the bridge.

5. A Incorrectly placing a lead or lead-equivalent thyroid collar in the path of the primary x-ray beam will block radiation from reaching the film. The result would be an area of no exposure that would appear clear, or radiopaque.

B It may be possible to image carotid artery calcifications when present on some panoramic images. Although these calcifications manifest in a variety of shapes and sizes, they typically appear posterior and slightly inferior to the angle of the mandible. However, the hyoid bone, a normal radiographic landmark, should not be confused with pathology.

C The cervical vertebrae of the spinal column are often imaged on a panoramic radiograph in the middle of the film as an increased radiopacity superimposed over the anterior teeth. The vertebrae may sometimes appear as ghost images at either end of the panoramic image, often posterior to or superimposed over the ramus of the mandible. The image of the hyoid bone should not be confused with the spinal column.

D Panoramic x-ray unit machine parts such as a chin rest, forehead rest, side positioning guides, and bite block may be imaged on the panoramic radiograph. However, the hyoid bone, a normal radiographic landmark, should not be confused with the machine parts.

(E) The bilateral faint, horseshoe-shaped structure observed inferior to the mandible on a panoramic radiograph is the hyoid bone.

6.   A Endodontic implants are placed through the root canal of an endodontically treated natural tooth and out the apex. Endodontic implants are not commonly used because of the potential for root fractures and resorption.

B Subperiosteal implants are inserted under the periosteum but over the bone.

C Transosteal implants, also referred to as a mandibular staple, are placed completely through the mandible from under the chin into the oral cavity.

(D) The radiographs reveal an endosteal or endosseous implant placed within the bone.

E A post-and-core restoration is not used as an implant. A post is placed into an endodontically treated root canal for the purpose of retaining a core buildup to support a crown.

7.   A Blade implants present with a unique larger sized shape used for a fibrous attachment to the bone. The use of blade implants has greatly declined.

(B) The radiographs reveal the typical cylinder shape of these dental implants.

C Transosteal implants utilize a mandibular staple implant that penetrates through the mandible from under the chin.

D Plate-form implants refer to those used to anchor transosteal implants.

E The radiographs reveal the typical cylinder shape and not a screw shape of these dental implants.

8.   A,D This normal appearance of the submandibular fossae regions should not be confused with pathology or radiographic error.

B Superimposition of several structures imaged in the same place would produce a lighter, or more radiopaque result and not this radiolucent appearance.

(C) On most panoramic radiographs, a negative shadow occurs where there is an absence of superimposition of structures. In the anterior region of the panoramic image there is superimposition of the anterior jaws and teeth with the spinal column and back of the skull. On the left and right sides of the panoramic image there is superimposition of the left and right jaws with the ghost images of the jaws of the opposite sides. In addition to the submandibular fossa region being less dense, there is a lack of superimposition of other structures, allowing more radiation to reach the film and create the darker areas noted.

E This normal appearance of the submandibular fossae regions should not be confused with accidental exposure of the film to white light. Additionally, it would be difficult to open the film cassette and expose this film in exactly this pattern.

9.   (A) The pulp of this tooth has produced reparative dentin in response to trauma, probably due to the size and location of the restoration. The pulp chamber of this tooth appears smaller because of the amount of this secondary dentin.

B Enamel pearls are found in the furca of multirooted teeth and not within the pulp chamber.

C Condensing osteitis is a bone condition and would be observed around the root apices of the affected tooth.

D Hypercementosis would appear as an excess growth of cementum, causing the roots to appear enlarged and bulbous.

E Dens invaginatus is essentially a tooth within a tooth, an invagination of enamel, dentin, and pulp within the pulp chamber of the maxillary lateral incisors. When present, it often occurs bilaterally.

10. A,B,C,E These conditions are not adverse reactions directly related to NSAIDs, acetaminophen, or topical trolamine salicylate.

(D) Nonsteroidal anti-inflammatory drugs (NSAIDs) are reported to cause xerostomia.

11.   A Wooden wedges specifically designed for oral self-care would most likely be a good choice to recommend for this patient to replace his, possibly incorrect, use of toothpicks.

      B Although his use of toothpicks should be evaluated for proper use, a holder designed specifically for oral self-care in conjunction with a wooden pick would most likely be more effective and less likely to damage the soft tissue structures of the periodontium than his use of toothpicks alone.

      C An end-tuft brush is probably the best choice of oral hygiene aids listed to recommend for this patient. End-tuft, or single tuft, brushes are adaptable for use in open contacts, wide embrasures, around and, when possible, under the fixed bridge and implant abutments without risk of harm to the tissues or restorations.

      (D) The interproximal brush is most likely to be constructed of nylon filaments wound around a metal wire core. Dental implants are easily scratched by this metal, therefore any oral hygiene aid should be inspected thoroughly for metal components before being recommended for the patient with dental implants.

      E Correct use of tufted floss can effectively remove plaque from multiple problem areas, such as implant abutments, fixed bridges, and open contacts. Although it may be unlikely that this patient will be able to fit the yarn portion of tufted floss under the implant superstructure, tufted floss products have a section of regular floss for interproximal plaque removal needs as well.

12.   A The joints affected by osteoarthritis may be aggravated by changes in body weight and pressure of the body weight on the affected region. The dental chair should be adjusted for the least amount of weight being placed on cervical spine C3 to C7 vertebrae. Although the patient may be questioned for feedback, a semisupine position is likely to be acceptable.

      B,C Providing physical supports and allowing for frequent position changes in the treatment chair will assist with making the patient comfortable for the duration of the appointment.

      D Scheduling short appointments will assist with managing patient comfort.

      (E) The patient with osteoarthritis is more likely to feel pain and stiffness in the morning or after a period of inactivity such as sleeping. Although not likely to last as long as the pain and stiffness experienced with rheumatoid arthritis, later in the day, after activity, may be a better time to schedule appointments for this patient.

13.   A One oral prophylaxis appointment is not likely to address the need for a thorough periodontal assessment and to perform nonsurgical periodontal therapy for this patient. Reevaluation of the pocket depths and bleeding should occur at an interval of 4 to 6 weeks.

      B Full-mouth disinfection is thought to assist with preventing the pathogens from unscaled regions from reinfecting scaled regions by removing as many pathogens from the oral cavity as possible at one time. Based on his periodontal status, this patient would not be a candidate for this procedure. Additionally, the long appointment may be difficult for this patient to tolerate.

      (C) Based on the periodontal status, amount and location of calculus, presence of complex restorations, and the patient's medical status, one 1-hour appointment for full-mouth debridement and one 45-minute appointment 7 to 10 days later to evaluate tissue response and to instrument if inflammation persists is appropriate. Reevaluation of the pocket depths and bleeding should occur at an interval of 4 to 6 weeks.

      D Based on his periodontal status, this patient would not be a candidate for two half-mouth periodontal debridement appointments. Additionally, the long appointments may be difficult for this patient to tolerate.

      E Scheduling four quadrant scale and root debridement appointments seems unnecessary given this patient's periodontal condition.

14.   A Area-specific curets are most often used for root debridement in periodontal pockets, and require frequent and time-consuming instrument changes to effectively debride all regions of the oral cavity. The amount and location of calculus in shallow pockets indicates that universal curets would be an effective and efficient choice for this patient.

      (B) For slight calculus and shallow pocket depths, the universal curet can be used to effectively remove supragingival and subgingival deposits in all regions of the oral cavity, eliminating the need to switch instruments.

      C The extended shanks of modified curets allow for debridement of root surfaces in deep periodontal pockets not observed in this patient. As with standard area-specific curets, modified curets require frequent and time-consuming instrument transfers.

      D Sickle scalers are used to debride superior to the gingival margin and would most likely not be effective in removing subgingival calculus for this patient.

      E Periodontal files are used to prepare large accumulations of calculus for removal by another instrument. This patient does not present with large deposits that would necessitate the use of periodontal files.

15.   (A) Dental implants are easily scratched by metallic instruments of a hardness greater than the implant material.

  B,C,D,E Instruments selected for use around dental implants should be softer than the implant material. Plastic, gold-tipped, nylon, or graphite instruments are indicated for use around dental implants.

16.   A,B Four to 6 weeks is an ideal reevaluation interval for all patients who initially present with inflammation or poor oral self-care. This patient was most likely scheduled within this time frame to evaluate initial placement of the dental implant, and for a reevaluation of dental hygiene treatment following the initial periodontal debridement appointment after not having professional care in the past 10 months. However, the interval time for his next appointment should be based on findings at the reevaluation appointment.

      C Following initial reevaluation and successful stabilization of the dental implant, it is recommended that periodontal maintenance appointments be scheduled for 3-month intervals for the first year after dental implant surgery.

      D Based on this patient's initial evaluation, reevaluation, and complex restorative treatment, 6 months will most likely be too long of an interval to maintain oral health.

      (E) This patient reports having dental implants placed 3 years ago. A personalized appointment plan based on his needs at each appointment may be developed at this time. His recommended recall interval should be based on evaluation of peri-implant and periodontal tissues, compliance with oral self-care recommendations, and effectiveness of biofilm control.

17.   A Evaluation of tissue response to periodontal debridement and implementation of oral self-care at 6 weeks is an appropriate interval in which to observe tissue healing. In fact, a generalized improved tissue condition is noted by the reduction in probing depths in other regions.

      (B) The best explanation for the localized lack of tissue response is that bacteria from the carious lesion observed radiographically on the distal of the mandibular left premolar may be causing continuous reinfection (seeding) of the gingiva in the adjacent area.

      C Exposure to ionizing radiation from diagnostic medical and dental radiation would not affect tissue healing.

      D Undetected systemic conditions that may influence gingival health would most likely have a generalized manifestation.

E Inappropriate toothpick use can result in trauma to soft tissue, and more frequently, damage to the papilla, but is less likely to increase the pocket depth observed at the reevaluation appointment. It is more likely that the caries present on the distal occlusal of the mandibular left premolar may be causing continuous reinfection of the periodontal tissues in this region.

18.   A,B Diseased tissue may not reveal changes in color or gingival contour.

(C) The best indicator of implant success is lack of mobility indicating that osseointegration was successful.

D Unless the baseline probing depths at the time of final delivery of the implant superstructure are available, probing depths at subsequent intervals cannot be reliable indicators of implant success or failure. Additionally, probing dental implants in the absence of conditions that evoke disease, such as bleeding and inflammation, is controversial in that peri-implant tissues adhere to the implant differently than periodontal tissues adhere to the tooth surface.

E In addition to the question of whether to probe around dental implants, bleeding may be related to probing force and wounding of the tissue, and therefore is not an ideal indicator of healthy or diseased peri-implant tissue.

19.   A Based on this patient's age and condition of his remaining unrestored teeth (the premolars), pit and fissure sealants would not be significantly beneficial.

B The direct, local application of chlorhexidine to the peri-implant tissues would better meet this patient's needs at this time. Fluoride application is not likely to remineralize the caries observed. If future development of new caries is observed, or recurrent or root caries present in the future, a fluoride treatment may be indicated.

(C) Directly applying chlorhexidine to the peri-implant tissues via an end-tuft brush or tufted floss can effectively minimize biofilm accumulation and reduce inflammation.

D This patient's dental implant–supported superstructure does not leave much room to safely direct oral irrigation under the restorative superstructure and not at the peri-implant tissues. Directly applying a chemotherapeutic agent, such as chlorhexidine, with an end-tuft brush is the better recommendation in this case.

E Potassium oxalate is an ingredient in desensitizing agents and does not appear to be indicated for use by this patient.

20.   A Although this patient is currently taking a medication that puts him at risk for xerostomia, he is not likely to develop a severe case, nor is he to remain on the drug for very long, as it is prescribed for short-term use in response to acute pain.

(B) Acidic fluoride may corrode titanium implants. Only neutral sodium fluoride at low concentrations should be recommended.

C,D,E These agents, although not necessarily recommended at this time, present no contraindications for use by this patient.

21.   (A) A slim diameter, or periodontal tip, insert is made of a metal harder than the dental implant. Because of the potential to scratch the surface of the implant, the use of metal instruments is contraindicated.

B Although some studies contraindicate the use of the air polisher on dental implants, others have found it to be safe and effective at removing deposits. Appropriately directing the spray away from the gingival margin with a light, sweeping motion would not be contraindicated. In this list of devices, the metal slim diameter ultrasonic tip is the more obvious contraindication.

C Tin oxide appropriately applied with a rotary rubber cup is safe and effective at removing light stain from dental implants.

D Using a specially designed plastic tip sleeve over a sonic or ultrasonic instrument allows the safe use of these instruments for removing deposits from dental implants.

E Nonabrasive paste applied with dental tape is especially useful for removing stains from surfaces not easily accessible by other means.

22. A,B,C,E Even though all three—dentist, dental hygienist, and patient—play a role in helping to establish an effective oral self-care routine, it is the patient who is ultimately responsible for his oral health.

D The dental hygienist and dentist are responsible for providing the information and education the patient needs to develop his goals for oral health; and both are responsible for providing supportive care as needed. However, the patient is ultimately responsible for maintaining his oral health.

23. A Immediately following placement of the final restoration of the dental implant superstructure, radiographs should be taken every 3 months for the first year.

B Bitewing radiographs are recommended every 6 to 18 months for adult recall patients who present with signs, symptoms, or risk factors for caries. This recommendation for detecting caries should not be confused with the recommendation for radiographs to evaluate dental implants.

C After the first year of placement of the dental implant, radiographs should be taken once a year. Findings should be compared with the baseline images.

D Bitewing radiographs are recommended every 24 to 36 months for adult recall patients who present with no signs, symptoms, or risk factors for caries. This recommendation for detecting caries should not be confused with the recommendation for radiographs to evaluate dental implants.

E After the first year of placement, radiographs should be taken once a year to evaluate dental implants even when there are no signs or symptoms of failure. Radiographs should not wait until problem signs are observed clinically.

24. A The patient's medical condition must be assessed to determine if conditions exist that will contribute to implant surgery failure. Conditions that contribute to poor healing or rejection of the implant such as diabetes and immunocompromising diseases would contraindicate the placement of implants.

B The patient must present with the psychological ability to undergo treatment for placement of dental implants, and be motivated to learn and use meticulous oral self-care skills.

C Because of the relationship between smoking and periodontal health and healing, osseointegration of the implant is likely to be jeopardized in a smoker. Smoking will play a role in the decision to treatment plan for placement of an implant.

D A thorough assessment of the bone in the site selected for placement of the implant is paramount. The bone height, width, contour, and density must be able to support the implant.

E DNA testing for periodontal pathogens continues to be developed and implemented. However, genetic testing would not likely be considered before placement of a dental implant.

25. A,C,D,E These design features all provide a harbor for the accumulation of biofilm and debris and make access for effective self-care difficult.

B The left side of the implant consists of a cantilever pontic that is attached to the fixed bridge on only one side. This cantilever design should not be considered a mistake in design.

CASE K SPECIAL NEEDS PATIENT JOHNNIE JOHNSON

1.   **A** Nicotine stomatitis is characterized by red raised dots at the openings of minor salivary gland ducts on the hard palate. Cigarette smoking is associated with these lesions and should be distinguished from the other conditions.

  B Hyperkeratosis presents as white lesions on the oral mucosa.

  C Pyogenic granuloma presents as a single red lesion on the oral mucosa.

  D Kaposi's sarcoma is purplish in color and is found on the hard palate or gingiva.

  E Although burn trauma from hot foods may appear similar, this patient's history of tobacco use should be taken into consideration.

2.   A The free or marginal gingiva appears as the gingival crest nearest the incisal or occlusal edge of the tooth and is covered by the oral epithelium.

  B The paler pink attached gingiva is differentiated from the alveolar mucosa by the mucogingival line.

  C The masticatory mucosa covers the gingiva and hard palate.

  D The alveolar mucosa lines the inner surface of the lips and cheeks. This tissue is not attached to the underlining structures, and blood vessels located beneath make this area appear redder in color than the nearby masticatory mucosa.

  E The junctional epithelium is not visible clinically as it is located at the base of the sulcus.

3.   A Glass ionomers are often used as a caries preventive sealant or as a cervical restoration in the older patient with a high risk of root caries. Multipurpose composite restorations provide better esthetics than glass ionomers and better meet the need for restoring the large caries affecting this patient's anterior teeth.

  B Acrylic and silicate resins were first introduced as dental restorations in 1878. These materials proved to have dimensional instability that led to staining and recurrent caries. The use of these materials has been replaced by composites.

  C Porcelain bonding is dental ceramic used to fabricate veneers, or nonmetal crowns. Porcelain veneers are manufactured in a dental laboratory and require significant tooth preparation before placement.

  D Dental ceramics refers to restorations that use nonmetallic materials such as porcelain to make crowns, onlays, inlays, and veneers. These restorations are manufactured in a dental laboratory and require significant tooth preparation before placement.

  E These teeth exhibit multipurpose composite restorations that can provide this patient with a cost-effective tooth-colored restoration for esthetic purposes. Multipurpose composites are ideal for anterior restorations because occlusal forces are less than those in posterior regions.

4.   A Use of multiple antacids is not a risk factor for oral cancer. If chewable and formulated with sugar, use of these products throughout the day may increase this patient's risk for caries.

  B Research provides strong evidence for the relationship between smoking and alcohol ingestion and the development of squamous cell carcinoma.

  C,D Xerostomia conditions and high pulse and respiration rate are not risk factors for oral cancer.

  E Rampant caries with abscesses may be creating a low grade infection. However, caries would not be considered a risk factor for oral cancer.

5. A,B,C,E Each of these conditions (hand tremors, rapid pulse rate, xerostomia, and swollen parotid glands) are indicative of a heavy alcohol user.

(D) This patient reports using over-the-counter medications to alleviate his stomach pain. Although his use of these products is frequent, it is in response to stomach irritation most likely caused by excessive alcohol use and not as a result of alcohol-induced craving.

6. (A) Chronic alcohol use frequently causes benign bilateral parotid swellings called sialadenosis. Reduced salivary output or xerostomia allows for the overgrowth of oral microorganisms leading to caries. However, dry mouth conditions are not responsible for the spread of caries from tooth to tooth. Carious lesions begin within the enamel and progress into the tooth tissue.

B,C,D,E These answers are not correct.

7. A Cigarette smoking can contribute to changes in the appearance of the tissues in the oral cavity. However, the most common effect on the papillae of the tongue is staining.

B,D The excessive use of some medications, such as antacids, and alcohol may interfere with the normal absorption and metabolism of folate resulting in a folic acid deficiency. Although the use of these drugs plays a role in creating the condition for the effect on the tongue, the direct cause is the folic acid deficiency itself.

(C) The burning sensation symptoms and the red tip and lateral borders of the tongue indicate a folic acid deficiency.

E A geographic tongue occurs in some patients as a normal condition. The papillae on the dorsum of the tongue in certain regions appear smooth and less raised. This pattern changes over time. There is no pain or loss of taste sensation associated with this condition.

8. (A) The extent of caries involvement evident on this tooth is most likely causing pulpal necrosis resulting in the inflammatory lesion that appears as a radiolucency at the apex indicating a periapical abscess.

B Condensing osteitis is a condition of the supporting bone and appears radiopaque.

C When inflammation becomes chronic, granulation tissue begins to infiltrate the lesion and entrapped epithelial tissue may result in the formation of an apical cyst. Although it is difficult to distinguish between a periapical abscess and cyst radiographically, the term *residual cyst* would not be applied here because the affected tooth is present. A residual cyst is left intact when the affected tooth is extracted.

D If this radiolucency had been a normal anatomic landmark, such as the lingual foramen, it would appear separated from the tooth by the appearance of an intact lamina dura. Additionally, the lingual foramen is often imaged encircled by the radiopaque genial tubercles.

E When imaged on a radiograph, the mental foramen usually appears near the apices of the mandibular first and second premolars. The mental foramen is distinguished from an abscess by the presence of an intact lamina dura separating the radiolucent mental foramen from the apex of the tooth it appears near.

9. A,B,C Caries is evident clinically and radiographically on the maxillary right lateral and central incisors and the maxillary left central incisor.

(D) The mandibular left central incisor appears sound both clinically and radiographically.

E The mandibular left lateral incisor presents with composite restorations, which appear defective on the mesial-incisal surface.

10. A,B,D,E   Both the statement and reason are correct and related.

(C)   Non-alcohol-containing preprocedural mouth rinses are recommended for the alcoholic patient and the patient with xerostomia.

11.   A   Sunlight exposure is essential for vitamin D absorption.

B,C   Foods such as organ meats and green vegetables contain folic acid. However, excessive use of alcohol tends to result in poor appetite for food. This patient may be more likely to follow protocol for taking a supplement while being counseled to develop a plan for an improved diet.

D   Multiple vitamins can be recommended as well, but a folic acid supplement specifically targets this patient's deficiency.

(E)   Oral signs and symptoms of folate deficiency include a red, sore, and burning tongue. The best way to treat this patient's deficiency is with a 1 mg folic acid supplement three times a week.

12.   A   The cost of chronic alcohol use and excessive drinking can impact an individual's finances by reducing the amount of money available to spend on dental treatment.

B   Chronic excessive drinking can lead to apathy regarding health issues and an inability to keep appointments and follow through with treatment.

(C)   The excessive use of alcohol is not associated with respiratory conditions that would interfere with treatment.

D   When chronic alcoholism is suspected, bleeding problems may result from liver impairment.

E   Emotional instability during appointments may result when this patient is under the influence of alcohol or as the result of alcohol withdrawal.

13.   A   Alcohol consumption may result in poor self-care, but is not cariogenic. Consumption of alcohol mixed with beverages containing sucrose can supply fermentable carbohydrates for acidogenic bacteria to metabolize. However, the alcohol is not cariogenic.

(B)   Saliva contains peroxidases, lysozymes, and specific antibodies that have anti-cariogenic properties. A deficiency of saliva allows for the overgrowth of bacteria that leads to caries development.

C   Lack of professional care did not cause the caries, but has allowed the caries process time to progress to this advanced stage.

D   Tobacco use plays a role in periodontal disease, but is not cariogenic.

E   Although poor oral self-care is a contributing factor to the accumulation of biofilms, xerostomia plays the key role in the caries process. Additionally, this patient presents with a fairly adequate ability to remove bacterial plaque.

14.   (A)   Because this patient exhibits signs of recent alcohol consumption and based on his reported lifestyle, alcohol withdrawal syndrome may manifest during treatment. Alcohol withdrawal may occur within a few hours after the last drink. In fact, this patient already exhibits hand tremors, nervousness, and a rapid pulse rate, all indicative of alcohol withdrawal syndrome.

B,C,E   Nothing in this patient's health history increases his risk of a possible airway obstruction, adrenal crisis, or asthma attack.

D   Although he has not indicated an allergy or past allergic reaction to agents that may be used by the dental hygienist in the treatment of his oral condition, there remains the potential of an anaphylactic reaction to a drug or agent. However, he does not present with an increased risk over that of the general population.

15.   A This patient recognizes and admits that the appearance of his teeth may be preventing him from securing better disk jockey jobs, which indicates his interest in achieving appropriate knowledge regarding the care of his oral health.

      B This patient recognizes and admits that the condition of his smile is affecting his life and has made this appointment based on this primary concern.

      C,E The nervous behavior observed is more likely physical in nature, and probably related to alcohol withdrawal. Given the evidence of extensive dental treatment in the past, fear of additional dental treatment is probably not the primary reason for the broken appointments.

      (D) Not keeping scheduled appointments is typical behavior for the alcohol abuser. Because this patient's lifestyle revolves around drinking it becomes a priority for him. The difficulty for the alcohol abuser comes from having to make appointments ahead of time. Because drinking and a drinking lifestyle take priority he cannot guarantee that he will be able to keep a scheduled appointment on any given day in the future.

16.   A The maxillary left canine/premolar area would be an ideal location to attain leverage for instrumentation.

      B Using the palm of the hand to fulcrum on the patient's chin is an accepted extraoral fulcrum for the maxillary left posterior facial aspects when conditions compromise an intraoral fulcrum.

      (C) Because of the advanced state of dental caries, the maxillary left central and lateral incisors are not the best choice for a stable finger rest. These teeth have the potential to fracture with the applied pressure.

      D Fulcruming with the ring finger resting on the index finger of the nondominate hand is an acceptable advanced fulcrum technique that can help stabilize the instrument for access to these posterior root surfaces.

17.   (A) Phase I, the initial nonsurgical phase of periodontal therapy, consists of procedures that are designed to control or eliminate the etiologic factors of the disease process. Education and plaque control instruction occur at the beginning of this phase followed by scaling and root debridement. The purpose of Phase I therapy is to bring this patient's periodontal disease under control.

      B Phase II or the surgical phase of periodontal therapy involves regenerative techniques to help restore periodontal tissues that have been lost because of disease. Therapy usually involves restoration and replacement of lost teeth.

      C If required, the surgical intervention of periodontal disease performed in Phase II will identify teeth that can be saved through restorative therapy. In Phase III, restorative care takes place on those teeth deemed periodontally sound. Ideally, periodontal disease risk and contributing factors have been identified and eliminated or controlled and self-care has been established setting the stage for restorative therapy and finally for periodontal maintenance.

      D Following stabilization of the periodontal condition and restoration of a functioning dentition, the patient will remain in Phase IV Maintenance Therapy for a lifetime to continuously monitor his periodontal health.

18.   A Peridex (chlorhexidine) has demonstrated antiplaque and antigingivitis properties and is especially useful for patients with periodontal disease. However, its 11.6% alcohol content contraindicate its use for this patient. More importantly, a fluoride supplement would better meet this patient's needs.

      B,D Research on the active ingredient in Viadent, sanguinarine, and the active ingredient in Scope, cetylpyridinium chloride, has been inconclusive on the ability of these agents to reduce plaque and gingivitis. However, this patient's needs indicate that a fluoride supplement would be a better recommendation. Additionally, the alcohol content of Viadent at 5.5% and of Scope at 18.9% contraindicate use by this patient.

C Essential oils, such as those found in Listerine mouth rinse, have been shown to reduce plaque and gingivitis. However, the high alcohol content (26.9%) contraindicate the use of this product for this patient. More importantly, a fluoride supplement would better meet this patient's needs.

(E) Caries prevention appears to be this patient's greatest need. Gel-Kam, a brush-on self-care stannous fluoride gel, would be the best recommendation because it has been shown to be effective in reducing gingivitis as well. Additionally, each of the other antiplaque and antigingivitis agents contain alcohol, which should not be recommended given this patient's history of excessive alcohol consumption.

19. A This patient has a moderate buildup of subgingival calculus. Tartar control toothpaste is effective at reducing the buildup of supragingival accumulation only. More importantly, controlling this patient's caries should be the primary concern.

(B) This patient's caries activity prompts the use of fluoride varnish.

C All sites that are usual candidates for pit and fissure sealants appear to have restorations and/or caries activity.

D At the reevaluation appointment, most deep pockets have responded to treatment. Those probing depths at the reevaluation appointment that remain at 5 to 6 mm are in the region of the third molars. These readings most likely indicate pseudopocketing that would not benefit from locally delivered antimicrobial therapy.

E The burning tongue sensation and loss of papillae experienced by this patient is most likely due to a deficiency in folate. Antifungal agents would not be indicated treatment.

20. A,B The use of ultrasonic and sonic scalers may damage composite restorations and should be avoided.

(C) The method chosen to remove stains should not cause harm to the surface of the restoration. The rubber cup polishing method is a reasonable choice to selectively polish to remove stains. Choosing the least abrasive grit capable of removing the stains will help avoid scratching the restorations.

D Toothbrush polishing is a safe alternate to other polishing methods. However, it is unlikely to remove stains, especially those caused by smoking. Tartar control toothpaste is no more effective at removing stains than other toothpastes currently available. The purpose of tartar control toothpaste is to reduce buildup of supragingival calculus by interfering with the attachment process.

E Research has demonstrated that air abrasion polishing can be harmful to composite restorations and suggests caution when using this method. Because this patient's new anterior composite restorations are so large and cover a significant percentage of the tooth surface, it may be difficult to avoid prolonged exposure to the abrasive. The rubber cup method of polishing would be the better choice in this case.

21. A Rampant, severe caries and xerostomia make the use of fluorides essential for this patient.

B,C Tobacco use in conjunction with alcohol consumption dramatically increases this patient's risk of oral cancer. A tobacco cessation program should be discussed with this patient along with a discussion regarding the role alcohol plays in oral health.

(D) Tooth whitening products are not indicated when the patient presents with severe carious lesions. Also, the use of whitening products following restoration of his anterior teeth is not recommended. The whitening products will not change the shade of the composite dental materials with which this patient's anterior teeth were restored.

E Following an explanation of the cause of his burning tongue sensation and the role alcohol plays in nutritional deficiencies, a nutritional counseling session is recommended.

22.   (A) This patient currently exhibits alcohol withdrawal symptoms, which could escalate into confusion and distortion affecting his decision making regarding consent to dental treatment and his ability to undergo treatment. A physician's examination may indicate that this patient should be referred for medication, counseling, and/or psychiatric intervention during modification of his alcohol use to stabilize his condition.

B,D,E   Once a medical examination has been done and his physical condition is stabilized, referral should be made to address his nutritional status. Additionally, counseling in smoking cessation and recovery groups such as Alcoholics Anonymous can be recommended.

C   This patient's dental conditions are considered chronic and he is not in pain. Although his oral exam indicates that he is in need of extensive dental treatment, his lack of a diagnosis concerning his stomach pain and his unchecked excessive alcohol consumption make extensive, invasive dental treatment risky at this time.

23.   A   Safe treatment of this patient today requires knowing if he is still under the influence of alcohol.

B,C,E   Identification of excessive use of alcohol can better prepare the dental hygienist to plan safe treatment for this patient. Treatment planning should be based on accurate information regarding the patient's health behaviors.

(D) The health history should include questions that lead to more information regarding safe treatment of this patient and accurate recommendations and referrals for improved oral and general health. Knowing the type of alcohol this patient consumes does not add to this base knowledge.

24.   A   The dentist and the oral health care team is under obligation to inform the patient of all treatment options available and then allow the patient to make his own decisions based on knowledge provided regarding the advantages and disadvantages of each treatment. Once the patient–professional relationship has been established there is a responsibility to honestly disclose all available treatment options.

(B) There is often more than one treatment option for many dental situations. In this case, ideal treatment may indeed be crown restorations for these teeth. However, the choice to use composite restorations is adequate. The patient has a right to make a choice to sacrifice the best dental treatment for himself to use his financial resources on other nondental needs.

C   When the dental hygienist is in a position to assist with case presentation, a collaborative effort can be made to help provide the patient with many of the details he will need to decide on which course of treatment he will consent to. However, the decision to proceed with one treatment or another should be made by the patient.

D   Porcelain veneer crowns or full porcelain-fused-to-metal crowns would most likely provide improved stability for the anterior teeth affected by the rampant, severe caries. Although the composite restorative dental materials adequately restored these teeth, crowns may have provided an improved esthetic appearance.

E   There is no indication that this patient is not capable of understanding the need for comprehensive restoration of these badly decayed teeth.

25.   A   Because the patient is not currently inebriated and has decision-making capacity, he is able to give informed consent to be treated today.

B   Admitting to excessive drinking would impact treatment today if this patient was currently inebriated. Moreover, although this patient has admitted to heavy drinking, it is unclear at this point as to whether he views this as a problem.

C   Having liability insurance does not excuse a practitioner from providing negligent or substandard care. If this patient was determined to be inebriated at today's appointment, then treatment would be postponed to a time when he could make sound decisions and provide informed consent.

D   Because this is not an emergency procedure in which the patient cannot give informed consent, the dental hygienist is not using the right of therapeutic privilege.

(E)   Because the patient has decision-making capacity, he is able to give informed consent. Decision-making capacity is a standard that varies with the level of risk to the patient. Because scaling and root debridement involve a low level of risk (compared to the higher level of risk of periodontal surgery), the patient's level of understanding and reasoning is adequate.

CASE L SPECIAL NEEDS PATIENT THOMAS SMALL

1.   A   A papilloma is a benign tumor often described as cauliflower-like in appearance and often found on the soft palate or tongue.

B   Neurofibroma, a benign tumor of nerve tissue, is most often discovered as a nonulcerated mass on the lateral border or the tongue.

(C)   Because this finding is noted to be hard upon palpation, and no signs of pathosis are present on the radiographs, a bony exostosis is concluded.

D   Chronic irritation of the oral mucosa can result in frictional hyperkeratosis, a thickened response of the tissue to this trauma.

E   Lipoma, a benign tumor of mature fat cells, often appears as a yellowish mass of enlarged tissue in the vestibule or on the buccal mucosa.

2.   A,B   A possible adverse effect of this patient's medications is dryness of the oral cavity. This dryness may be extended to the mucosa covering of the lips. Combined with mouth breathing, the habitually parted lips have become thickened and cracked.

C,E   This patient has developed a habit of licking and sucking on his lips, which keeps them constantly bathed in saliva. Evaporating moisture adds to the drying effect of these tissues.

(D)   Although a person with a seizure disorder may accidentally bite the lips during convulsions, the dry, chapped appearance of this patient's lips do not indicate a traumatic injury.

3.   A   Linear gingival erythema is a type of necrotizing ulcerative gingivitis observed in the HIV-positive patient that is characterized by an intense red color of the free gingival margin.

(B)   Gingival enlargement is a side effect of many anticonvulsant drugs such as phenytoin. This enlargement makes plaque biofilm control difficult, resulting in gingival inflammation that may contribute to further enlargement.

C   Gingival enlargement sometimes occurs in patients not taking anticonvulsant drugs as an inherited condition. However, the gingival enlargement observed in this patient is most likely influenced by the anticonvulsant drugs he is taking to manage his seizure disorder.

D   Necrotizing ulcerative gingivitis is characterized by a grayish pseudomembrane overlaying the free gingival margin and necrotic, or punched-out papillae. Pain is associated with this infection, not expressed by this patient.

E   A primary infection of the herpes virus often manifests as acute herpetic gingivostomatitis, characterized by oral vesicles and ulcers and intense pain, not expressed by this patient.

4.   (A)   Food and debris can easily become trapped under the opercula covering the partially erupted mandibular third molars, precipitating pericoronitis.

B   Osteomyelitis develops acutely or chronically and involves an inflammation of the bone following trauma or surgery or as an extension of another infection, such as a periapical abscess. There is nothing in this patient's medical or dental history or clinical exam that indicate risk of osteomyelitis.

C Melanosis is the normal physiologic pigmentation of the oral mucosa often associated with dark-skinned individuals although not evident here.

D If a salivary gland becomes damaged, the mucous salivary secretions may enter the surrounding tissues, creating a swelling called a mucocele. The most common site of occurrence is the lower lip.

E Taurodontism refers to a developmental anomaly where the tooth exhibits an elongated (bull-like) pulp chamber. This anomaly is not considered a risk to oral health and the impacted, partially erupted mandibular third molars do not appear to present with this anomaly.

5. A The normal appearance of the mandibular canal should not be mistaken for a bone fracture.

B Nutrient canals appear as thin radiolucent lines, usually running in a vertical position when observed in a radiograph of the mandible.

C,D The oblique ridge and mylohyoid line should not be confused with the appearance of the mandibular canal. If observed in this region, the oblique ridge and mylohyoid line would most likely appear slightly more distinct with an increased radiopacity. Additionally, the radiolucency outlined by the paired faint radiopaque lines observed in this radiograph is the characteristic appearance of the mandibular canal.

(E) The paired parallel radiopaque lines outlining this radiolucency indicate the presence of the mandibular canal, which appears to traverse the body of the mandible.

6. A Although it may be difficult to identify foreign objects stuck to the film emulsion from this photograph, the characteristic lightening-patterned radiolucency that results from exposure to static electricity should not be confused with other conditions that affect the quality of the radiograph.

(B) Static electricity created a white light spark that resulted in an exposure of the film with a lightening-patterned line of radiolucency.

C Roller marks that result when automatic processor rollers are contaminated, or when a film gets stuck between the rollers for a period of time, appear as a thick horizontal or vertical band of uniform radiolucency corresponding to where the roller contacted the film.

D Depending on the chemical, either developer or fixer, an accidental chemical splash will appear radiolucent or radiopaque, respectively. The thin artifact observed here is characteristic of exposure to static electricity and should not be confused with an accidental chemical splash.

E Scratching the emulsion results in white marks on film representing where the emulsion is missing.

7. A The image of teeth, including the enamel, dentin, and pulp chambers, can be identified in these radiographs and should not be confused with the presence of tori.

B Dens invaginatus often affects the maxillary lateral incisors bilaterally. When present, dens invaginatus appears as an invagination of tooth structure within the pulp chamber.

C An enamel pearl, when present, will appear as a smooth, round extension of enamel within the furcation area of a multirooted tooth.

(D) The radiographs reveal supernumerary teeth (fourth molars).

E As observed on the radiographs, this patient's maxillary third molars are erupted. The impacted teeth imaged here are supernumerary.

8.   A Although this patient's medications have controlled his seizure episodes for the past 8 months, treatment armamentarium should include devices that will help manage and respond to the possible incidence of a generalized tonic-clonic convulsion.

    B To help minimize the risk of a seizure episode during dental hygiene treatment, appointments should be made within a few hours of taking the medications designed to control them.

    C The patient should be questioned about any known precipitating factors regarding his seizures and he should be instructed to report these sensations if they manifest during the appointment.

    D Should a seizure occur, the patient should be monitored for respiratory difficulty as it may be necessary to administer oxygen.

    (E) Based on this patient's medical conditions, preparations should be made for a possible seizure. Administration of a bronchodilator would be appropriate for an asthmatic attack.

9.   **(A)** During a seizure, the patient's movements become spastic and generalized muscle rigidity will cause uncontrolled forceful movements of his limbs and head. The primary task of management during this stage must be to protect the patient from injury. The treatment chair should be positioned in a supine, protected position, and the instrument tray and other equipment moved out of the way. However, no attempt should be made to move this patient out of the treatment chair and onto the floor

    B,C,D,E These answers are incorrect.

10.   A,E Vital signs and airway should be monitored to avoid escalation of the emergency.

    (B) Given this patient's medical history, uncontrolled muscle motor movements will mostly likely indicate the onset of an epileptic seizure. The patient should not be forcibly restrained. Passive restraint may be applied, only if the patient is in danger of contacting objects in the area that may cause injury, or if the patient is in danger of falling out of the treatment chair.

    C Placing the patient in a supine position in the treatment chair can help to provide support throughout the seizure.

    D Equipment should be removed from the area to prevent injury to the patient during uncontrolled forcible movements.

11.   A Coronal polishing with a power-driven handpiece may create noise that could have the potential to exacerbate a seizure. However, the louder and higher pitched noise output of the ultrasonic scaler listed here should be considered more of a risk.

    B Local delivery of subgingival irrigants with a pulsating syringe is not likely to create the loud noise associated with precipitating this patient's seizures. The louder and higher pitched noise output of the ultrasonic scaler listed here should be considered more of a risk. Irrigation using a handheld syringe is not likely to produce loud noises that are suspected of exacerbating this patient's seizures.

    (C) Because this patient's epileptic seizures are exacerbated by monotonous and loud noises, it may be prudent to forego the use of an ultrasonic scaler.

    D,E Root planing with handheld instruments and toothbrush deplaquing are not likely to create the loud noise associated with precipitating this patient's seizures.

12.   A,E The use of disclosing solution and demonstration of oral hygiene instructions using the patient's own mouth is a sound strategy for explaining self-care techniques. Using a handheld mirror or projecting the images on a computer monitor assists in the demonstration of appropriate techniques. However, the first step in gaining patient interest would be to address his primary complaint—the lack of a toothbrush at home.

B Giving this patient a brochure that he can take home can help remind him of the need for self-care. However, the first step in gaining patient interest would be to address his primary complaint—the lack of a toothbrush at home.

C This patient's chief concern is that he does not have a toothbrush. His concern indicates that he knows taking care of his oral health is important. His probable response to oral hygiene instructions will be that he has not been able to perform adequate self-care because his toothbrush is missing. The best approach to home care instruction is to provide him with a new toothbrush. Providing a toothbrush with his name on it will further motivate this patient by addressing his chief concern first.

D When the opportunity presents, including a patient's caregiver in oral hygiene instructional services for the patient with mental retardation can lead to increased effectiveness and improved outcomes. However, it is highly unlikely that the social services case worker lives at the care facility with this patient. Additionally, the first step in gaining this patient's interest in improving oral self-care would be to address his primary complaint—the lack of a toothbrush at home.

13. A There is nothing in this patient's medical history that would indicate a need for antibiotic prophylaxis.

  B The possible side effects of the multiple anticonvulsant drugs this patient is taking include increased incidence of postscaling gingival bleeding and delayed healing time. Given the severity of the gingival inflammation and the spontaneous gingival bleeding that this patient presents with, a pretreatment bleeding time might be prudent before subgingival instrumentation.

  C There is nothing in this patient's medical history that would necessitate the administration of an analgesic drug. Additionally, it is possible that phenytoin (Dilantin) will increase the likelihood of acetaminophen hepatoxicity, and therefore concurrent use of these drugs should be avoided.

  D Using an alcohol-containing mouth rinse should be avoided in the patient with evidence of dry mouth.

  E Given the severity of the gingival inflammation and the spontaneous gingival bleeding that this patient presents with, a pretreatment bleeding time might be prudent not only before subgingival instrumentation but also before subgingival irrigation.

14. A A score of 0 indicates that the tooth is plaque free.

  B A score of 1 indicates slight plaque biofilm, detectable by swiping a hand instrument across the tooth.

  C A score of 2 indicates biofilm accumulation is observable visibly as a thin film.

  D The Plaque Index of Silness and Löe measures the amount of plaque biofilm at the gingival margin. A score of 3 indicates heavy accumulation.

15. A The initial colonization of bacteria on the teeth surfaces consists of 75% to 80% gram-positive cocci. The plaque observed in this region is thick and has accumulated a high concentration of bacteria capable of producing gingival inflammation.

  B Increasing numbers of gram-positive filamentous forms and short rods indicate that the plaque has gone undisturbed for about 1 to 2 days. The thickened, matured plaque observed in these regions has been undisturbed for over a week, and is producing gingival inflammation.

  C Plaque that remains undisturbed for 4 to 7 days develops an increasing number of rods, filamentous forms, and fusobacteria. Although the biofilm observed in these regions is thick at the gingival margin, the severity of gingival inflammation indicates the presence of vibrios and spirochetes.

  D Gram-negative and anaerobic organisms begin to colonize plaque that remains undisturbed for 1 to 2 weeks. However, the severity of gingival inflammation in these regions indicates an older biofilm of vibrios and spirochetes, along with cocci and filamentous forms of bacteria, which have become densely packed causing the severe gingivitis.

(E) The significant gingival inflammation observed indicates the presence of mature plaque biofilm containing gram-negative motile rods and spirochetes.

16. A,B,C,E Subgingival irrigation, polishing, toothbrushing, or applying fluoride will not remove this calculus deposit.

(D) The photographs reveal a partially supragingival calculus deposit. This deposit must be removed with the use of a universal curet.

17.   (A) A curved sickle scaler is ideal for removing supragingival calculus from this region.

B A file scaler is used when the calculus deposits are large or burnished and can not be readily removed with the curved or straight sickle scaler. The file scaler can be used to crush gross deposits for easier removable by other instruments.

C The hoe scaler is used to break up gross deposits for easier removal by other instruments. However, the wide straight cutting edge of the hoe scaler makes its effective and safe use in this region difficult.

D The purpose of the chisel scaler is to remove large deposits from proximal surfaces of anterior teeth that are accessible as a result of missing interdental gingival.

18.   (A) Anticonvulsants taken by this patient are partly responsible for his gingival enlargement. Although meticulous home care will likely reduce the gingival inflammation caused by the accumulation of bacterial plaque at the gingival margin, the fibrotic enlargement caused by the anticonvulsants will probably remain. Additionally, research has shown that initial probing depths of 1 to 3 mm are not likely to demonstrate a reduction in probe readings at the reevaluation appointment and that probing depths of 4 to 6 mm will most likely demonstrate only a 1 mm reduction in probe readings at the reevaluation appointment.

B Research has indicated that deep pockets depths of 7 mm or greater usually show the greatest reduction, 1.5 mm to 3 mm at the reevaluation appointment.

C A reduction in pocket depths of 4 to 5 mm is unrealistic given this patient's initial 2 to 6 mm measurements.

D Reduction in probing depths is an expected outcome of nonsurgical periodontal therapy. Even if the patient's home care does not improve significantly, instrumentation will have disrupted the bacterial flora of the pockets. New biofilm accumulations at the reevaluation appointment will consist mainly of gram-positive bacteria that is more like those microbes found in healthy sites.

19.   A To gain maximum benefits from a fluoride mouth rinse, proper swishing mechanics must be followed. Using the correct swishing methods and holding the solution in the mouth for the required length of time may be too demanding for this patient, and may lead to decreased compliance. Additionally, the risk of accidental swallowing would need to be assessed.

B The custom tray application procedure may be too demanding for this patient, and may lead to decreased compliance.

(C) Using a fluoride application that utilizes brushing, a skill this patient can be encouraged to improve, can help with patient compliance. Additionally, although stannous fluoride does not have the American Dental Association Seal of Acceptance for reducing plaque and gingivitis, it is often used in periodontal therapy as an antiplaque and antigingivitis agent, a use which may benefit this patient.

D This patient, like all patients whether at risk for caries or not, should be encouraged to use a fluoride dentifrice. Because patients at risk for caries will benefit from more than one method of fluoride use, recommending the use of a stannous fluoride gel is the best choice from this list.

E Dietary fluoride supplements are usually prescribed for children aged 6 months to 16 years, whose water supply is not fluoridated at an optimal level. Although most fluoride supplements are chewed and swished for a topical effect, they are also swallowed for a systemic influence on the developing dentition.

20.   A   This patient presents with risk factors for caries, including clinically visible caries, poor self-care, and a tendency toward xerostomia, making him a candidate for fluoride. A varnish application that requires less need for isolating the teeth and drying would be an ideal method of delivery.

(B)   Removing diseased tissue from the lining of periodontal pockets during scaling and root debridement exposes the pocket wall to possible invasion of polishing paste particles. During polishing, particles can become lodged in the tissue and may delay healing. Additionally, polishing should be postponed when the gingival tissues are spongy and bleed easily.

C,D,E   Provided there are not complications with this patient's medical history and no contraindications to treatment are noted, probing, scaling, and root planing should begin as soon as possible.

21.   (A)   Most seizures last between 1 and 2 minutes. When uncontrolled movements end, the muscles relax and the patient falls into a deep sleep, and usually requires several hours of rest. However, status epilepticus results in reoccurring seizures or a seizure that becomes prolonged. Seizures lasting longer than 5 minutes should be suspected of developing into life-threatening status epilepticus and emergency medical assistance should be summoned.

B,C,D,E   Because seizures usually last 1 to 2 minutes, a seizure lasting longer than 5 minutes should be suspected of developing into life-threatening status epilepticus and emergency medical assistance should be summoned.

22.   A,B,C   Learning as much as possible about the type of seizure, frequency, and degree of control will assist the dental professional with the decision to provide treatment and with managing a medical emergency.

D   Knowing precipitating factors will allow the dental professional to adequately prepare for a medical emergency.

(E)   Assessing this patient's mental status is not a prerequisite for treatment. However, knowing about any warnings or preseizure changes in the patient's emotions would be helpful information. Emotionally, some patients may demonstrate an increased sense of irritability right before an impending seizure.

23.   (A)   This patient communicates well and appears capable of understanding the need for his own oral self-care. Additionally, he is able to perform simple skilled work to maintain his job at the grocery store.

B   Adults with moderate retardation are less able to perform self-care without assistance, and are more likely to be able to perform unskilled work only with direct supervision.

C   Severely retarded adults are less likely to be employable and although can adapt to daily routines, need supervised self-care.

D   Profoundly retarded individuals require close supervision and daily assistance with self-care.

24.   A   Dental hygiene treatment of this patient will require his cooperation. All aspects of treatment, and hence, the informed consent, must be explained to the patient, and he should be given the opportunity to ask questions, and agree or disagree with procedures. However, his mother is his legal guardian and therefore, her signature must be obtained on the informed consent form.

B   Although this patient's case worker has brought him to the appointment today, it is not likely that she has legal authority to consent to his treatment. Her agreement with his legal guardian, his mother, is most likely limited and would not be likely to give her permission to consent to dental treatment. Because his mother is known to be his legal guardian, her consent must be obtained.

C This patient's mother is his legal guardian. Permission to treat him must be secured from his mother.

D This patient's mother has most likely made an agreement with the group home director to allow the case worker to transport him to his appointment today. However, as his legal guardian, his mother is responsible for signing the informed consent form.

E Although the dental hygienist works with the dentist in providing treatment recommendations and developing a dental hygienist diagnosis, the dentist cannot allow treatment of this patient without the patient's legal guardian, his mother, providing informed consent.

25.   A A patient who is legally competent is an individual who has not been through a legal process to be declared incompetent and/or who has not legally granted authority to another for the purpose of decision making. A person may have varying degrees of decision-making capacity and not all legally competent individuals have decision-making capacity. However, this patient's mild mental retardation limits his decision-making ability.

B A patient may have impaired decision-making capacity, although maintaining a legally competent status. However, this patient and his mother have been through a legal process granting her legal guardianship.

C A patient who has been through a legal process to be declared incompetent may still have decision-making capacity. For example, a person entering a life-threatening medical operation may take legal action to grant another authority to carry out his wishes should the patient become incapacitated.

D This patient's mother is his legal guardian and as such, has the responsibility for making competent decisions regarding his treatment. Given his mental retardation, this patient is considered to have impaired decision-making capacity.

CASE M MEDICALLY COMPROMISED PATIENT NANCY FOSTER

1.   A Although it may occur at any age, Type I diabetes usually has a sudden onset during puberty, where insulin-producing beta cells in the pancreas are destroyed. This patient is dependent on exogenous insulin for survival as a result of this complete lack of insulin production, evidenced by her use of a continuous subcutaneous infusion pump.

B Patients with Type 2 diabetes exhibit an insulin resistance rather that a lack of insulin-producing beta cells in the pancreas. The disease onset usually occurs over a long period of time in individuals with a genetic propensity for the disease and/or as a result of a sedentary lifestyle and high-fat diet that leads to obesity. Although some individuals with Type 2 diabetes are treated with exogenous insulin, many others can manage their disease through lifestyle changes such as diet and exercise or with oral hypoglycemic medications.

C Gestational diabetes refers to an alteration in glucose tolerance observed during pregnancy.

D Other specific types of diabetes not linked to Type 1, Type 2, or gestational diabetes include drug- or chemical-induced diabetes, genetic defects of beta cell function, and pancreatic diseases, none of which is evident in this patient's health history.

2.   A,B Insulin resistance and inadequate insulin secretion is typical of Type 2 diabetes. Many Type 2 diabetics manage their disease through lifestyle changes such as diet and exercise or with oral hypoglycemic medications.

C When insulin-producing beta cells in the pancreas are destroyed, the patient must depend on exogenous insulin for survival. This patient's use of a continuous subcutaneous insulin infusion pump indicates that her pancreas no longer contains insulin-producing beta cells.

D Obesity is a major risk for diabetes across all age groups. However, this patient's weight is within the acceptable range (10th percentile) for females at her height and age.

E Although the risk factors for diabetes may include a high-fat diet and being overweight, sucrose consumption is not a direct cause of diabetes.

3. A A numerical score of 0 indicates no evidence of fluorosis.

B The anterior teeth present with a parchment-white color confined to the incisal edges. Additionally the parchment-white color presents in the posterior teeth as "snowcapping" where the fluorosis is confined to the cusp tips, indicating a numerical score of 1.

C A numerical score of 2 indicates fluorosis that presents as a parchment-white color covering at least one-third of the tooth surface but less than two-thirds.

D A numerical score of 3 indicates fluorosis that presents as a parchment-white color covering at least two-thirds of the tooth surface.

E A numerical score of 4 indicates fluorosis that has begun to show evidence of brown staining of any of the preceding levels.

4. A Changes in salivary flow are not directly affected by periodontal disease. Diabetes does pose a significant risk for periodontal disease; and periodontal disease has been linked with altering blood glucose levels that make control of the disease difficult.

B Although many medications have adverse effects on salivary flow that results in xerostomia, insulin is not one of these.

C Excessive fluid loss through an increased volume of urine produced by the diabetic patient can be expected to reduce secretion of saliva and result in xerostomia.

D Depending on the type of food ingested, salivary flow can actually be stimulated to increase with mastication.

E This patient's self-care, although not the cause of xerostomia, can play an important role in maintaining oral health in the presence of reduced salivary flow.

5. A The risk of dental caries increases as a result of increased glucose in parotid saliva during uncontrolled periods.

B During periods of hyperglycemia body fat is metabolized resulting in weight loss.

C,E Hyperglycemia increases pulse rate and lowers blood pressure.

D Congenitally missing teeth is unrelated to poor glycemic control. The most likely reason that this patient is missing her first premolars and third molars is because of orthodontic intervention.

6. A,B Patients with uncontrolled diabetes often have a reduced level of polymorphonuclear leukocytes, the first line of defense in an immunoinflammatory process, increasing the risk of gingivitis and periodontal disease for diabetic patients.

C Decreased salivary flow in the diabetic patient often leads to xerostomia that has a high risk of being accompanied by burning mouth syndrome.

D Decreased salivary flow often leaves the diabetic patient susceptible to opportunistic bacterial and fungal infections.

E Dentinal hypersensitivity is not a possible risk factor for the patient with diabetes. Additionally, nothing in this patient's assessment indicates her developing dentinal hypersensitivity. Each of the other oral manifestations listed here are potential risks for the diabetic patient during uncontrolled glycemic periods.

7. A An embossed film identification dot is found in one corner of an intraoral radiographic film. This raised bump is used to determine the film's orientation when viewing the radiographic image after processing. During film packet placement intraorally, the embossed dot is positioned at the incisal or occlusal edge of the teeth being imaged. This placement helps to place the inevitable distortion of the

radiographic image caused by the bump in the film in an area so as not to interfere with important radiograph interpretation, especially near the tooth apex.

B,C,D,E The unique round appearance of the film identification dot should not be confused with a composite restoration, attrition, calculus, or caries. The typical location of the film identification dot in this corner would further indicate that this finding is not a composite restoration, attrition, calculus, or caries.

8. A Overlapped interproximal spaces would appear as an increased radiopacity between the teeth as a result of the superimposition of the images of adjacent teeth.

(B) A diagnostic-quality periapical radiograph should image the entire tooth from incisal or occlusal edge to the apex and include approximately 2 to 4 mm of supporting bone beyond the apex.

C Cone cutting error occurs when the film packet is not centered within the beam of radiation. Cone cutting error presents as a clear or radiopaque area representing no exposure.

D Herringbone is the name given to the visual pattern of the lead foil imaged onto the film where the film packet is placed in the oral cavity backward and exposed through the lead foil. Although still a relevant term, many films available today contain various patterns, such as the tire track pattern used by Kodak films.

E There is a possibility that a film holding device may be imaged onto the resultant radiograph. The radiopacity of this image depends on the material (metal or plastic) of the film holder. However, the radiopacity of the film holder used imaged on this film does not interfere with the diagnostic quality of the radiograph and is not considered an error.

9. A Decreasing the vertical angulation would result in a further loss of image in the region of the teeth apices. If the patient could not tolerate biting further down on the bite block of the film holding device, increasing the vertical angulation could be used to image more of the apical region.

B Shifting the horizontal angulation to the mesial or to the distal would be the corrective action for overlapping error.

(C) The most likely reason that the apices were not imaged onto the film was that the patient was not fully occluded on the bite block of the film holder. The location of the image of the metal section of the film holder device on the radiograph further indicates that the occlusal edges of the teeth were not closed as far as possible on the bite block causing the loss of the image of the teeth apices.

D Reversing the film packet when placing into the oral cavity is the corrective action for a backwards film placement. There is no evidence, underexposure with an image of the pattern of the lead foil, to indicate that this film was placed into the oral cavity backwards.

E Centering the film within the x-ray beam is the corrective action for cone cut error. The radiopaque area at the edge of this film represents the metal portion of the film holding device and should not be confused with cone cut error.

10. A The nasal septum is the bony wall separating the paired radiolucent ovals of the nasal cavity. The nasal septum appears radiopaque.

B Although nutrient canals will appear radiolucent when imaged on a radiograph of the maxilla, they are most often visible as faint lines within the walls of the maxillary sinus. The normal appearance of the midpalatine suture in this region of the palate should not be mistaken for a nutrient canal.

C,D The appearance of the midpalatine suture in this region is typical and should not be mistaken for bone loss or a palatal fracture.

(E) The midpalatine suture is an opening in the bone that allows more x-rays to pass through to the film, increasing radiolucency. The appearance of the midpalatine suture in this region is typical and should be identified as normal radiographic anatomy.

11.   **(A)** The radiographs reveal a distal radiolucency indicating a Class II classification. Class II caries are cavities in the proximal surfaces of posterior teeth. Early Class II caries are most often detected on radiographs.

      B Class III caries are cavities in the proximal surface of incisors or canines.

      C Class IV caries are cavities in the proximal surface of the incisors or canines that also involves the incisal angle.

      D Class V caries are cavities in the smooth surface of the cervical third of the facial or lingual surfaces of the teeth.

      E Class VI caries are cavities in the incisal edges of anterior teeth or in the cusp tips of posterior teeth.

12.   A A microdont is a tooth that appears smaller than normal. The maxillary lateral incisors and the maxillary and mandibular third molars are the teeth most commonly affected.

      B The most common occurrence of a supernumerary tooth is the mesiodens, an extra tooth that erupts between the maxillary central incisors.

      C Secondary dentin occurs in response to trauma or as a natural aging process. Secondary dentin cannot be distinguished radiographically from primary dentin. The addition of secondary dentin, deposited within the pulp chamber, appears as a reduction in the size of the pulp chamber.

   (D) The smooth, round appearance of the radiopacity observed in the furcation area of this molar tooth is characteristic of an enamel pearl.

      E Pulp stones would appear as calcifications within the pulp chamber.

13.   **(A)** The maxillary right second premolar presents with an abnormal bend in what is normally a straight tooth root.

  B,C,D,E These teeth all present with normal appearing tooth root structures.

14. A,C,D Hyperglycemia, where there is an accumulation of ketone bodies in the blood (ketoacidosis), results in diabetic coma. Hyperglycemia refers to a very high level of glucose in the blood. This occurance is unlikely in this patient who uses an insulin pump to deliver regular insulin doses. Additionally, the onset of hyperglycemia builds slowly over a period of time, most likely causing the patient to feel too ill to keep the dental hygiene appointment. For this reason, diabetic coma is less likely to occur during treatment.

   (B) The most likely emergency situation regarding this patient would result from hypoglycemia or insulin shock. Hypoglycemia occurs when the patient has received a dose of insulin but failed to eat a meal. The onset is usually acute. This patient is receiving regular insulin through the use of an insulin pump. She must balance this with regular meals, which she has admitted to having trouble managing.

15. A,B,D,E Each of these is a symptom of hypoglycemia.

   (C) Numbness or a tingling of the extremities referred to as paresthesia is not a symptom of hypoglycemia.

16.   A Oral antibiotic prophylaxis is sometimes suggested for the uncontrolled diabetic with significant chronic oral infections who requires extensive treatment. This patient's oral conditions and the instrumentation expected do not warrant premedication.

      B Having an ammonia capsule ready for use would be more likely to benefit management of the patient with syncope.

      C The insulin pump is not expected to interfere with treatment. More importantly, the insulin pump provides this patient with a continuous, precisely measured base dose of insulin, and can be programmed to deliver a bolus dose prior to meals. It should not be disconnected.

D   Patients with diabetes may be treated in the same manner as nondiabetic patients. A semisupine chair position is not required for management of this patient.

(E) The most likely emergency would result from hypoglycemia, or insulin shock, where the patient has received a dose of insulin without eating regular meals. When symptoms of hypoglycemia present, while the patient is conscious, she can be given oral sugar such as orange juice or sugary cake frosting to reverse the hypoglycemic condition. When unsure if the patient's symptoms indicate hypo- or hyperglycemia, administering oral sugar is still the recommendation. If the condition is hyperglycemia, the sugar will not reverse the condition, but neither will it harm the patient.

17.   A   Increased glucose levels often found within the gingival crevicular fluid of diabetics allows bacteria to thrive. Therefore, one must consider this patient's diabetes to have the potential to affect tissue response to plaque microorganisms.

B   Nonplaque-induced gingival disease results from viral or fungal infections, allergic reactions or dermatologic diseases, or mechanical trauma. Given this patient's medical history, one can assume that her gingival disease will be affected by diabetes.

C   The insulin taken by this patient does not play a role in classification of her gingival condition as other drugs, such as those taken to manage seizure disorders.

(D) Although plaque has initiated the gingivitis, this patient's diabetes can be expected to play a role in modifying the disease.

E   Gingival lesions such as those related to lichen planus and lupus would be considered nonplaque-induced gingival manifestations of systemic conditions.

18.   A   The body's inflammatory response to invasion of bacterial plaque is responsible for producing redness and edema, along with varying degrees of heat, pain, and reduced function. The red and edematous gingiva observed in this region is the result of an increased blood flow as the inflammatory process reacts to the invasion of bacterial plaque.

B,D   The body's inflammatory response to invasion of bacterial plaque is responsible for producing redness and edema, along with varying degrees of heat, pain, and reduced function. The role of phagocytes, usually leukocytes, in the inflammation process is to ingest and digest invading bacteria. While performing this function, phagocytes in turn may create more inflammation as they die and spill their contents into neighboring regions.

(C) Prostaglandins play a role in activating alveolar bone destruction in periodontitis by stimulating osteoclasts, cells responsible for bone destruction. Based on this patient's assessment data, her periodontal status is gingivitis without bone loss.

E   The body's inflammatory response to invasion of bacterial plaque is responsible for producing redness and edema, along with varying degrees of heat, pain, and reduced function. Plasma proteins and leukocytes leak from the blood vessels into the surrounding tissue resulting in redness and edema, leading to the production of heat, pain, and reduced function.

19.   (A) The uncontrolled diabetic patient is more susceptible to contracting infections in general, and is therefore considered to be at high risk for developing periodontal disease. However, if the diabetes is well controlled, the risk for periodontal disease is reported to be about the same as that of nondiabetics.

B,C,D   These answers are incorrect.

20.   A   A change in body weight is not expected to affect the healing of the gingiva.

B   The etiology of the gingival inflammation observed at the initial appointment was plaque-induced and not from trauma of a nail biting habit. Therefore, cessation of her nail biting habit is not expected to have an affect on gingival healing.

C   Maintaining ideal glucose levels will help prevent an increase in risk for peri-odontal disease. However, changing between self-injections and the continuous subcutaneous infusion pump method of insulin delivery is not expected to af-fect the healing of the gingiva.

D   The use of whitening products will not improve gingival health.

(E) The goal of periodontal debridement and improved self-care has produced the desired outcome of improved health of this tissue.

21.   A   It is very likely that this patient will be able to improve self-care. Given the gin-gival assessment at the 6-week reevaluation appointment, a 3-month recall should be recommended.

(B) Recent studies have indicated that even in well-controlled diabetics, gingivitis has a tendency to develop more frequently than in nondiabetic patients. Given this patient's gingival assessment in response to the slight generalized plaque detected, she should be encouraged to keep 3-month recall appointments.

C   Because gingivitis has a tendency to develop more frequently in the diabetic pa-tient, especially when glycemic control fluctuates, and given this patient's gingi-val assessment at the initial appointment, a 3-month recall should be established.

D,E Nine- and 12-month recall intervals would not benefit this patient.

22.   (A) The maxillary right second molar presents with deep fissures and pits that would most likely benefit from the placement of a sealant.

B,D,E The maxillary right first molar and the mandibular left and right first molars all have amalgam restorations on the occlusal surfaces.

C   The dental chart and radiographs reveal caries on the maxillary left first molar that contraindicates placement of a sealant.

23.   A   This patient's dentition does not present with conditions that would prompt recommending an end-tuft brush.

B   Although a tooth whitening product may indirectly assist in better home care, by motivating the patient to follow meticulous self-care, the use of self-applied fluoride will provide a more important benefit for this patient.

C   Diabetics regularly obtain in-depth dietary assessment and counseling for their glycemic control. The dental hygienist's role would be to support the patient in following her recommended diet.

(D) Xerostomia and elevated levels of glucose in saliva put this patient at risk for caries.

E   Although products can be introduced to help this patient improve self-care, the use of self-applied fluoride will provide a more important benefit for this patient.

24.   A   Although the presence of gingival inflammation observed at this patient's ini-tial appointment would contraindicate the use of a whitening product at that time, inflammation does not affect whitening results.

B   Nail biting will not affect the outcome of tooth whitening.

(C) Fluorosis does not respond well to whitening procedures.

D   Although diabetes may affect how this patient responds to healing, this medical condition will not affect the outcome of tooth whitening.

E   The placement of posterior occlusal sealants will not be an esthetic considera-tion when considering the use of whitening agents.

25.   A,B To prevent a medical emergency from arising during treatment, a patient re-ceiving insulin to manage their diabetes should be questioned regarding main-tenance of regularly scheduled doses and possible insulin reactions that might occur today.

C,D To prevent a medical emergency from arising during treatment, a patient receiving insulin to manage diabetes should be asked questions to determine the blood glucose level at the time of treatment and to ensure that the patient has eaten regular meals before the appointment and encouraged to eat following the appointment.

E Although unexplained weight loss or gain can play a role in helping to identify patients who have not yet been diagnosed with diabetes, this patient's current weight will not impact safe dental hygiene treatment at today's appointment.

CASE N MEDICALLY COMPROMISED PATIENT BRIAN BARTLETT

1. A,B,C These answers are incorrect.

D Insulin resistance in the presence of normal, decreased, or increased insulin production is typical of patients with Type 2 diabetes.

2. A For an adult, systolic readings less than 120 mm Hg and diastolic readings less than 80 mm Hg are considered within normal limits.

B For an adult, systolic readings between 120 and 139 mm Hg and diastolic readings between 80 and 89 mm Hg are considered prehypertensive.

C For an adult, systolic readings between 140 and 159 mm Hg and diastolic readings between 90 and 99 mm Hg are classified as stage 1 hypertension.

D For an adult, systolic readings greater than 160 mm Hg and diastolic readings greater than 100 mm Hg are classified as stage 2 hypertension.

3. A,B,C,E The body mass index (BMI) is used to determine whether an adult is at a healthy or unhealthy body weight. The formula used to determine BMI is based on an individual's weight and height. This allows for a more precise estimation of unhealthy body fat. Body fat has been linked to an increased risk for developing diabetes, hypertension, and high cholesterol or dyslipidemia leading to coronary artery disease.

D A decreased pain threshold is not known to be directly related to obesity or conditions of being overweight.

4. A Dry mouth and/or taste disturbance are not adverse oral effects of the antidiabetic medication Avandamet.

B,C Dry mouth is an adverse oral effect of most antihypertensives and diuretics, including Avapro and Zaroxolyn.

D Taste disturbance is an adverse oral effect of Zocor.

5. A Enlarged gingiva would most likely result in a free gingival margin position located coronally, increasing toward the incisal edges of these teeth.

B The gingival margin in this region has migrated apically to reveal the root surfaces of these teeth. Recession refers to this apical migration of the gingiva.

C Cratering often refers to papillae that no longer fill in the spaces between the teeth.

D Clefting refers to a more localized condition of recession, in which a wedge-shaped slit forms.

E Hyperplastic refers to an increase in cells that results in a thickening of the tissues.

6. A The composite restoration present on the occlusal surface of the maxillary right second molar should not be mistaken for a temporary restoration.

B The photographs and radiographs indicate the presence of a temporary restoration on the distal occlusal surfaces of the maxillary right first premolar.

C The radiographs reveal the probable presence of caries on the mesial surface of the maxillary right canine that should not be mistaken for a temporary restoration.

D   The radiographs reveal the probable presence of recurrent decay around the restoration on the mesial surface of the maxillary left lateral incisor that should not be mistaken for a temporary restoration.

E   The composite restoration present on the distal surface of the maxillary left canine should not be mistaken for a temporary restoration.

7.   A   Gingival abrasion due to incorrect toothbrushing technique can result in gingival recession.

B   An abnormal frenal attachment position contributes to gingival recession.

(C)   Gingival recession is not an adverse effect of this patient's medications.

D   Teeth that are rotated, tilted, or otherwise malaligned in the arch can contribute to the etiology of gingival recession.

E   Plaque-related gingivitis is a common etiology for gingival recession.

8.   A   Exposed cemental root surfaces are more likely to be difficult for the patient to clean and are therefore more likely to accumulate biofilm.

B,C   Exposing the root surfaces increases the risk for cemental wear, thus increasing the risk of sensitivity for these teeth.

D   Recession that exposes the root surfaces to the conditions in the oral cavity is likely to increase the risk of root decay for these teeth.

(E)   Nothing in this patient's assessment would put these teeth at an increased risk for trauma.

9.   (A)   The crowding of the premolars in this region of the arch will result in overlapped images on the radiograph, representing the superimposition of the adjacent teeth.

B   Although incorrect horizontal angulation does result in overlapped images, the cause of this overlapping is the malaligned teeth.

C   Excessive vertical angulation would have resulted in cutting off the occlusal edges (periapical radiographs) and unequal distribution of the arches (bitewing radiographs) where more of the maxilla and less of the mandible would be imaged.

D   Cone cut error would have resulted if there was inadequate coverage of the film with x-ray beam.

E   Not placing the film packet parallel to the tangent of adjacent teeth can result in overlapping of the images. This may occur if the film holder is not retained in proper position by the patient. However, this overlap error is the result of the anatomic location of the teeth in this region and not from incorrect film packet retention by the patient.

10.   A   Accidentally tearing the film packet and exposing the film to white light will cause an area of blackness on the film. However, the thin radiolucent line observed in this example is characteristic of a film packet that has been bent.

(B)   Bending the film packet will result in a radiolucent crease mark where the film emulsion is damaged. Carelessly positioning the film packet into the film holder increases the likelihood of bending the film.

C   Certain chemicals and products have the potential to contaminate radiograph film. Films should not be touched, or if unavoidable, should only be contacted by the edges to avoid leaving fingerprints. However, the thin radiolucent line observed in this example is characteristic of a film packet that has been bent.

D   Static electricity will produce a white light spark that has the potential to create a radiolucent artifact on the film. However, the thin radiolucent line observed in this example is characteristic of a film packet that has been bent.

E   A herringbone image refers to the pattern embossed into the lead-foil packaged in the back of the film packet. When the film packet is positioned into the oral cavity backwards, the lead foil absorbs most of the primary beam resulting in an underexposed image that, when viewed on a view box, reveals the herringbone pattern characteristic of the film's manufacturer. Herringbone error should not be confused with a bent film artifact.

11. A The radiolucency observed on the mesial surface of the maxillary right canine is indicative of caries.

B The radiolucency observed on the mesial surface of the maxillary left lateral incisor, apical to the radiopaque restoration, is indicative of recurrent decay.

C The radiolucency observed on the mesial surface of the maxillary left first molar is indicative of caries.

D The radiolucency observed on the distal surface of the mandibular left first premolar, outlining the radiopaque metal restoration, is indicative of recurrent decay.

(E) The mandibular right first premolar does not exhibit caries radiographically. The radiolucent fissures observed between the cusps on the occlusal surface of posterior teeth should be not confused with caries.

12. A Local infiltration, where anesthesia is deposited near the terminal nerve endings at the specific site for instrumentation, is recommended when scaling an individual tooth or individual root surface.

B Field block, where anesthesia is administered near the tooth roots, provides pain control for an area of one or two teeth.

(C) A regional nerve block, where anesthesia is deposited near the trunk of a major nerve, is recommended when anesthesia is required for an entire quadrant.

D A supraperiosteal injection is more often used on the maxilla. Multiple supraperiosteal injections would be required to scale an entire quadrant, increasing the risks associated with injections and potentially increasing the dosage of anesthesia. A nerve block would be the better choice.

E An intraligamentary injection, also called a periodontal ligament injection, administers the anesthetic to the supporting bone to provide anesthesia to one tooth. An intraligamentary injection is administered with a specially designed syringe and is used when a nerve block in the mandible is not desired.

13. A The middle superior alveolar nerve block provides anesthesia to the maxillary premolars.

B The posterior superior alveolar nerve block provides anesthesia to the maxillary molars.

C The greater palatine nerve block provides palatal anesthesia from the canine distally to the molars.

(D) An inferior alveolar nerve block deposits anesthesia at the trunk of the inferior alveolar and lingual nerves to provide anesthesia to the mandible.

14. (A) This patient's antihypertensive medication may produce orthostatic or postural hypotension that results in syncope when he stands up too quickly. Allowing the patient to rise slowly may help to prevent a sudden drop in arterial blood pressure and avoid this medical emergency.

B A diabetic coma emergency is more likely to occur in Type 1 diabetics. Diabetic coma is the result of too little insulin and develops over time. A diabetic coma emergency is not likely to be exacerbated by the position of the treatment chair.

C The sudden onset of hypoglycemia, which results from too much insulin, is more common in Type 1 diabetics. A hypoglycemic emergency is not likely to be exacerbated by the position of the treatment chair.

D There is nothing in this patient's health history that would indicate possible respiratory difficulty.

E A reaction to an overdose of anesthesia is not likely to be influenced by the position of the treatment chair.

15. A The use of lidocaine HCl 2% without epinephrine does not provide the length of anesthesia required for a typical quadrant scaling appointment. Additionally, without a vasoconstrictor, there is likely to be an increase in bleeding during instrumentation.

B The duration and depth of pain control with lidocaine HCl 2% with epinephrine 1:50,000 and lidocaine HCl 2% with epinephrine 1:100,000 is similar. However, lidocaine HCl 2% with epinephrine 1:100,000 contains half the dose of vasoconstrictor making it less likely to elicit an adverse response in this patient with hypertension.

C The duration and depth of pain control achieved with lidocaine HCl 2% with epinephrine 1:100,000 is ideally suited to nonsurgical periodontal therapy. The addition of the vasoconstrictor will provide profound anesthesia for the time required for scaling, and when injected directly into the region, can help control bleeding during instrumentation. When considering this patient's hypertension, which is secondary to the underlying diabetes, the use of epinephrine is considered safe if the maximum recommended dosing for a medically compromised patient is followed.

D The short duration and less profound anesthesia produced by mepivacaine HCl 3% without a vasoconstrictor is not recommended for nonsurgical periodontal therapy. Mepivacaine HCl 3% without a vasoconstrictor is often used for short dental procedures on children.

E Bupivacaine HCl 0.5% with epinephrine 1:200,000 is more often used for extensive periodontal surgeries including implant surgical procedures when the duration of anesthesia needed is lengthy. Bupivacaine HCl 0.5% with epinephrine 1:200,000 is also used to manage postoperative pain associated with these surgical procedures.

16. A Early chronic periodontitis presents with slight bone loss as determined by probing depths of 2 to 3 mm representing 1 to 2 mm total loss of attachment.

B The probing depths, location of the free gingival margin, and localized furcation involvement and mobility indicate an increased amount of bone loss classifying this patient's periodontal status as moderate chronic periodontitis. The periodontal status of patients who present with generalized probing depths of 4 to 5 mm representing 3 to 4 mm total loss of attachment are classified as moderate periodontitis.

C Advanced chronic periodontitis presents with major bone loss as determined by probing depths of 4 to 5 mm representing 3 to 4 mm total loss of attachment.

D Aggressive periodontitis is characterized by localized or generalized rapid, destructive bone loss that presents in otherwise healthy patients.

E This term refers to regions of disease that do not respond to treatment.

17. A The Gracey 7/8 is designed for instrumention in the anterior regions.

B Although a rigid instrument is ideal for removing tenacious deposit, the Gracey 9/10 is designed for instrumentation of the premolar teeth and for the direct facial and lingual surfaces of the molars.

C The Gracey 11/12 is designed to be used on the mesial and distal surfaces of the anterior teeth and the mesial, facial, and lingual surfaces of the posterior teeth.

D The Gracey 15/16 is designed to be used on the mesial, facial, and lingual surfaces of the posterior teeth.

E The Gracey 17/18 is designed to be used on the distal surfaces of the maxillary and mandibular posterior teeth. The extended shank of this instrument will allow better access to the base of this deep pocket.

18.   A   Total loss of attachment is calculated by adding, and not by subtracting, the loss observed from recession to the measurement of the pocket depth.

B   To determine the total loss of attachment, the 2 mm facial surface probing depth must be added to the 4 mm recession measurement.

C   Total loss of attachment is calculated as the sum of the measurement (in millimeters) of the loss observed from the CEJ (clinically observable because of recession) to the free gingival margin and the measurement (in millimeters) of the depth of the pocket. In this case, 4 mm is given as the measurement of recession (from the CEJ to the free gingival margin) on the facial surface of the mandibular right central incisor. To this 4 mm, the probing depth (pocket measurement) in this region of 2 mm is added for a total loss of attachment (sum) of 6 mm.

D   Adding the 2 mm probing depth measurement to the 4 mm of recession equals a 6 mm total loss of attachment.

19.   A,D   These brown discolored areas represent demineralized enamel and possible caries that should not be scaled or polished.

B   Tooth whitening should not be applied to these brown discolored areas as they represent demineralized enamel and possible caries.

C   These brown discolored areas represent demineralized enamel and possible caries. Although the caries will need restoration, application of fluoride can help to inhibit the demineralization process and possibly enhance remineralization of some of the defects.

E   These brown discolored areas represent demineralized enamel and possible caries. There is no benefit to be gained from burnishing these areas with a desensitizing agent.

20.   **A**   Although polishing should be postponed when a patient presents with a communicable disease to avoid producing contagious aerosols, this patient does not present with a communicable disease.

B   This patient presents with areas of demineralized enamel that are at an increased risk for caries. Removing the fluoride-rich outer layer of enamel by polishing these teeth should be avoided.

C   This patient presents with several teeth affected by cemental caries that should not be subjected to unnecessary polishing.

D   Polishing may force microorganisms into spongy, bleeding tissue and potentially elicit an inflammatory response. Polishing near soft, spongy gingiva should be avoided.

E   The medications this patient takes puts him at risk for xerostomia, and increases his risk for caries. Removing the fluoride-rich outer layer of enamel by polishing should be avoided when conditions exist that increase the patient's risk of caries.

21.   A   To maintain even blood glucose levels throughout the day, the diabetic is advised to eat small, frequent meals and snacks. Additionally, small, frequent meals may help prevent hunger that can stimulate overeating and lead to weight gain.

B   Counting carbohydrates is an accepted method for helping the diabetic to maintain even blood glucose levels throughout the day.

C   To maintain optimum glucose control, the diabetic is advised to limit alcohol intake. Eliminating the calories from alcohol may help this patient better achieve his goal of weight loss.

D   Fats are high in calories. Consuming less fats, especially less saturated fat, is not only recommended for diabetic patients, but also plays a major role in helping to manage unhealthy cholesterol levels.

E   Sucrose may be consumed as part of an overall healthy diet. Diabetics no longer have to completely eliminate sugar from their diet.

22. A Chewing gum can help stimulate salivary flow. Additionally, the use of gum sweetened with xylitol has been shown to be cariostatic. However, given the evidence of areas of demineralized enamel and caries, home fluoride rinses are the best choice from this list.

B,C Although the medications this patient has recently started taking are known to produce xerostomia, this patient is not experiencing dry mouth conditions that would prompt the use of a saliva substitute or the need for frequent sips of water. Additionally, the areas of demineralized enamel and caries indicate that home fluoride rinses are the best choice from this list.

(D) Home fluoride rinses should be recommended for this patient. Even though he has not complained of dry mouth, his medications, which he has only recently started taking, have an adverse effect of creating dry mouth conditions. Xerostomia may have already played a role in this patient's oral condition as observed by the presence of several areas of demineralization and caries, making home fluoride rinses a good recommendation.

E Limiting salt will not improve salivary flow or dry mouth conditions.

23. A Diets high in carbohydrates put this patient at risk for caries, especially if medications are reducing his production of saliva.

(B) Crowded and malaligned teeth will most likely present a challenge for thorough oral self-care, by creating areas where plaque removal is difficult. However, poor oral hygiene self-care habits are not the cause of this patient's crowding and malaligned teeth.

C Research has linked diabetes and periodontal diseases, suggesting that control and management of both these diseases are interrelated.

D Research has linked periodontal diseases with coronary artery disease (CAD) suggesting that bacterial by-products from periodontal disease may enter the bloodstream causing the liver to produce proteins that inflame arteries or result in the formation of clots.

E Xerostomia is an adverse oral effect associated with most antihypertensives and diuretics, including Avapro and Zaroxolyn taken by this patient.

24. A Assisting this patient in staying motivated to follow a healthy diet that includes limiting high-carbohydrate snacking and adding fruits and vegetables into his daily diet may assist in reducing his risk for caries and indirectly help to improve his periodontal disease, respectively. However, improving his periodontal condition is not a catalyst for weight reduction.

(B) This patient's physician is aware of research that indicates a possible link between the inflammatory condition of periodontal disease and glycemic control. Diabetes and periodontal diseases have the potential to influence each other. As chronic diseases, both diabetes and periodontitis require collaborate efforts between oral health care professionals and the patient's physician to provide this patient with comprehensive health care.

C Improving this patient's periodontal condition through nonsurgical periodontal therapy may play a role in helping to control his diabetes. Because high blood pressure is often associated with diabetes, it may be expected to improve if glycemic control improves. However, the most likely primary concern of his physician is the concurrent chronic inflammatory affect his periodontal condition has on control of his diabetes.

D Restoring his oral health may have an effect on his ability to control his diabetes. However, weight reduction and lifestyle changes will most likely play a larger role in helping this patient manage his need for medications.

E Periodontal disease has not been linked with cholesterol levels.

25. A If the original treatment plan to which the patient has given informed consent changes, treatment should be stopped to discuss the alternate or additional treatment procedures. Therefore, if this patient had not given consent to use a

topical anesthetic, treatment should be stopped, the patient allowed to sit up, and a discussion should take place regarding his anesthesia options. Written informed consent should be obtained.

B   Obtaining verbal consent may appear easier than having to interrupt treatment, sit the patient up, and allow time for questions. However, informed consent requires that the patient be given sufficient information about a treatment or procedure before providing written permission.

(C)   Because the treatment planned changed, additional written informed consent must be secured. The patient must be provided with an opportunity to ask questions. Stopping treatment and sitting the patient upright will facilitate a direct discussion and allow the patient to make an informed choice.

D   Sitting the patient up and allowing time for questions can occur in the dental chair. Although a patient can request the option to think over the treatment plan, rescheduling the patient is not required.

CASE O   MEDICALLY COMPROMISED PATIENT EILEEN OLDS

1.   A   Centric relation refers to an unstrained occlusal position where the arches may be moved freely from side to side.

B   Open bite refers to a lack of contact between the maxillary and mandibular teeth when the arches are closed together.

(C)   The left and right maxillary central incisors should contact one another at the mesial surface. The term *diastema* is used to describe the space created when adjacent teeth in the same arch do not contact.

D   Parafunctional refers to a deviation from a normal functioning occlusion.

E   Fremitus refers to vibrations that may be detected when a tooth prematurely contacts a tooth in the opposing arch.

2.   (A)   The radiographs further confirm that this bony exostosis is a torus mandibularis.

B   A polyp refers to a soft tissue swelling or mass that is not hard when palpated. Additionally, the radiographs confirm the presence of bilateral tori.

C,E   A salivary gland that becomes blocked may swell into a mucocele or a ranula that would not be hard upon palpation. Additionally, the radiographs confirm the presence of bilateral tori.

D   A cyst would not be hard upon palpation. Additionally, the radiographs confirm the presence of bilateral tori.

3.   A   Knife-like describes marginal gingiva that lies flat against, and fits snugly around, the teeth. Knife-like marginal gingiva is usually associated with healthy tissues.

B   Cratered papillae appear scooped out, or concave in the interproximal regions.

C   Blunted papillae are flat and do not fill in the interproximal area.

D   Rolled usually refers to a thickened marginal gingiva that appears as a collar around the tooth.

(E)   This enlargement of the papilla is referred to as bulbous.

4.   A   A developmental anomaly that changes the shape of the tooth should not be confused with this heavy buildup of dental calculus.

B,C   The heavy buildup of dental calculus on the lingual surfaces of these teeth should not be confused with restorative materials such as those used to stabilize periodontally involved teeth or composite restorations.

(D)   The mineralized biofilm in this region has built up into a tenacious mass of dental calculus that almost completely covers the lingual surfaces of these teeth.

E   Hypercementosis is most often observed on radiographs as an excessive buildup of cementum on the roots of the effected tooth. Excessive buildup of cementum should not be confused with this excessive buildup of dental calculus.

5.   A   This patient's height and body weight indicate the use of a regular adult-size cuff.

   (B) Compression of the arteriovenous shunt must be avoided. Therefore, the blood pressure cuff must not be placed over this patient's right arm. This patient's height and body weight indicate the use of a regular adult-size cuff applied to the left arm.

   C   Compression of the arteriovenous shunt placed in this patient's right arm must be avoided. Therefore, the blood pressure cuff must be placed over this patient's left arm.

   D,E The adult thigh-size cuff applied to the leg is not necessary. This patient's height and body weight indicate the use of a regular adult-size cuff.

6.   A   The infraorbital foramen is located just inferior to the border of the orbit. An intraoral radiograph will not be in a position to record an image of this landmark.

   (B) This oval radiolucency located between the right and left maxillary central incisors demonstrates the characteristic appearance of the incisive foramen.

   C   The incisive fossa appears as a diffuse radiolucency between the central and lateral incisors.

   D   The canine fossa appears as a diffuse radiolucency between the lateral incisor and the canine lateral to the canine eminence.

   E   The nasal fossa, or cavity, appears as paired radiolucent ovals separated by the bony nasal septum. If imaged on an intraoral radiograph, the nasal fossa appears superior to the maxillary anterior teeth roots.

7.   A,D Osteosclerosis and condensing osteitis are forms of ossification where dense bone forms resulting in an increased radiopacity. These conditions occur within the bone, and should not be confused with the bony exostoses of tori. Additionally, the photographs indicate the presence of significantly sized bilateral tori that are expected to be imaged on the radiographs.

   B   Hypercementosis represents an excessive formation of cementum along the root of a tooth. The radiopaque appearance of hypercementosis would be surrounded by the radiolucent periodontal ligament space, separating the condition from the bone.

   (C) Mandibular tori represent a localized overgrowth of bone, resulting in an increased radiopacity often imaged on radiographs. This round, cotton-ball appearance is characteristic of tori. Additionally, the photographs indicate the presence of significantly sized bilateral tori that are expected to be imaged on the radiographs.

   E   Touching the film emulsion is not likely to produce radiopaque artifacts on the image unless the finger is contaminated with a chemical or product that is likely to damage the film emulsion in this manner. Fixer contamination may produce radiopaque artifacts. However, this round, cotton-ball appearance is characteristic of tori and should not be confused with film artifacts. Additionally, the photographs indicate the presence of significantly sized bilateral tori that are expected to be imaged on the radiographs.

8.   (A) The crowns of the maxillary right first premolar and first molar appear to have been severely broken down, leaving retained root tips.

   B   The crowns of the maxillary right first premolar and first molar are missing. The retained root tips of these severely broken down teeth should not be confused with the presence of extra, or supernumerary teeth.

   C   Retained root tips from these severely broken down teeth should not be mistaken for a smaller than normal sized tooth, referred to as a microdont.

   D   Dental implants may be placed into the alveolar bone ridge to help restore missing teeth. Additionally, because they are made of metal, implants will appear distinctly radiopaque. Surgically placed dental materials should not be mistaken for natural teeth roots that were retained when the crowns of these teeth fractured off.

E   Retention pins are used to provide support for restorative materials such as amalgam, composite, and crowns. Retention pins are placed within the dentin and because they are made of metal, appear distinctly radiopaque.

9. A,B,C   Careless film storage, handling, exposure, and processing technique can result in the formation of a cloudy gray appearance, called film fog, that diminishes image contrast and makes interpretation of the radiographs difficult. Film fog may result when films are stored near stray radiation and under conditions of high humidity and heat.

D   Film fog can result when excessive physical pressure is applied to the film. Stacking film boxes such that the physical pressure created exerts enough force can result in film fog.

(E)   Long wavelengths of orange/red light is considered relatively safe for processing radiographic films and storing film under these conditions is not likely to produce film fog.

10.   A,E   This patient's lack of professional dental hygiene care has contributed to the accumulation of significant calculus and periodontal disease that has resulted in loss of alveolar bone support for the teeth. However, the ground glass appearance of the trabecular bone, the disappearance of the lamina dura, and the narrowing of the pulp chambers are all characteristic of renal osteodystrophy.

B   Although the medications taken by this patient have multiple adverse effects on the oral cavity, the ground glass appearance of the trabecular bone, the disappearance of the lamina dura, and the narrowing of the pulp chambers are all characteristic of renal osteodystrophy.

C   Habitually chewing on ice may contribute to occlusal trauma that could play a role in periodontal disease and the resultant loss of alveolar bone support. However, the ground glass appearance of the trabecular bone, the disappearance of the lamina dura, and the narrowing of the pulp chambers are all characteristic of renal osteodystrophy.

(D)   The bone disease osteodystrophy develops when the kidneys fail to regulate blood levels of calcium and phosphate. The resultant demineralization of the bone often appears radiographically as a decrease in trabeculation, loss of lamina dura, and pulp chamber narrowing.

11.   A   Currently, there is no consensus on the need for prophylactic premedication for patients with ESRD who are receiving hemodialysis who do not have known cardiac risk factors. Instead the determination for premedication is made on an individual basis. This patient's nephrologist should be contacted to determine the need for antibiotics prior to scaling.

B   Patients with ESRD have abnormal bleeding tendencies that result from altered and decreased platelets. Additionally, the use of heparin in dialysis procedures will further increase this patient's risk for bleeding during oral procedures. Therefore, her nephrologist should be contacted to determine blood clotting time before scaling.

(C)   This patient presents with moderate xerostomia. Her medical condition, the medications she is taking, and the restrictions on her oral intake of fluids all present a challenge when considering the usual recommendations to combat dry mouth. However, adequacy of salivary flow would not be a contraindication to quadrant scaling that must be discussed with her nephrologist.

D   The adequacy of control of this patient's high blood pressure should be discussed with her nephrologist to determine whether scaling may be performed.

E   In addition to avoiding or reducing the dosage of drugs that are excreted by the kidney, the interactions of the multiple medications taken by this patient must be considered before introducing another drug. Additionally, hypertension will most likely prompt the use of local anesthetics with a reduced dose and possibility with a reduction of epinephrine. Because the need for pain control may not be evident until after treatment has started, it may be prudent to anticipate this need and contact her nephrologist before initiating scaling.

12. A,C,D These answers are incorrect.

B Because the anticoagulant heparin is used during hemodialysis, quadrant scaling appointments for this patient should be scheduled on the days in between her dialysis sessions to avoid bleeding complications. Scheduling dental surgical procedures on the day after the last day of the week of hemodialysis will allow an extra day clotting time before this patient returns for her next dialysis session on Monday.

13.   A,B Antihypertensives including Vasotec and Cozaar can be expected to contribute to xerostomia; and some antihypertensives, such as Vasotec, have been shown to alter taste as well.

C Diuretics, such as Lasix, can be expected to contribute to dry mouth conditions.

D Procrit, taken to treat anemia related to this patient's ESRD, is the only medication on this list that does not contribute to dry mouth or taste disturbances.

E Many antidepressants, such as Prozac, contribute to xerostomia and taste disturbance.

14.   A A power toothbrush may be the best recommendation from this list for helping this patient to improve her oral hygiene.

B This patient presents with areas of open contracts that prompt the recommendation of an interproximal brush.

C This patient should be encouraged to add the use of dental floss to her daily oral self-care routine.

D The use of a toothpick-in-holder may help this patient to remove biofilm at or just apical to the marginal gingiva.

E Floss threaders are used to gain access to areas under fixed prostheses. This patient does not present with conditions that prompt the use of a floss threader.

15.   **A** A pallor in the mucosa of patients with ESRD is usually the result of anemia and the decreased production of erythropoietin by the kidneys.

B Mucosal pallor is not related to hypertension.

C Most patients with ESRD develop anemia caused by the kidney's decreased erythropoietin production. Mucosal pallor of patients with ESRD is therefore the result of anemia.

D Dialysis can help to improve anemia and its oral manifestations.

E Periodontal disease is more likely to be associated with erythema.

16.   A The saliva of patients with ESRD contains a high urea content that contributes to the development of an ammonia odor to the breath.

B Increased salivary urea levels in patients with ESRD appear to induce the formation of dental calculus.

C Because this patient presents with caries, a moderate risk for future caries exists. However, in spite of poor oral self-care and lack of professional care for several years, rampant caries is not highly likely. In fact, studies have indicated that patients with ESRD may have a low caries incidence because of salivary changes related to their disease.

D Many patients with ESRD develop renal osteodystrophy with resultant demineralization of bone.

E Bleeding tendencies exhibited by the patient with ESRD may be evident as increased gingival bleeding.

17. A A sonic scaler may not have the power to adequately remove the heavy calculus.

B The ultrasonic scaler would be the best choice for initial treatment of the heavy supragingival calculus.

C,E Scalers and curets will most likely play a role in debridement. However, the heavy calculus accumulation would best be initially treated with the ultrasonic scaler.

D The use of the chisel scaler is limited to the specific area for which it is designed. The chisel scaler is used primarily to remove calculus from the proximal surfaces of the anterior teeth when the interdental papillae are missing. Although the chisel scaler may play a role in debridement of the maxillary central incisors where a diastema presents, its use would be limited because most of the other regions exhibit intact papillae.

18. **A** The beavertail tip is designed to remove heavy, supragingival calculus and with its broad, flat design, is an ideal choice for this region.

B Although the standard-diameter universal tip is designed to remove medium to heavy calculus deposits, the broad, flat tip of the beavertail is the best choice for removing deposit from the lingual surfaces of these teeth.

C The standard-diameter triple bend tip is designed to fit around line angles, and into interproximal areas. Although it may be used to access the proximal surfaces of these teeth, the beavertail tip design makes it the better choice for initial removal of the heavy supragingival calculus from these lingual surfaces.

D,E Slim-diameter tips are designed to remove light calculus deposits and would not be effective at initial debridement of the calculus present on these teeth.

19. A The significant bone loss observed in the radiographs of this region indicate that once the heavy bridge of calculus is removed, these teeth are likely at risk for mobility.

B As calculus is removed and inflamed tissue shrinks, the teeth root surfaces in this region are likely to be exposed, increasing the risk for dentinal sensitivity.

C Based on the location of the gingival margin before scaling, there is likely to be significant gingival recession after the calculus and endotoxins are removed from these teeth prompting the shrinkage of these edematous tissues.

D Because these teeth do not present with fractures or a condition that puts them at risk for fractures such as caries, attrition, or erosion before scaling, the risk of tooth fractures is not likely to increase as a result of scaling.

E As tissue shrinkage takes place, recession and papillary shape changes can result in the appearance of a longer clinical crown.

20. A This patient initially presented motivated to improve her oral health to gain access to the kidney transplant wait list. It is highly unlikely that she would have lost sight of this goal after scaling appointments. It is more likely that the presence of heavy calculus at the initial appointment prevented the probe from accessing the base of the pockets to record a true reading.

B Although this patient's medical conditions may play a role in the healing process, it is more likely that eliminating her oral infections will lead to improved overall health. Additionally, it is more likely that the presence of heavy calculus at the initial appointment prevented the probe from accessing the base of the pockets to record a true reading.

C Although an adverse oral effect of ESRD is a tendency for higher accumulations of dental calculus, it is more likely that the presence of heavy calculus at the initial appointment prevented the probe from accessing the base of the pockets to record a true reading.

D   Although probing with greater than 10 to 20 g of pressure may produce probe readings that are greater than the actual depth of the pocket, it is more likely that the heavy accumulation of calculus prevented accurate readings at the initial appointment.

(E) The presence of heavy calculus most likely limited access to the base of the pockets resulting in probe readings that did not represent the actual depth of the pockets at the initial appointment.

21.   A,D   This patient is on a salt restrictive diet contraindicating the use of sodium bicarbonate in the air-powder polisher and saline in oral irrigation.

B,E   Caution should be used when prescribing medications for the patient with ESRD. Drugs metabolized and/or eliminated by the kidneys, such as tetracycline and doxycycline, are potentially nephrotoxic and should be avoided. The use of aspirin and ibuprofen should be avoided because of their risk of sodium and water retentive properties, and the risk of hemorrhage.

(C) This patient presents with caries indicating her moderate risk for future occurrences. Additionally, removal of the heavy calculus and the expected tissue shrinkage following debridement will most likely expose more of the tooth surface to caries susceptibility. Exposing the root surface also has potential for increasing tooth sensitivity. Therefore, this patient would benefit from a fluoride varnish treatment.

22.   A   Although Listerine® Antiseptic (essential oils) can help destroy the bacteria associated with halitosis and biofilm, the alcohol content of Listerine® Antiseptic may exacerbate this patient's dry mouth conditions.

B   The active ingredient chlorhexidine gluconate found in the product PerioGard® should be used for a limited time, specifically treating gingivitis and would not be recommended for long-term daily oral self-care. Additionally, the adverse effects of chlorhexidine gluconate use are similar to the adverse effects this patient already experiences from her medical conditions and/or the medications she is taking. These adverse affects include an increase in calculus formation and taste alterations. The possible superficial desquamation of the oral mucosa may be exacerbated by her dry mouth condition. Additionally, chlorhexidine gluconate presents the adverse effect of staining exposed tooth root surfaces.

(C) Biotene Mouthwash (lactoperoxidase enzyme) is alcohol and sugar free, and formulated specifically for patients with a serious illness or whose medical condition is compromised by medication use. Biotene Mouthwash provides relief of dry mouth conditions.

D   Although Scope (cetylpyridinium chloride) may help manage halitosis, the alcohol content may exacerbate this patient's dry mouth conditions.

E   This patient does not appear to have a high caries risk, in spite of poor oral self-care practices. Studies have indicated that patients with ESRD may have a low caries incidence because of salivary changes related to their disease. Using a product such as Oral-B Fluorinse (0.2% sodium fluoride) may be recommended; however, the use of a daily mouth rinse that provides relief of dry mouth conditions is the best choice from this list.

23.   A   The maxillary right first molar and first premolar have fractured off at or very near the gingiva. The remaining teeth roots should be referred for evaluation for extraction. Testing these fractured teeth for vitality would not add to this diagnosis.

B   The maxillary left and mandibular right second molars have clinically detectable caries. The decay is not apparent on the radiographs indicating that the lesions have not advanced into the pulp. Furthermore, these teeth are asymptomatic negating the need to test for vitality.

C The maxillary right and left central incisors are periodontally involved; however, because they are asymptomatic, pulp vitality testing would not be indicated.

(D) The radiographs reveal a mixed radiopaque/radiolucent lesion apical to the mandibular right and left central and lateral incisors. These teeth should be tested for vitality to distinguish periapical cemental dysplasia (PCD) from periapical abscess.

E The mandibular right first molar and first premolar appear to be supererupted. Given that these teeth are asymptomatic, a pulp vitality test would not add information to further diagnose this condition.

24.   A Tartar control toothpastes can help prevent the additional buildup of supragingival calculus, but will not prevent subgingival dental calculus buildup.

(B) The active ingredient in most tartar control toothpastes, such as pyrophosphate, triclosan, or zinc citrate, inhibits calculus crystal growth and helps prevent attachment of supragingival dental calculus to the tooth.

C,D Tartar control toothpastes can help prevent the additional buildup of supragingival dental calculus but they cannot remove dental calculus once it has attached to the tooth surface.

25.   (A) Studies have demonstrated an increased incidence of hepatitis among patients receiving hemodialysis. It is illegal and unethical to refuse to treat this patient because she has, or is at risk for, hepatitis. In fact, all patients should be treated with standard infection control precautions. Dental health care professionals should take steps to receive recommended immunizations.

B,C,D These answers are incorrect.